D1450326

*The Clinical Management of*

# Itching

*The Clinical Management of*

# Itching

### Alan B. Fleischer, Jr., MD
Wake Forest University School of Medicine, Winston-Salem, NC, USA

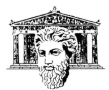

# The Parthenon Publishing Group
## International Publishers in Medicine, Science & Technology

NEW YORK                                                                LONDON

**Library of Congress Cataloging-in-Publication Data**

Fleischer, Alan B.
   The clinical management of itching / by Alan B.
   Fleischer, Jr.
     p.    cm.
   Includes bibliographical references and index.
   ISBN 1-85070-779-0
   1. Itching. I. Title.
   [DNLM: 1. Pruritus. WR 282 F596c 1997]
RL721.F56 1997
616.5 --dc21
DNLM/DLC
for Library of Congress          97-25928
                      CIP

**British Library Cataloguing in Publication Data**

Fleischer, Alan B.
   The clinical management of itching
   1. Itching   2. Pruritus
   I. Title
   616.5
   ISBN 1-85070-779-0

Published in the USA by
The Parthenon Publishing Group Inc.
One Blue Hill Plaza
PO Box 1564, Pearl River
New York 10965, USA

Published in the UK and Europe by
The Parthenon Publishing Group Limited
Casterton Hall, Carnforth
Lancs., LA6 2LA, UK

Copyright © 2000 Parthenon Publishing Group

Printed and bound by
T.G. Hostench S.A., Spain

# Contents

# Dedication

This book is dedicated to Anne's patience, love and understanding; to Gerrit's keen insight, and to the bright eyes of Sarah and Rebecca. Without the nurturing of my devoted parents, my extended family, and my superb mentors, this book would not have been possible. This book is also dedicated to itching people worldwide

A.B. Fleischer, Jr., MD

# Foreword

Itching, or pruritus, is that unpleasant sensation that provokes an urge to scratch. In a broad sense, itching is a primary sensory modality by which the central nervous system interacts with its environment. Itching generally involves a complex series of interactions between the skin, inflammatory processes, cutaneous nerves and the central nervous system.

Since itching is a common complaint in a vast number of dermatologic diseases, the organization of chapters within this text is based upon convenience. Within chapters and sections, for lack of a better schema, topics are often presented in alphabetic order.

The reader should note that all itching diseases are not presented equally. Those that are particularly common and cause great morbidity (e.g. atopic dermatitis and urticaria) are discussed more than unusual or uncommon causes of itching. Certain topics around which vast libraries can be built, such as contact dermatitis, are presented in a superficial fashion. The interested reader can always read entire texts on this subject. For the itch trivia master, truly obscure and arcane diagnoses are presented and constitute some of the author's favorite material.

This is not the first text to deal with itching. Wolstenholme and O'Connor published *Pain and Itch; Nervous Mechanisms* in 1959. Keele and Armstrong published *Substances Producing Pain and Itch* in 1964. Also in 1964, Musaph published *Itching and Scratching*. Gatti and Serri first published *Prurito Nella Practica Medica* in 1984, and recently Bernhard published *Itch: Mechanisms and Management of Pruritus* in 1994. Although the serious student of itching will want to obtain all of these references, the present text is designed to give the interested clinician rapid access to information about itching and itching diseases. The format is unusual, i.e. an outline form, for the sole purpose of condensing material and making the text more useful for the busy clinician.

On a linguistic note, whenever possible I have substituted the words 'itch' and 'itching' for 'pruritus' and 'pruritic'. Although they are equivalent in denotation, the latter terms are more difficult to pronounce and are frequently misspelt. A Medline search from 1966 to 1996 revealed 189 citations for 'pruritis', some by noted authorities. This text includes four of these citations with the original incorrect spelling. At my discretion, I have also taken the liberty of translating titles of published papers in many languages into English.

For the clinician, learning about itching diseases can be amusing and rewarding. Hopefully, itching patients will benefit from your lifelong learning.

Alan B. Fleischer, Jr., MD
Wake Forest University
School of Medicine
Winston-Salem, NC

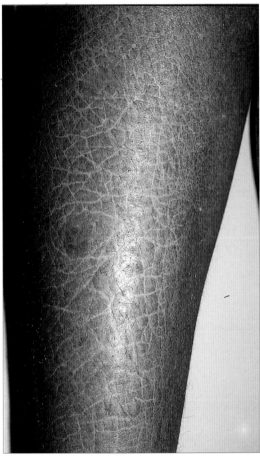

**1** Asteatosis in a patient with hypothyroidism

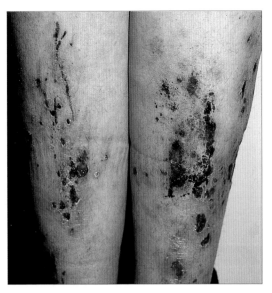

**3** Neurotic excoriations in a patient who denied that she touched or scratched the skin

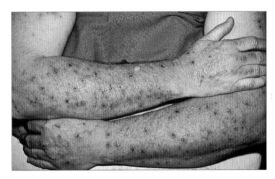

**4** Neurotic excoriations in a patient with obsessive–compulsive disorder

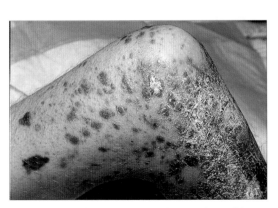

**2** Widespread Kaposi sarcoma in a patient with acquired immunodeficiency syndrome

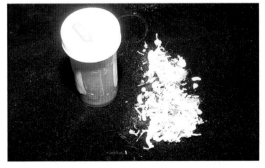

**5** Monosymptomatic hypochondriasis. A patient brought in samples of 'worms' that were infesting her skin, which were small bits of scale, crust, and paper fibers. The patient's mother sent a letter corroborating her account of 'worms'

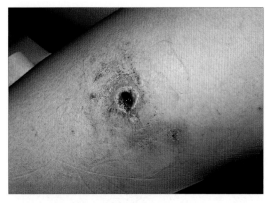

**6** This patient with monosymptomatic hypochondriasis was convinced that an infectious organism infested her skin

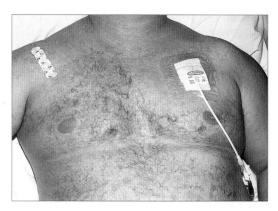

**9** An itchy eruption of graft versus host disease following bone marrow transplantation

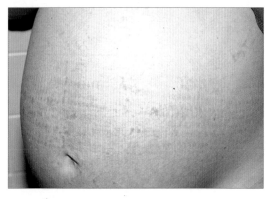

**7** Polymorphous eruption of pregnancy. This woman in her third trimester of pregnancy presented an extraordinarily itchy condition characterized by small, erythematous macules and papules on the trunk

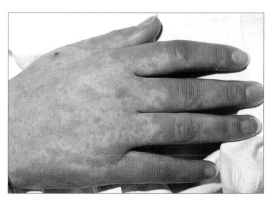

**10** Juvenile rheumatoid arthritis may present with an itchy eruption

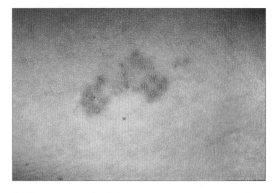

**8** Herpes gestationis in a pregnant woman can be quite itchy (Figure courtesy of David Crosby, MD, Medical College of Wisconsin, USA)

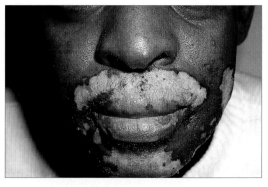

**11** Lesions of chronic cutaneous lupus erythematosus are frequently noted to itch, particularly if they are rapidly advancing

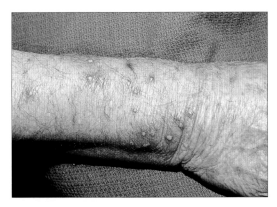

**12** Folliculitis may present with characteristic folliculocentric pustules and intense itching

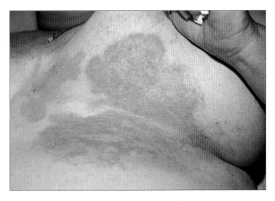

**13** Intertriginous dermatitis in the inframammary fold

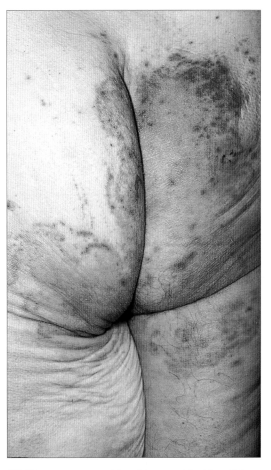

**15** Tinea can present in widespread fashion; this patient rapidly responded to systemic therapy

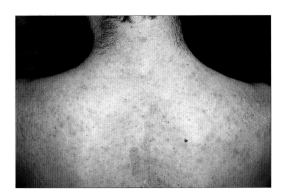

**14** Secondary syphilis presented in this patient with an itchy, generalized, scaling eruption

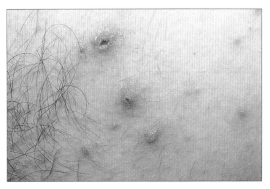

**16** Varicella is commonly an itching disease which presents with umbilicated vesiculopustules

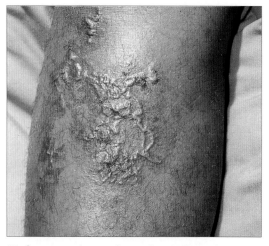

**17** Cutaneous larva migrans in a patient who attempted unsuccessful self-treatment with mercurochrome

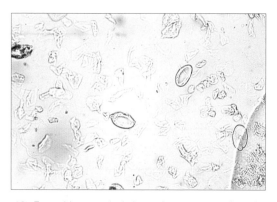

**18** *Enterobius vermicularis* or pinworm eggs found by examination of the perianal area

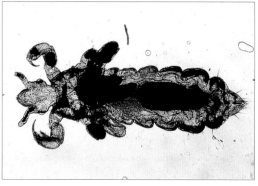

**19** *Pediculus humanus capitis,* the head louse, is recognized by its elongated body

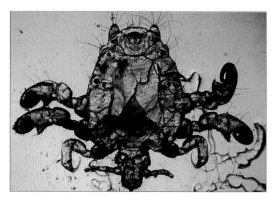

**20** *Pthirus pubis,* the crab louse, has a wide, short body

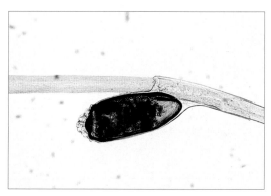

**21** A nit from a patient with pediculosis

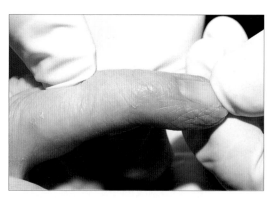

**22** This patient has a typical scabies burrow on the finger

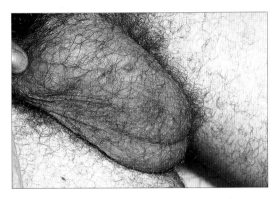

**23** Scrotal inflammatory nodules characteristic of scabies

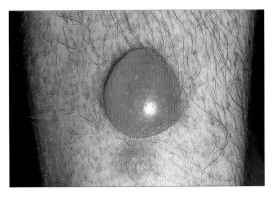

**26** Bullous insect bites can be so intense as to mimic an autoimmune blistering disorder

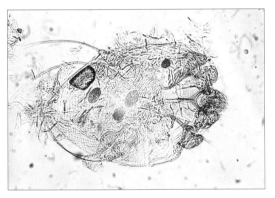

**24** *Sarcoptes scabiei* found during microscopic examination of burrow contents

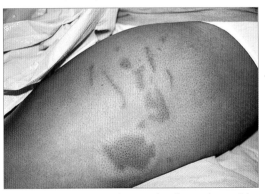

**27** Jellyfish can cause impressive linear dermatitic patches reminiscent of allergic contact dermatitis

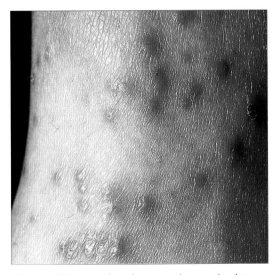

**25** Insect bite reactions in an outdoor enthusiast

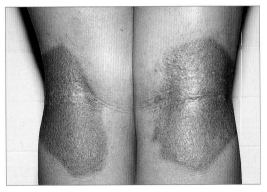

**28** Atopic dermatitis can present with lichenified plaques in the antecubital and popliteal fossae

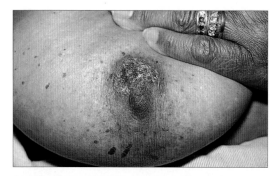

**29** Nipple dermatitis in an adult with atopic dermatitis

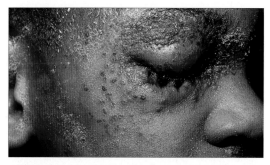

**30** Kaposi varicelliform eruption or eczema herpeticum in a patient with poorly controlled atopic dermatitis

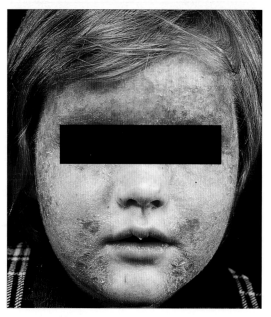

**31** This child has atopic dermatitis and has a poorly defined immunodeficiency syndrome with failure to thrive

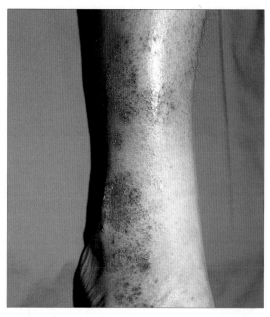

**32** Irritant contact dermatitis of the legs to chronic asteatosis and the repeated application of alcohol

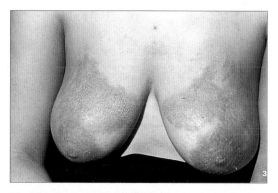

**33** Allergic contact dermatitis due to elastic in a brassiere

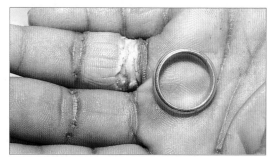

**34** Irritant contact dermatitis in a patient whose skin underneath her ring was chronically macerated

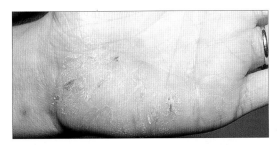

**35** Irritant hand dermatitis in a patient whose employment required exposure to solvents

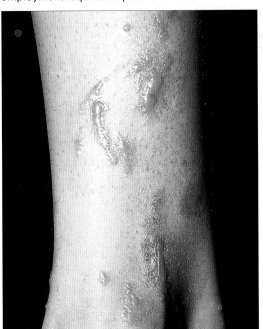

**36** Allergic contact dermatitis due to exposure to poison ivy

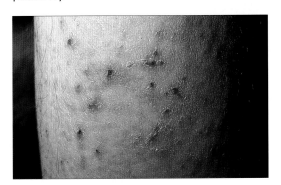

**37** Fiberglass dermatitis may present as an extraordinarily itchy disease

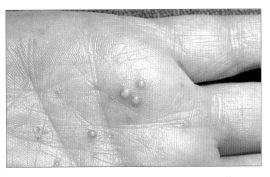

**38** Dyshidrotic dermatitis presenting as small palmar vesicles and pustules

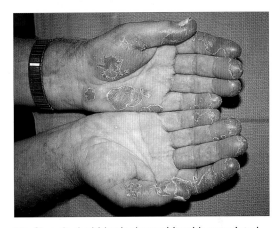

**39** Chronic dyshidrotic dermatitis with associated scale and fissuring

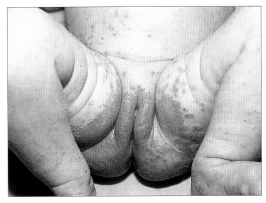

**40** Diaper dermatitis can be extraordinarily symptomatic, especially in patients with atopic dermatitis

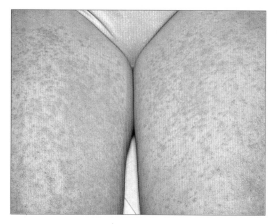

**41** Polymorphic light eruption on the legs of a young woman

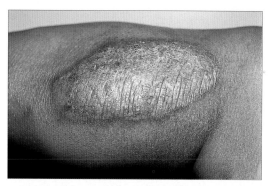

**42** This plaque of lichen simplex chronicus has been present for several years and the patient acknowledges scratching and rubbing it for hours

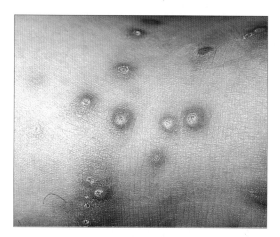

**43** Idiopathic prurigo nodularis

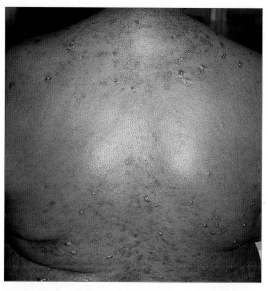

**44** Prurigo nodularis displaying the 'butterfly sign' where relative sparing is found on the upper back in areas inaccessible to scratching behavior

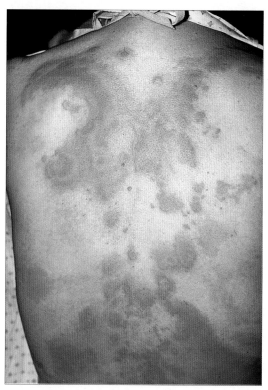

**45** Acute urticaria probably secondary to medication demonstrating primary lesions and dermatographism in areas scatched

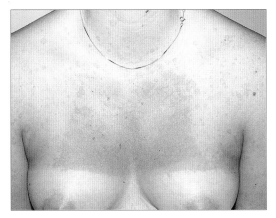

**46** Solar urticaria which was reproducible by phototesting

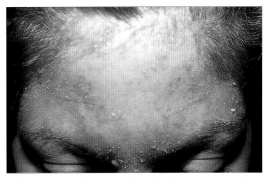

**49** Seborrheic dermatitis on the face and extending into the scalp of a young woman

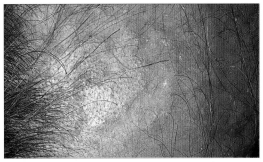

**50** Seborrheic dermatitis may present with unusual annular patterns on the scalp

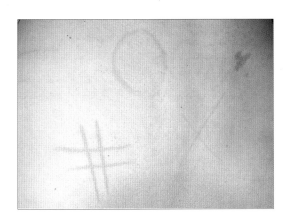

**47** Symptomatic dermatographism

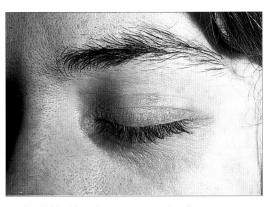

**48** Eyelid itching due to neomycin allergy

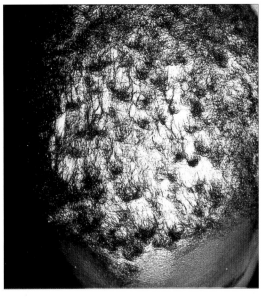

**51** Severe seborrheic dermatitis

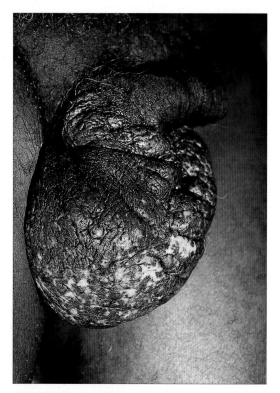

**52** Scrotal lichenification due to lichen simplex chronicus of the entire scotum

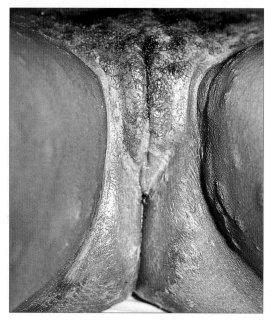

**53** Allergic contact dermatitis due to self-treatment with multiple allergens

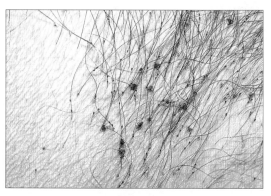

**54** Pediculosis should not be overlooked as a potential cause of vulvar itching

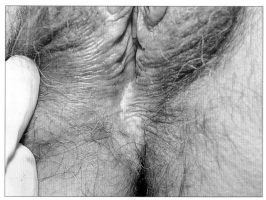

**55** Lichen sclerosis in an older woman with typical white, atrophic areas

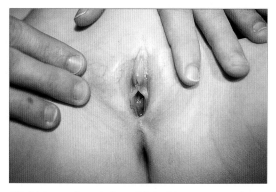

**56** Lichen sclerosis in a child with vulvar itching

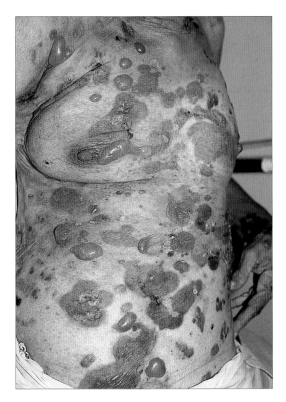

**57** Bullous pemphigoid may be inordinately itchy

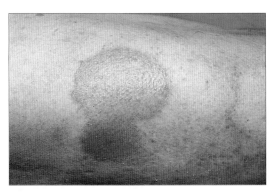

**58** Cutaneous T-cell lymphoma may present as plaques, patches and tumors

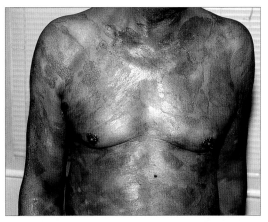

**59** Cutaneous T-cell lymphoma has a multitude of presentations

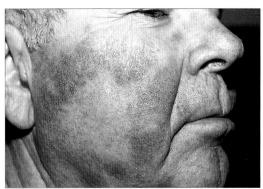

**60** Cutaneous T-cell lymphoma often has a violaceous look to the erythematous eruption

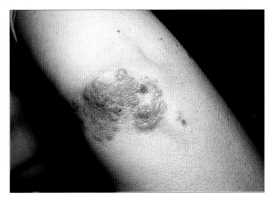

**61** Dermatitis herpetiformis occasionally presents with vesicles, but these are often scratched away

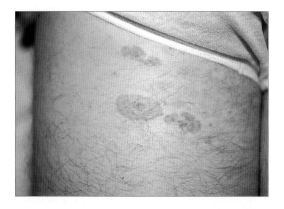

**62** Dermatitis herpetiformis can also present with erythematous patches

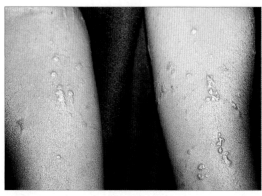

**64** Traumatic spread of the lichen planus may occur due to scatching behavior

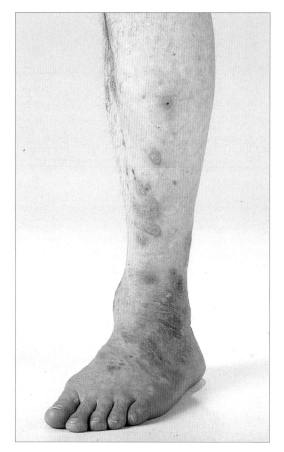

**63** Lichen planus is notoriously itchy, yet excoriations are rarely seen

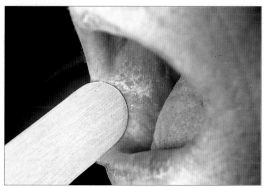

**65** The diagnosis of lichen planus can often be confirmed by finding lacy white lines on the oral mucosa

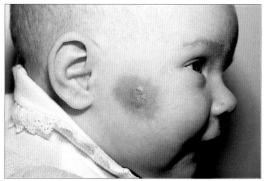

**66** Mastocytosis can be confirmed by stroking the lesions, resulting in urtication and occasional vesiculation

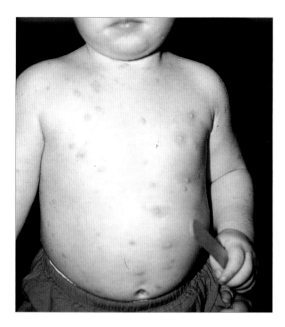

**67** Urticaria pigmentosa with typical brown papules and plaques

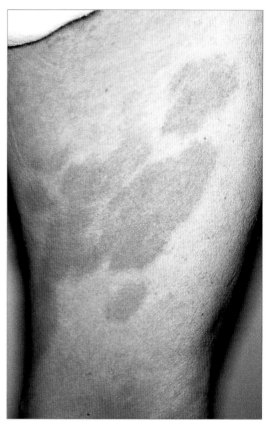

**69** This patient with highly pruritic large plaque parapsoriasis may eventuate in cutaneous T-cell lymphoma

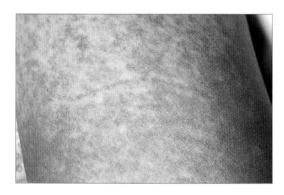

**68** Telangiectasia macularis eruptiva perstans

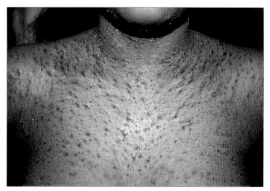

**70** Pityriasis rosea can become highly inflammatory and symptomatic

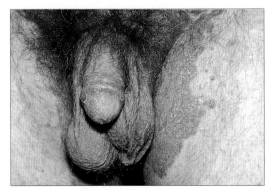

**71** Psoriasis may present with scattered pruritic papules

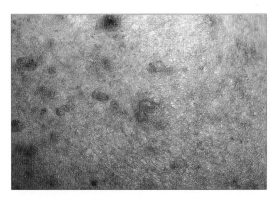

**74** Transient and persistent acantholytic dermatosis

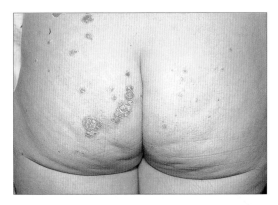

**72** Psoriasis may also be exacerbated by chronic scratching behaviour, resulting in lichenified psoriasis

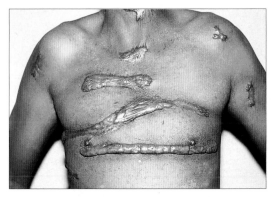

**75** Keloids may present with striking itching during the active growth phase

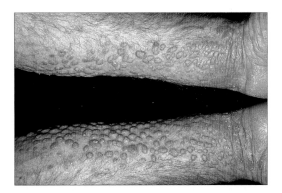

**73** Itching psoriasis

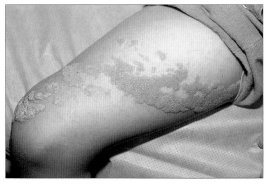

**76** Inflammatory linear verrucous epidermal nevi

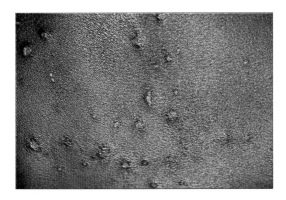

**77** Subacute prurigo with evident excoriations

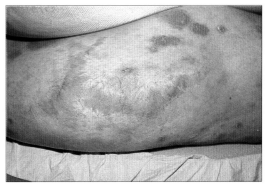

**79** Cutaneous atrophy from prolonged use of potent topical corticosteroid agents

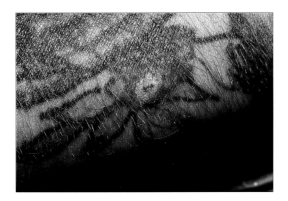

**78** Tattoo iching

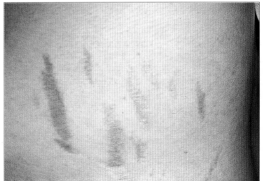

**80** Cutaneous atrophy from prolonged use of potent topical corticosteroid agents

# Science of itching

Although its incidence and prevalence are unknown, itching may be one of the most common human sensations

The itch receptor is a free unmyelinated nerve ending – possibly distinguishable from pain receptors – which enters the spinal cord, has controlled connections with fibers that ascend the ipsilateral spinothalamic tract, and then subsequent higher processing begins in the thalamus

## Epidemiology of itching

Because most people do not present to physicians for each arthropod assault or other minor condition, the incidence and prevalence of itching remains unknown. However, it is reasonable to assume that all humans itch at some point in their lives.

- Insect bites, viral exanthems, and contact dermatitis are universal human experiences

Itching is likely to be more common in certain populations.

- Within elderly populations, itching may be experienced by 30–60% within any one week period[1]
- Within certain countries in which filariasis and other pathogens are common, i.e. Nigeria, generalized itching may be present in nearly 7% of dermatology patients[2]

Specific itching conditions such as aquagenic itching may be under-recognized merely because no one asks about the symptom or because it is generally of little clinical significance[3].

- In one study[4], 4.5% of an unselected population reported aquagenic itching

Given the small amount known about itching, there is a fertile field for research addressing the epidemiology of itching.

## Neuroanatomy and neurologic processes

### Neuroanatomy

Itch sensation arises from the superficial layers of skin and mucous membranes.

### Itch reception and transmission

The itch receptor is a free unmyelinated nerve ending that may be distinguishable from pain receptors. Itch stimuli enter into the central nervous system (CNS) via unmyelinated C-fibers and possibly A-δ fibers. The axon enters through the dorsal horn for spinal dermatomes or the trigeminal equivalent of the brain stem for head and neck itching, and, after synaptic connection within the ipsilateral gray column of the spinal cord, processing and control of the transmission occurs prior to crossing the midline (see below). After synaptic transmission with the next neuron, the fiber ascends within the contralateral anterolateral spinothalamic tract[5,6].

- Destruction of the spinothalamic tract inhibits distal perception of itch
- The next synapse occurs within the thalamus where higher processing is initiated
- Functional positron emission tomography studies[7] suggest that the next areas related to itching and the urge to scratch include

the anterior cingulate cortex, the supplementary motor area, the premotor area, and the inferior parietal lobule

## Itch versus pain sensations

The intensity hypothesis holds that itching appears to be mediated by low-level stimulation of pain fibers, whereas pain results from intense stimulation of the same fibers[6].

- Counter to this hypothesis is the finding that direct recordings from C-fibers of itch and pain stimuli show similar impulse rates
- Also countering this hypothesis is the finding that direct electrical itch stimulation of fibers does not produce pain when the stimulation rate increases

The specificity hypothesis suggests that itching occurs when single unmyelinated C fibers are stimulated – two fiber populations have been identified, the majority of which mediate pain and a minority which mediate itch[6,8].

- Counter to this hypothesis is the finding that C-fibers which are responsive to histamine pruritogenesis also respond to pain-inducing chemical mediators
- Also countering this hypothesis has been the variable ability of investigators to induce itching with microstimulation of single fibers

The selectivity hypothesis suggests that itch-mediating fibers are a subpopulation of C-fibers with appropriate central connections for mediating itch[6].

- A required subhypothesis is that when large numbers of C-fibers are stimulated, pain sensations from the majority of fibers mask the itch sensation[9]
- This hypothesis also explains psychophysiologic data indicating that pain inhibits itch, and pain is not perceived at the time itch is perceived[10]

This hypothesis helps to explain how scratching, with stimulation of large numbers of A-δ and C-fibers, can mask itching

- The selectivity hypothesis also helps explain how opiate drugs may improve pain and cause itch
- Further supporting the separation of pain from itch is the finding that topical corticosteroid agents such as clobetasol can decrease histamine-induced itch but not thermal sensation or pain[11]

## Gate theory of itch control

Melzack and Wall[12] proposed the gating of pain sensations wherein simultaneous firing of multiple other neurons inhibits the perception of sensation from smaller pain neurons. If pain and itch are mediated by the same or similar nociceptor nerves then control mechanisms should be identical or similar. Gating of itch stimuli appear to be controlled by both descending inhibitory and excitatory pathways[13].

- Enkephalins are produced by spinal interneurons which appear to be sensory modulatory compounds
- Leu-enkephalin and met-enkephalin may stimulate CNS opioid receptors and regulate both pain and itch signals

Exogenous opioids administered in small quantities to spinal levels in spinal anesthesia relieve pain and can stimulate itch. Inattention and emotional state could enhance or impede perception through descending modulatory mechanisms.

## Neural modulation of inflammation and itching

Skin injury is able to evoke afferent impulse to the CNS, and the peripheral nervous system can evoke neuroeffector responses which contribute to inflammation and thus itch[14].

- The cutaneous flare response is eliminated by degeneration of local nerve fibers following nerve injury; yet it persists if injury is recent
- Afferent nociceptor nerve fibers have close relationships with mast cells
- Neuropeptides synthesized in the neuron cell body are preferentially transported to the periphery
- Neuropeptides are orders of magnitude more potent than histamine in inducing wheal and flare responses (see discussion of neuropeptides below)
- Neuropeptides likely contribute to itching because neuropeptide levels are affected in a wide variety of pruritic dermatoses including atopic dermatitis, psoriasis and others[15]
- Clearance of psoriasis following nerve sectioning and absence of contact dermatitis after peripheral nerve damage are intriguing reports which link the nervous system to inflammatory itching diseases and their perpetuation

## Itch mediators

### Cytokines and other inflammatory mediators

Since the majority of itching skin diseases are inflammatory or allergic, it is reasonable to assume that release or activation of inflammatory mediators can stimulate itch receptors. This stimulation probably plays an essential role in itch pathophysiology.

Interleukins, especially interleukin-1 and interleukin-2, may cause cutaneous inflammation and itching in minute concentrations[16]. Skin concentrations of prostaglandin E are elevated in atopic dermatitis and UVB-induced inflammation[17].

- Prostaglandin E can enhance itching induced by intradermal histamine and serotonin injection, but alone is a weak pruritogen[18, 19]
- Pretreatment with antihistamine before prostaglandin E injection did not inhibit itching, suggesting that it is mainly potentiating non-histaminic itch mediators
- Aspirin and other non-steroidal anti-inflammatory agents which affect prostaglandin synthesis relieve clinical pain but not itching

Preliminary studies show other lymphokines may be involved in the pathogenesis of clinical itch.

- Corticosteroid agents decrease expression of a broad range of inflammatory mediators and reduce itch in many clinical states
- Cyclosporin A, an inhibitor of lymphokine production, reduces itch in atopic dermatitis[20,21]
- Tacrolimus, another anti-inflammatory agent, also seems to decrease itching

Platelet activating factor, released by several inflammatory cells, produces dose-dependent flare and itching responses which are inhibited by a local antihistamine agent.

- Platelet activating factor-induced itching is indirect and mediated by its ability to release histamine from mast cells

### Endopeptidases and other proteases

Several exogenous endopeptidases, such as trypsin and chymotrypsin, may induce itch, presumably via peptide products of proteases[22].

- Kallikrein can elicit a burning itch sensation
- This hypothesis has been limited by the fact that no itch-mediating peptide protease product has been isolated from the human skin[23]

## Histamine

Histamine plays a primary role in the itches of urticaria, mastocytosis and a few select conditions, but its mediation of itching in other conditions is suspect[24, 25].

There are three types of histamine receptors, but only $H_1$ and $H_2$ receptors have thus far been identified in the skin, and $H_2$ receptors do not appear to mediate itch[26].

Histamine induces itch when injected intradermally, and this injection is accompanied by wheal and flare[27].

- Note that most skin cases of itching are not accompanied by wheal and flare response
- Moreover wheal and flare phenomena last an hour or less, compared with most itching disease, where they may persist for hours to days

$H_1$ blocking agents decrease itching in most cases of urticaria and mastocytosis, but in most tested non-urticarial conditions they produce a poor therapeutic response.

- Newer multifunctional antihistamines such as cetirizine and loratidine are exceptions to this rule, as are therapeutic responses to the sedation of some antihistamines

    These agents may have additional non-antihistaminic therapeutic effects such as inhibition of leukocyte migration and mast cell stabilization

## Kinins

Bradykinin causes intense pain, but is weakly pruritogenic[18, 23].

## Neuropeptides

There are over 50 described neuropeptides, and these have been found in the central nervous system as well as in unmyelinated cutaneous sensory nerve fibers[3,28]. Itching results from intradermal injection of several peptides with neurotransmitter functions, such as vasoactive intestinal polypeptide, neurotensin, secretin, and substance P[29-32].

Although it is not clear that it is the only or main neuropeptide that mediates itching, the undecapeptide substance P has been studied more intensively than other neuropeptide itch transmitters[33]. Substance P is synthesized in dorsal root ganglia of nociceptor C fibers and is transmitted peripherally to the nerve endings[34].

- Substance P is an 11-amino acid peptide that is demonstrated in normal skin and increased amounts in itchy skin diseases
- Substance P releases histamine with resultant whealing and itch, but does not release other mast cell products such as prostaglandin D2

The role of neurogenic peptides in clinical itching has yet to be elucidated, and specific neuropeptide antagonists may offer a promising therapeutic approach to itching[20, 35].

## Opioid peptides

Centrally, opioids appear to play a major role in control mechanisms.

- Opioid peptides appear to be involved in the central transmission and regulation of itching[36]
- Systemic opiates such as morphine and codeine and epidural morphine may induce intense itching in the absence of demonstrable skin changes
- Plasma from patients with cholestatic itching causes facial scratching when introduced into the medullary dorsal horn of monkeys, and this scratching is abolished by administering the opioid receptor antagonist, naloxone[37]

    Itching in clinical disease has shown variable response to naloxone, indicating that this may only be one component of the control mechanism

Nalmefine, another opioid antagonist, has shown some promising therapeutic response in clinical itching

- Of unknown significance is the finding of elevated serum-endorphins in itchy atopic patients[36]

Peripherally, opioids appear to potentiate itch but do not seem directly responsible.

- Although opioids may promote histamine release by mast cells, e.g. exacerbating urticarial itch, opioid peptides do not generally cause any release of histamine when injected alone

When injected with histamine, opioids enhance the ability of histamine to induce itching

## Physical mediators

Although not true chemical mediators in the traditional sense, certain physical conditions modify itching response.

- Cooling the skin can diminish experimentally induced itching
- Heating may reduce or aggravate itching[38]
- Vibration at 100 Hz reduces itch intensity[39]
- Transcutaneous electrical nerve stimulation at 2 Hz reduces itching
- Paroxysmal itching in multiple sclerosis occurred at the onset of treatment with external pico tesla range electromagnetic fields[40]

## Serotonin

When intradermally injected, serotonin is a less potent itch inducer compared with histamine. It may synergize with prostaglandins to induce itch (in polycythemia rubra vera)[18].

Intravenous administration of the serotonin type 3 receptor antagonist ondansetron induces a marked relief of itching in cholestasis-associated itching[40].

## Immunology

Pruritic conditions such as insect bites, atopic dermatitis, and bullous pemphigoid are mediated in large part by immunologic responses. Type I (humoral immunity): antibodies manufactured by plasma and mast cells bind to antigens and immediately create an inflammatory response[42].

- Clinical significance in itching: a common mechanism in urticaria due to drugs and food[43, 44]
- Potential role in atopic dermatitis

Type III (cell-mediated immunity): cytotoxic T-cells and other T-lymphocytes attack victim cells, activate complement, and release inflammatory mediators including interferon.

- Clinical significance in itching: autoimmune blistering diseases, atopic dermatitis, tinea and viral diseases may itch due to activation of this inflammatory mechanism

Type III (immune complexes): these antibody–antigen complexes produce a cascade of reactions including activation of complement, lymphokines, and phagocytosis.

- Clinical significance in itching: serum sickness from a drug reaction

Type IV (delayed-type hypersensitivity): activated T-cells act via lymphokines to mediate a broad range of cellular responses.

- Clinical significance in itching: allergic contact dermatitis and atopic dermatitis[43–45]

## Complexities

More than one type of immunity is often responsible for the inflammatory response.

- Urticaria

Urticaria is usually a Type I reaction mediated by IgE antibodies, but it can be a Type III

5

reaction in which the antigen forms a comple-ment-fixing complex with antibody

It can also be non-immunologic, as in symp-tomatic dermatographism where pressure is a sufficient stimulus to create an inflammatory response

- Arthropod bites

An insect bite may produce direct effects of the toxin injected (generally non-immunolog-ic), or components of the toxin may promote lymphocyte and monocyte infiltration as a delayed-type hypersensitivity response, and local cell proliferation as a more general response to the local damage and inflammat-ory stimulus

When bitten initially by most arthropods, aside from symptoms from the physical skin damage, no reaction usually occurs

Only after repetitive exposure does one begin to develop hypersensitivity, manifest by a typical bite

With prolonged exposure an immediate weal reaction occurs, to be followed by the delayed papular reaction

Immunologic tolerance may occur with resul-tant lack of reaction

- Atopic dermatitis will be further discussed in chapter 6: The common dermatitis diseases.

## Lymphokines

Most evidence for involvement of lymphokines in itching comes from atopic dermatitis re-search. In atopic dermatitis, there is decreased interferon-$\gamma$ (IFN-$\gamma$) but high interleukin 4 (IL-4) production. The activities of IL-4 and IFN-$\gamma$ seem to regulate the amplitude of the IgE response. Patients with atopic dermatitis improve during systemic IFN-$\gamma$ therapy[45].

## Autoantibodies

Autoantibodies may play an important role in initiating inflammation in diseases such as bullous pemphigoid.

- However, autoantibodies such as those directed at the bullous pemphigoid antigen may occur in a wide variety of pruritic der-matoses, yet may have little significance[42]

Autoantibodies directed at the mast cell IgE receptor may induce chronic urticaria via hista-mine release and thereby indirectly mediate itching.

## Psychology

Although psychogenic itching is an uncommon diagnosis of exclusion, psychologic and social factors influence itch sensations[46–48].

- The role of the central nervous system mechanisms in itch mediation is poorly understood

In some surveys of dermatologic patients, at least one-third of the visits depend upon emotional factors; yet in only a few instances, such as factitial disease, do these play a primary and pathogenic role.

- Therefore, the assumption that patients with chronic itching must have primary psychopathology may be erroneous
- Nevertheless, even if patients have a primary cutaneous itching condition, psychiatric disease may contribute to the chronicity of the itching

## Psychologic concepts that play important roles in itching

Perceived stress has an extremely important impact on itch perception. The concept of psy-chologic stress is easier to understand than to define, but is best understood as abnormal or extreme adjustment in the physiology of a person to cope with adverse effects of the environment[49].

- Stress may also include distress
- Stress clearly makes itching worse

   In a study of subjects suffering from psoriasis and atopic dermatitis, perceived itch was enhanced in those with atopic dermatitis in response to stress[50, 51]

   The impact of stress among patients with chronic diseases such as atopic dermatitis and psoriasis may differ from the normal population[52]

Patients' social support and social relations are also important in disease mediation.

- Intractable atopic dermatitis has been reported to be exacerbated by an impaired parent–child relationship[48, 53]

## Somatization

Emotionally distressed patients are more likely to present to clinicians with physical symptoms than to complain about psychological or social problems[54,55].

- Somatizing patients have psychologic symptoms but these are overshadowed by physical complaints, such as itching, which allow those reluctant to accept the stigma of mental illness still to occupy the 'sick role'

## Psychopathology and itching

### Depression and anxiety

Depression and anxiety are the most common psychologic disorders which contribute to itching. In one study[56], the degree of depressive psychopathology in psoriasis was found to correlate with itch severity. Depression seems to modulate itch severity in itchy conditions including psoriasis, atopic dermatitis, and chronic idiopathic urticaria.

- In one study[57], using a standardized instrument (Beck Depression Inventory), significantly more patients with generalized itching had depressive symptomatology (32.4%) than dermatology controls (13.2%), and more patients with chronic urticaria had depressive symptomatology (14.7%) than controls (4.4%)
- In addition to a small, select group of patients with overt depression, many patients with chronic itching have subclinical reactive depression or anxiety disorders, often in response to major life stressors[58–60]

In patients with itching psoriasis, psychiatric and possibly sleep pathologic factors rather than primary dermatologic factors determined the wakenings from sleep as a result of itching[61].

- The act of scratching itself can cause sleep disturbance which may contribute to psychiatric disease

Certain patients with anogenital itching may be more likely to have concurrent psychiatric disease.

### Obsessive–compulsive disorder

In one survey of randomly selected patients who presented with one of several chronic pruritic conditions attending a dermatology clinic[62], 14% had previously undiagnosed obsessive–compulsive disorder. Obsessive–compulsive behaviors including ritual hand washing and obsessive scratching or picking behavior can exacerbate many inflammatory skin diseases that have itching as a major component.

### Psychotic disorders

Psychotic delusions about their skin may manifest as itching in delusions of parasitosis wherein patients may envision common or exotic parasites infesting the skin.

- A delusion is a false belief that cannot be corrected by argument or persuasion and may or may not be founded logically[63, 64]

   Bernhard et al.[65] give as an example 'telepathic pruritus' which was reported in a paranoid schizophrenic man with the delusion that two other men used mental telepathy to make him itch

Localized itching may also be a sign of psychiatric disease[48]

- Chronic hand dermatitis in those with handwashing rituals due to obsessive–compulsive disorder
- Anogenital itching as a sign of obsessive–compulsive disorder, depression, erotic fantasies, sexual dysfunction, guilt and shame

## Scratching

Since the definition of itching revolves around the desire or act of scratching, this behavior must be closely allied with the sensation[66]. Scratching may be either a spinal reflex function activity or a neurobehavioral manifestation of a tic.

- As noted above, functional positron emission tomography studies suggest that the areas related to itching and urge to scratch include the anterior cingulate cortex, the supplementary motor area, the premotor area, and the inferior parietal lobule

Scratching clearly occurs during sleep and profoundly interferes with normal sleep patterns.

- In one study[68], nocturnal scratching and sleep was studied with 17 overnight polygraphic records of the scratch bouts and EEG of severely itchy patients

Patients spent little time in deep orthodox sleep (stages 3 and 4), which was absent from 7 of the 17 records

Bouts of scratching were found to occur in all stages of sleep but were most numerous in stage 1 (light orthodox sleep)

Sleep tended to remain stable for the 40 seconds immediately before a bout of scratching but had often changed to a more superficial stage by the time the bout had ceased, implying perhaps that scratching itself was the event linked most closely with arousal

- In another study[69], the total scratch time of nocturnal itching in atopic dermatitis was found to vary from 7 minutes to nearly 5 hours

The mechanisms by which itching is abated by scratching are uncertain.

- Since the sensation of itching is reinforced by facilitating circuits in the relay synapses of the spinal cord, the prolonged scratch-induced relief could be due to temporary disruption of these circuits
- Alternatively, scratching could simply damage sensory nerve endings, repair occupying several minutes
- Scratching behavior has been ingeniously quantified by motion detectors and utilized as an indirect, objective method of quantifying itch using motion detectors[70, 71]
- Although little objective information exists, personal experience suggests that scratching relieves itching

## References

1. Beauregard S, Gilchrest BA. A survey skin problems and skin care regimens in the elderly. *Arch Dermatol* 1987;123:1638–43
2. Olumide YM, Oresanya F. Generalized pruritus as a presenting symptom in Nigeria. *Int J Dermatol* 1987; 26:171–3
3. Logan RA, Fehrer MD, Steinman HK. The prevalence of water-induced itching. *Br J Dermatol* 1984; 111:734–6
4. Potasman I, Heinrich I, Bassan HM. Aquagenic pruritus: prevalence and clinical characteristics. *Israel J Medical Sciences* 1990;26:499–503
5. Denman ST. A review of pruritus. *J Am Acad Dermatol* 1986;14:375–92

6. Ekblom A. Some neurophysiologic aspects of itch. *Sem Dermatol* 1995;14:262–70

7. Hsieh JC, Hägermark Ö, Ståhle-Bäckdahl M, *et al.* Urge to scratch represented in the human cerebral cortex during itch. *J Neurophysiol* 1994;72:3004–8

8. McMahon SB, Koltzenburg M. Itching for an explanation. *Trends Neurosciences* 1992;15:497–501

9. Koppert W, Reeh PW, Handwerker HO. Conditioning of histamine by bradykinin alters responses of rat nociceptor and human itch sensation. *Neuroscience Letters* 1993;152:117–20

10. Handwerker HO, Forster C, Kirchhoff C. Discharge patterns of human C-fibers induced by itching and burning stimuli. *J Neurophysiol* 1991;66:307–15

11. Yosipovitch G, Szolar C, Hui XY, *et al.* High-potency corticosteroid rapidly decreases histamine-induced itch but not thermal sensation or pain in human beings. *J Am Acad Dermatol* 1996;35:118–20

12. Melzack R, Wall P. Pain mechanisms: A new theory. *Science* 1965;150:971–983

13. Vuadens P, Regli F, Dolivo M, *et al.* Segmental pruritus and intramedullary vascular malformation. *Schweizer Archiv Neurol Psychiatrie* 1994;145:13–6

14. Fantini F, Magnoni C, Pincelli C, *et al.* Neurogenic inflammation and the skin: neural modulation of cutaneous inflammatory reactions. *Eur J Dermatol* 1995;5:349–57

15. Giannetti A, Fantini F, Cimitan A, *et al.* Vasoactive intestinal poypeptide and substance P in the pathogenesis of atopic dermatitis. *Acta Derm Venereol* 1992;176(Suppl):90–2

16. Dowd PM, Camp RDR, Greaves MW. Human recombinant interleukin-1 is proinflammatory in normal human skin. *Skin Pharmacol* 1988;1:30–7

17. Greaves MW, McDonald-Gibson W. Itch: role of prostaglandins. *Br Med J* 1973;3:608–9

18. Greaves MW, Shuster S. Responses of skin blood vessels to bradykinin (histamine), and 5-hydroxytryptamine. *J Physiol* 1967;193:255–67

19. Hägermark Ö, Strandberg K. Pruritogenic activity of prostaglandin E2. *Acta Derm Venereol* 1977;57:37–43

20. Hägermark Ö. Peripheral and central mediators of itch. *Skin Pharmacol* 1992;5:1–8

21. Hägermark Ö, Wahlgren CF. Some methods for evaluating clinical itch and their application for studying pathophysiological mechanisms. *J Dermatol Sci* 1992;4:55–62

22. Shelley WB, Arthur RP. Studies on Cowhage (Mucuna pruriens) and its pruritogenic proteinase mucunain. *Arch Dermatol* 1955;72:399–406

23. Denman ST. A review of pruritus. *J Am Acad Dermatol* 1986;14:375–92

24. Misch KJ, Greaves MW, Black AK. Histamine and the skin. *Br J Dermatol* 1983;109 (Suppl 25):10–3

25. Greaves MW. Introduction to the pharmacology and physiology of itch. *Proc Roy Soc Med* 1975;68:529

26. Davies MG, Greaves MW. The current status of histamine receptors in human skin: therapeutic implications. *Br J Dermatol* 1981;104:601–6

27. Hägermark Ö. Itch mediators. *Sem Dermatol* 1995;14:271–6

28. Fjellner B, Hägermark Ö. Studies on pruritogenic and histamine-releasing effects of some putative peptide neurotransmitters. *Acta Derm Venereol* 1981;61:245–50

29. Fjellner B, Hägermark Ö. Experimental pruritus evoked by platelet activating factor (PAF-acether) in human skin. *Acta Derm Venereol* 1985;65:409–12

30. Foreman JC. Substance P and calcitonin gene-related peptide: effects on mast cells and in human skin. *Int Arch Allergy Appl Immunol* 1987;82:366–71

31. Wallengren J, Hakanson R. Effects of substance P, neurokinin A and calcitonin gene-related peptide in human skin and their involvement in sensory nerve-mediated responses. *Eur J Pharmacol* 1987;143:267–73

32. Wallengren J, Ekman R, Moller H. Substance P and vasoactive intestinal peptide in bullous and inflammatory skin disease. *Acta Derm Venereol* 1986;66:23–8

33. Jorizzo JL, Coutts AA, Eady RAJ, *et al.* Vascular responses of human skin to injection of substance P and mechanism of action. *Eur J Pharmacol* 1983;87:67–76

34. Teofoli P, Procacci P, Maresca M, *et al.* Itch and pain. *Int J Dermatol* 1996;35:159–66

35. Giannetti A, Girolomoni G. Skin reactivity to neuropeptides in atopic dermatitis. *Br J Dermatol* 1989;121:681–8

36. Georgala S, Schulpis KH, Papaconstantinou ED, *et al.* Raised beta-endorphin serum levels in children with atopic dermatitis and pruritus. *J Dermatol Sci* 1994;8:125–8

38. Fruhstorfer H, Hermanns M, Latzke L. The effects thermal stimulation on clinical and experimental itch. *Pain* 1986;24:259–69

9

37. Bergasa NV, Thomas DA, Vergalla J, *et al.* Plasma from patients with the pruritus of cholestasis induces opioid receptor-mediated scratching in monkeys. *Life Sci* 1993;53:1253–7

39. Ekblom A, Hansson P, Fjellner B. The influence of extrasegmental mechanical vibratory stimulation and transcutaneous electrical nerve stimulation on histamine-induced itch. *Acta Physiol Scand* 1985; 125:541–5

40. Sandyk R. Paroxysmal itching in multiple sclerosis during treatment with external magnetic fields. *Int J Neurosci* 1994;75:65–71

41. Schworer H, Ramadori G. Treatment pruritus: a new indication for serotonin type 3 receptor antagonists. *Clin Investigator* 1993;71:659–62

42. Rieckhoff-Cantoni L, Bernard P, Didierjean L, *et al.* Frequency of bullous pemphigoid-like antibodies as detected by western immunoblot analysis in pruritic dermatoses. *Arch Dermatol* 1992;128:791–4

43. Wahlgren CF. Itch and atopic dermatitis: clinical and experimental studies. *Acta Derm Venereol* 1991;165 (Suppl):1–53

44. Leung DY. The immunologic basis of atopic dermatitis. *Clin Rev Allergy* 1993;11:447–69

45. Reinhold U, Kukel S, Brzoska J,*et al.* Systemic interferon gamma treatment in severe atopic dermatitis. *J Am Acad Dermatol* 1993;29:58–63

46. Fried RG. Evaluation and treatment of "psychogenic" pruritus and self-excoriation. *J Am Acad Dermatol* 1994;30:993–9

47. Koblenzer CS. Psychosomatic concepts in dermatology. A dermatologist-psychoanalyst's viewpoint. *Arch Dermatol* 1983;119:501–12

48. Koblenzer CS. *Psychocutaneous Disease.* Orlando: Grune and Stratton, 1987

49. Arnetz BB, Fjellner B, Eneroth P, *et al.* Endocrine and dermatological concomitants of mental stress. *Acta Derm Venereol* 1991;156 (Suppl):9–12

50. Panconesi E. Psychosomatic dermatology. *Clinics in Dermatol* 1984;2:94–179

51. Panconesi E, Hautmann G. Psychophysiology of stress in dermatology. The psychobiologic pattern of psychosomatics. *Dermatol Clin* 1996;14;399–421

52. Ehlers A, Stangier U, Gieler U. Treatment of atopic dermatitis: a comparison of psychological and dermatological approaches to relapse prevention. *J Consult Clin Psychol* 1995;63:624–35

53. Koblenzer CS, Koblenzer PJ. Chronic intractable atopic eczema. Its occurrence as a physical sign of impaired parent-child relationships and psychologic developmental arrest: improvement through parent insight and education. *Arch Dermatol* 1988;124: 1673–7

54. Murphy M. Somatization: embodying the problem. *Br Med J* 1989;298:1331–2

55. Mechanic D. Social psychologic factors affecting the presentation of bodily symptoms. *N Engl J Med* 1972;286:1331–9

56. Gupta MA, Gupta AK, Schork NJ, *et al.* Depression modulates pruritus perception: a study of pruritus in psoriasis, atopic dermatitis, and chronic idiopathic urticaria. *Psychosomatic Med* 1994;56:36–40

57. Sheehan-Dare RA, Henderson MJ, Cotterill JA. Anxiety and depression in patients with chronic urticaria and generalized pruritus. *Br J Dermatol* 1990; 123:769–74

58. Gieler U, Ehlers A, Hohler T, *et al.* The psychosocial status of patients with endogenous eczema. A study using cluster analysis for the correlation of psychological factors with somatic findings. *Hautarzt* 1990; 41:416–23

59. Laihinen A. Assessment of psychiatric and psychosocial factors disposing to chronic outcome of dermatoses. *Acta Derm Venereol* 1991;156(Suppl):46–8

60. Musaph H. Psychodynamics in itching states. *Intern J Psycho-Analysis* 1968;49:336–40

61. Gupta MA. Evaluation and treatment of 'psychogenic' pruritus and self-excoriation. *J Am Acad Dermatol* 1995;32:532–3

62. Hatch ML, Paradis C, Friedman S, *et al.* Obsessive-compulsive disorder in patients with chronic pruritic conditions: case studies and discussion. *J Am Acad Dermatol* 1992;26:549–51

63. Koo J, Gambla C. Delusions of parasitosis and other forms of monosymomatic hypochondriacal psychosis. *Dermatol Clin* 1996;14:429–38

64. Shelley WB, Shelley ED. Delusions of parasitosis associated with coronary bypass surgery. *Br J Dermatol* 1988;118:309–10

65. Bernhard JD, Gardner MR. Nonrashes.6. Telepathic pruritus. *Cutis* 1990;45:59

66. Procacci P, Maresca M. A philological note on some words concerning itch and related cutaneous sensations. *Pain* 1993;55:137–8

67. Hsieh JC, Hägermark Ö, Ståhle-Bäckdahl M, *et al.* Urge to scratch represented in the human cerebral cortex during itch. *J Neurophysiol* 1994;72: 3004–8

68. Aoki T, Kushimoto H, Hishikawa Y, *et al.* Nocturnal scratching and its relationship to the disturbed sleep of itchy subjects. *Clin Exp Dermatol* 1991;16: 268–72

69. Ebata T, Aizawa H, Kamide R. An infrared video camera system to observe nocturnal scratching in atopic dermatitis patients. *J Dermatol* 1996;23: 153–5

70. Felix R, Shuster S. A new method for the measurement of itch and the response to treatment. *Br J Dermatol* 1975;93:303–12

71. Savin JA, Paterson WD, Oswald I. Scratching during sleep. *Lancet* 1973;2:296–7

# Measuring itching and scratching

# 2

Itching remains the primary symptom of inflammatory skin disease, and, as such, deserves special attention in any work on health-related quality of life in dermatology. However, itching, like pain, is a subjective symptom which cannot be verified by physical or biophysical examination

In order to address the issue of itching, we must first agree upon a definition.

- Greaves[1] stated that itching "can be defined subjectively as a poorly localized, non-adapting, usually unpleasant sensation which elicits a desire to scratch"
- In affected individuals, itching may be inconsequential, or extremely severe and occupy the individual's thoughts and actions around the clock

Little attention has been devoted to the issue of itching and health-related quality of life (HRQOL). Indirect reference is made to the relationship between itching and HRQOL[2-6], but these reports fail to substantiate this association.

## Measurement of itching

One of the difficulties in addressing this issue remains the difficulty in objectively assessing itching severity.

- A great deal of scholarly activity has focused on the issue of pain[7], but less is available to review for itching[8-11]
- Nevertheless, due to the work of a number of dedicated investigators, our understanding of itch measurement has progressed significantly in the past decade

Itching is not a monodimensional sensation.

- Accordingly, measurement of itching must take into account qualities of severity and duration, and subjective differences in determination of itching threshold

## Categorical scales

Categorical scales are commonly employed in itching research, and consist of discrete divisions of the measured dimension, such as: "Over the past week, I itched: never, rarely, occasionally, frequently, or always".

- This type of scale is a frequency assessment and is intuitively easy for literate adults to use

Similarly, a severity assessment can be used such as: "Over the past week, I had: no itch, some itching, considerable itching, or itching which could not have been worse".

- Both frequency and severity assessments measure related but distinct components to the itching phenomenon

Categorical scales can also be used to assess the impact of itching upon the life of affected patients.

- This more direct HRQOL measure theoretically combines intensity and frequency perceptions with the subjects' perceived impact on their lives

Consider the Behavioral Rating Scale developed by the author to describe the life-impact of itching[12].

■ As originated, this question reads "Over the past week, how would you describe the effect your itching has had on you?

    No itching

    Itching present, but easily ignored

    Itching present, cannot be ignored, but does not interfere with everyday activities

    Itching present, cannot be ignored, interferes with all tasks except taking care of basic needs such as toileting and eating

    Itching present, cannot be ignored, it interferes with all daily activities."

We assessed the intercorrelation between frequency and intensity of itching on visual analog scales (VAS) with the itching behavioral scale (Box 2.1) and found modest ($r=0.53–0.55$) but highly statistically significant correlations.

■ This finding suggests that intensity, frequency and the behavioral scales are overlapping, yet distinct, constructs

Another behavioral rating scale has been used by Pederson and colleagues[13] to assess itch relief from intervention. This scale used the following points:

■ I never itch
■ I itch rarely but never complain
■ I itch occasionally with mild annoyance
■ I itch often, it may be severe but I can be active and rest easily
■ I itch often, it may be severe and interferes with rest but not activity
■ I itch always, it is severe and it interferes with both rest and activity

This latter method also addresses clinimetric attributes beyond itch frequency or severity. Active treatment decreased itching scores, suggesting responsiveness of this scale. However no further validation studies have been performed.

Thus categorical scales can be used to describe itching frequency, severity, or life-impact. However, although a few preliminary validity studies have been performed on these techniques, no single instrument has been thoroughly validated. Although investigators analyze data from these categorical scales, there is no certainty that the difference between 'never itch' and 'rarely itch' is the same difference as

---

**Box 2.1** Examples of itch measurement instruments

Note that written itch instruments may have specified temporal intervals, e.g., now, over the past minute, over the previous week; or may lack this quantitative aspect

1. **4-point Intensity Rating Scale**
Over the past week, I had:
□ no itch; □ some itching; □ considerable itching; □ itching which could not have been more severe

2. **5-point Frequency Rating Scale**
Over the past week, I itched:
□ never; □ rarely; □ occasionally; □ frequently; □ always

3. **5-point Behavioral Rating Scale**
Over the past week, how would you describe the effect your itching has had on you?
□ no itching;
□ itching present, but easily ignored;
□ itching present, cannot be ignored, but does not interfere with everyday activities;
□ itching present, cannot be ignored, interferes with all tasks except taking care of basic needs such as toileting and eating;
□ itching present, cannot be ignored, it interferes with all daily activities

4. **11-Point Intensity Interval Scale**
Rate your itching intensity from zero to 10: _____

5. **100 mm Frequency Visual Analog Scale**
Over the past week how often did you itch?

|—————————————————————————|

never itched            always itched

---

between 'occasionally itch' and 'always itch'[10]. Investigators aware of this methodologic limitation should consider conservative data analysis.

## Interval scales

Itching can be described by choosing a number on a fixed and limited scale, such as 0 to 10. This technique has the theoretical advantage of a true ordinal scale with equidistant points between responses.

- Indeed, as the number of fixed points increases, e.g. 101 point scale, this scale can approach a continuous scale
- Response to this scale is intuitively easy, and relies less upon literary skill
- Both intensity and frequency can be measured by this technique

This process of reporting interval scale responses can also be cleverly automated, providing more information about the time-course of itching.

- Wahlgren *et al.*[8] evaluated the Pain-Track, a computerized system with a 7-step graded, fixed-point, non-verbal scale in experimental itching compared with the VAS
- This Pain-Track method allows frequent sampling, surveillance of compliance, and generates a large amount of data. Wahlgren *et al.*[8] demonstrated that the VAS produced a linear dose–response relationship with random injection order for itch latency, duration, maximal itch intensity, and 'total itch index.' The Pain-Track related to itch duration and 'total itch index', but not to other subjective variables
- Ståhle-Bäckdahl *et al.*[14] found that in patients undergoing maintenance hemodialysis, Pain-Track recordings showed that itching intensity was greater during dialysis than on days following dialysis, and that itching was worse at night; fluctuations in

itching were able to be detected by the Pain-Track and VAS data
- The Pain-Track has been successfully used in clinical studies to assess the comparative value of different antipruritic agents[11]. This finding supports the validity of the Pain-Track as a clinical measure

## Continuous scales

The VAS, as mentioned above, is the most common example[8].

- A VAS is a line of defined length (in most studies 100 mm) with descriptive anchors at the extremes, e.g., 'no itching' and 'itching as bad as it could be', or 'no itch' and 'maximum itch'
- Assuming a normal distribution of responses, the VAS allows investigators to produce continuous itching data for analysis and thus has methodologic advantages
- This data may be analyzed by parametric techniques and has the advantage of increased sensitivity
- Subjects unfamiliar with the VAS may be confused by this instrument and may require an example or detailed instructions

## Scratch behavior measurement

Scratch behavior reflects, in some fashion, itching sensation. Clinicians may be able to subjectively rate the number of excoriations or degree of lichenification[15].

- This rating is widely used clinically, but has not been validated and is not likely to be reproducible (consider the fact that some intensely itchy conditions such as urticaria rarely show lichenification)

The measurement of scratching behavior is problematic, and has been addressed in a variety of ways.

## Self-report of scratching behavior

Patients can be provided with hand-activated counters to record their scratching[16].

■ Although obsessive–compulsive patients may be able to record their number of scratches[17], the act of recording scratching behavior may alter the behavior itself

■ Moreover, nocturnal scratching cannot be recorded. Accordingly, other techniques have been developed

## Nocturnal bed movement

■ Felix and Shuster[18] measured whole body movement at night by a vibration transducer on a bed leg and measured limb movement with movement-sensitive meters

> They found that the subjective sensation of itch correlated with nocturnal scratching behavior. Increased itching severity is associated with an increase in number of scratching episodes but not scratching duration

Motion detection techniques can also demonstrate response to disease-specific therapy[19].

## Limb activity meters

Itchy patients tend to move their arms more than their legs, and careful analysis of both arm and leg movement can allow discrimination. A number of approaches have been used, each with relative merits[20–23].

■ Although limb activity meters may adequately demonstrate response to therapy and are reproducible, wiring and recording nightly from biophysical devices will always be intrusive and costly

■ One negative study utilized this technique to dissociate the etiology of itching in cholestatic liver disease from bile acid levels, a previously popular hypothesis[22]

■ Osifo[23] monitored scratching behavior with limb activity meters that were modified self-winding watches

This technique was used to evaluate the relative effect of antipruritic agents. These watches are not likely to be equally sensitive to all scratching behavioral movements; temporal recording of scratching is not possible

■ Rhythmic muscle potentials can be recorded at the same time as an electroencephalogram records sleep activity[24–26]

## Direct observation

■ Cornbleet[27] reported the results of his investigations in 1953 in which he directly observed patients and their scratching behavior.

> He found scratching occurred in bouts of multiple rhythmic strokes

> Given the intrusive nature and time requirements of this approach, this technique is unlikely to be repeated

■ Using different methods, Ebata and colleagues[28] recorded the total scratch time of nocturnal itching using infrared photographic monitoring sensitive down to zero ambient light levels

> In atopic dermatitis scratching time was found to vary from between 7 minutes to nearly 5 hours

■ Observation may miss scratching behavior underneath covers and this technique is extraordinarily expensive

## Itching as part of HRQOL indices

Within general medical research, HRQOL instruments such as the Brief Symptom Inventory[29] and SF–36[30] fail to mention itching. Thus, despite their broad use within disease and normative populations, these instruments rarely meet the needs of dermatologic investigators. More specific dermatologic instruments have been developed which utilize itching as part of their construct.

## Dermatology Life Quality Index (DLQI)

Finlay and Khan[31] incorporated itching into this dermatology-specific instrument.

- In order to decrease the number of questions, this index includes the question: "Over the last week, how itchy, 'scratchy', sore, or painful has your skin been?"
- The categorical responses include 'very much', 'a lot', 'a little' and 'not at all'
- Obviously, this question measures global skin symptoms including itching, but also including skin soreness and painfulness

Nevertheless, the DLQI as a whole suggests that patients with pruritic dermatoses (atopic dermatitis, psoriasis, and generalized itching) have lower HRQOL than those with nonpruritic dermatoses (acne, basal cell carcinoma, and viral warts).

## Children's Dermatology Life Quality Index (CDLQI)

This analogous instrument was subsequently developed by Lewis-Jones and Finlay[32] and contains the same global symptom question as noted above.

## Psoriasis-Related Stressor Scale (PRSS)

Based upon focus group sessions with patients and physicians, our group developed a 20-item scale, the PRSS, a measure of stressful aspects of psoriasis.

- Unlike the DLQI, this psoriasis-specific instrument inquires about itching itself, without mention of scratching, soreness, or pain
- Accordingly, the PRSS may be more useful for psoriasis which has itching as a major component, and is likely to be less useful for non-psoriatic skin disease
- The PRSS has undergone validation studies on a large group of psoriasis patients and

has been used to demonstrate HRQOL improvement in a clinical trial

## SCORAD

The European Task Force on Atopic Dermatitis developed a scoring index (SCORAD) for their target disease combining extent, severity and subjective symptoms[33].

- Unlike the Psoriasis Area Severity Index (PASI) which describes cutaneous disease severity[34] this global score incorporates both skin symptoms and disease severity into one index
- The itching question in this index is a VAS with anchors of 0 and 10. The VAS text asks the subject to describe the average itching severity for 'the last 3 days or nights'
- The SCORAD has been used to show HRQOL improvement in a clinical trial[35]

## Skindex

The Skindex is a 62-item, self-administered, survey instrument designed to assess skin disease health-related quality of life. It has had reliability and responsiveness validation[36].

- Itching is assessed as part of the physical discomfort component of the entire conceptual framework
- The question about itching is analogous to the 5-point Frequency Rating Scale as cited above: "My skin itches: never, rarely, sometimes, often, all the time."
- Itching and other components including skin irritation and pain explained only 5% of the common variance in the instrument, whereas feeling embarrassed, ashamed and humiliated explained 46% of this variance
- Thus itching apparently contributes to HRQOL as measured by the Skindex, but only explains a small proportion of the variance

# References

1. Greaves MW. Pruritus. In Champion RH, Burton JL, Ebling FJG, eds. *Textbook of Dermatology*, 5th edn. Oxford: Blackwell Scientific Publications, 1992:527–36

2. Turner IB, Rawlins MD, Wood P, *et al.* Flumecinol for the treatment of pruritus associated with primary biliary cirrhosis. *Alimen Pharmacol Ther* 1994;8:337–42

3. Ballinger AB, McHugh M, Catnach SM, *et al.* Symptom relief and quality of life after stenting for malignant bile duct obstruction. *Gut* 1994;35:467–70

4. Finelli C, Gugliotta L, Gamberi B, *et al.* Relief of intractable pruritus in polycythemia vera with recombinant interferon alfa. *Am J Hematol* 1993;43:316–8

5. Alarabi AA, Wikstrom B, Loof L, *et al.* Treatment of pruritus in cholestatic jaundice by bilirubin- and bile acid-adsorbing resin column plasma perfusion. *Scan J Gastroenterol* 1992;27:223–6

6. Lauterburg BH, Taswell HF, Pineda AA, *et al.* Treatment of pruritus of cholestasis by plasma perfusion through USP-charcoal-coated glass beads. *Lancet* 1980;2:53–5.

7. Jensen MP, Karoly P, Braver S. The measurement of clinical pain intensity: a comparison of six methods. *Pain* 1986;27:117–26

8. Wahlgren CF, Ekblom A, Hägermark Ö. Some aspects of the experimental induction and measurement of itch. *Acta Derm Venereol* 1989;69:185–9

9. Wahlgren CF. Itch and atopic dermatitis: clinical and experimental studies. *Acta Derm Venereol* 1991;165 (Suppl):1–53

10. Wahlgren CF. Measurement of itch. *Sem Dermatol* 1995;14:277–84

11. Hägermark Ö, Wahlgren CF. Some methods for evaluating clinical itch and their application for studying pathophysiological mechanisms. *J Dermatol Science* 1992;4:55–62

12. Fleischer AB Jr, McFarlane M, Hinds MA, *et al.* Skin conditions and symptoms are common in the elderly: the prevalence of skin symptoms and conditions in an elderly population. *J Ger Dermatol* 1996;4:78–89

13. Pederson JA, Matter BJ, Czerwinski AW, et al. Relief of idiopathic generalized pruritus in dialysis patients treated with activated oral charcoal. Ann Intern Med 1980;93:446–8

14. Ståhle-Bäckdahl M, Wahlgren CF, Hägermark Ö. Computerized recording of itch in patients on maintenance hemodialysis. *Acta Derm Venereol* 1989;69:410–4

15. Savin J. The measurement of scratching. *Semin Dermatol* 1995;14:285–9

16. Melin L, Frederiksen T, Noren P, *et al.* Behavioural treatment of scratching in patients with atopic dermatitis. *Br J Dermatol* 1986;115:467–74

17. Savin J. Neurotic excoriations – a quantitative approach to the effect of treatment. *Br J Clin Pract* 1970;24;451–3

18. Felix R, Shuster S. A new method for the measurement of itch and the response to treatment. *Br J Dermatol* 1975;93:303–12

19. Shuster S. Pruritus and its assessment as itch and scratch. *Acta Derm Venereol* 1991;156(Suppl):45

20. Summerfield JA, Welch ME. The measurement of itch with sensitive limb movement meters. *Br J Dermatol* 1980;103:275–81

21. Mustakallio KK. Scratch radar for the measurement of pruritus. *Acta Derm Venereol* 1991;156(Suppl):44

22. Bartholomew TC, Summerfield JA, Billing BH, *et al.* Bile acid profiles of human serum and skin interstitial fluid and their relationship to pruritus studied by gas chromatography-mass spectrometry. *Clin Sci* 1982;63:65–73

23. Osifo NG. The antipruritic effects of chlorpheniramine, cyproheptadine and sulphapyridine monitored with limb activity meters on chloroquine induced pruritus among patients with malaria. *Af J Med Sci* 1995;24:67–73

24. Savin JA, Paterson WD, Oswald I. Scratching during sleep. *Lancet* 1973;2:296–7

25. Monti JM, Vignale R, Monti D. Sleep and nighttime pruritus in children with atopic dermatitis. *Sleep* 1989;12:309–14

26. Brown DG, Kalucy RS. Correlation of neurophysiological and personality data in sleep scratching. *Proc Roy Soc Med* 1975;68:530–2

27. Cornbleet T. Scratching pattern. 1. Influence of site. *J Invest Dermatol* 1953;20:105–10

28. Ebata T, Aizawa H, Kamide R. An infrared video camera system to observe nocturnal scratching in atopic dermatitis patients. *J Dermatol* 1996;23:153–5

29. Derogatis LR, Spencer PM. *The Brief Symptom Inventory (BSI): Administration, Scoring and Procedures Manual.* Baltimore: Johns Hopkins Press, 1982

30. Julious SA, George S, Campbell MJ. Sample sizes for studies using the short form 36 (SF–36). *J Epidemiol Comm Health* 1995;49:642–4

31. Finlay AY, Khan GK. Dermatology Life Quality Index (DLQI) – a simple practical measure for routine clinical use. *Clin Exp Dermatol* 1994;19: 210–6

32. Lewis-Jones, Finlay AY. The Children's Life Quality Index (CDLQI): initial validation and subsequent use. *Br J Dermatol* 1995;132;942–9

33. Anonymous: Severity scoring of atopic dermatitis: the SCORAD index. Consensus Report of the European Task Force on Atopic Dermatitis. *Dermatology* 1993;186:23–31

34. Fredriksson T, Pettersson U: Severe psoriasis – oral therapy with a new retinoid. *Dermatologica* 1978; 157:238–44

35. Kowalzick L, Kleinheinz A, Neuber, *et al.* Low dose versus medium dose UVA–A1 treatment in severe atopic dermatitis. *Acta Derm Venereol* 1995;75:43–5

36. Chren MM, Lasek RJ, Quinn LM, *et al.* Skindex, a quality-of-life measure for patients with skin disease: reliability, validity, and responsiveness. *J Invest Dermatol* 1996;107:707–13

# Evaluation of the itching patient   3

There is no single evaluation style or technique that is best suited for every clinician and patient, thus this should only serve as a guide for evaluation. For the experienced clinician, the vast majority of patients require only a cursory history, limited physical examination confined to the skin, and no laboratory evaluation. A small number of patients need further evaluation including a more detailed history, a thorough examination beyond the skin, and select laboratory studies (see also chapter 8: Urticarial diseases for disease specific questions)

No matter how thorough, history, physical examination and laboratory evaluation do not always allow the clinician to develop a definitive diagnosis. There is always a place for empiric treatment approaches when other diagnostic maneuvers fail

## History

History may provide keen insight into the disease process. Ideally, a few select questions may help the clinician narrow the diagnosis.

**Is the itching localized or generalized? Where exactly do you itch?**
- Local itching is usually of exogenous etiology, whereas occasionally generalized itching is of endogenous etiology
- Inquiring about the exact location(s) helps focus the patients, as some patients itch only on their scalp and distal legs, yet claim to itch 'everywhere'

**What sensation do you feel in your skin?**
- Most patients describe itching and may be mystified by this question. Others will describe crawling, burning itch. Other patients will describe no itch, but describe a burning sensation
- These latter patients often have 'itching' skin conditions, but other physicians have never asked them about the sensation
- Some with burning actually have dysesthesia rather than itching and the approach to these patients is entirely different

**Is anyone else in your immediate family affected?**
- When multiple family members are affected, serious consideration of scabies and other parasites should be given
- Many other itching conditions may be shared including atopic dermatitis, psychoses, etc.

**Is there a relationship with your occupation?**
- Chronic hand dermatitis or latex allergy may be found in health care workers, insulation workers may acquire fiberglass dermatitis, etc.

**Is there any recent history of travel?**
- Parasitic infections from amoebiasis to onchocerciasis may be acquired in this small, interconnected world

**Have you been exposed to any animals?**
- Pets may harbor relatively asymptomatic ectoparasites, fungi, and other itch inducers

**Any history of exposure to irritating chemicals or plants?**
- Repetitive exposure to solvents and other harsh chemicals can cause cutaneous irritation, as may allergy to plants

### How do you bathe?

- Hot water, harsh soaps and detergents, and prolonged soaking may all dry the skin and predispose the patient to irritant dermatitis
- Itchy patients may feel they are unclean and thus redouble their efforts to cleanse their skin, in the process creating severe irritant contact dermatitis
- Bathing may induce aquagenic itching

### What cosmetics, toiletries, and fragrances do you use, and have these changed recently?

- Allergic or irritant reactions are possible reactions to the multitude of topically applied products

### What are you using on your skin to treat this condition?

- Patients may be using perfectly reasonable emollients and topical remedies that only rarely sensitize
- They may also be using a number of irritants and allergens that are exacerbating their condition
- The author has been told of multiple agents that patients have used for self-treatment including application of alcohol, ammonia, bleach, gasoline, ice water, neomycin, permethrin, scalding hot water, and urine

### Have you started any new drugs in the past few months?

- Adverse drug reactions may be delayed by weeks and may not have any associated rash
- Even drugs related to known drug allergens can be problematic, e.g. sulfa moiety-containing diuretics in sulfa antibiotic-allergic patients
- Non-prescription agents may cause cutaneous drug reactions, as may illicit drugs

### What is your personal theory as to why you itch?

- This is the author's favorite question, which most commonly produces no useful information but there are exceptional cases

- When an interesting answer is produced, more insight is produced by this question than any other
- Exercise-induced itching and other idiosyncratic itching disorders may be elicited this way
- One patient related that his itching began when he was fishing on a nuclear power plant lake and believes that he was bitten by 'nuclear mosquitoes'
- Another patient with neurotic excoriations displaying extensive linear excoriations and subungual blood told me that she itched, but she never touched her skin; she suddenly starts bleeding for no apparent reason

### Do you scratch at night while you try to go to sleep, or wake up scratching?

- Whereas psychogenic itching rarely interferes in sleep, most itching conditions cause nocturnal itching
- This question helps therapeutically, as an affirmative answer can be an indication to prescribe sedating agents at bedtime

### Have you been under a great deal of stress lately?

- 'Stress' has many meanings to clinicians and patients alike, but this may give insight into initiation of the disease process

### Do you have a prior history of this type of itching occurring before?

- This may give etiologic and therapeutic clues, e.g. seasonal itching in the summer due to solar pruritus or recurrent asteatotic dermatitis in the winter

## Past medical history

A history of atopy predisposes the patient to a large number of irritant reactions with intensified itch response. A past history of thyroid disease, cancer, or other systemic disease associated with itching may indicate recurrence.

## Review of systems

Ideally, a complete review of systems is performed. Although essentially any systemic disease can cause itching of unknown etiology, those questions relating to the liver, thyroid gland, and systemic malignancy are most likely to yield useful information.

## Family medical history

A history of atopic disease in the family may help establish the diagnosis in a patient with no personal history. As noted above, a history of others currently itching is extremely useful.

## Social history

A history of intravenous drug abuse or high risk sexual behavior should prompt the clinician to consider testing for human immunodeficiency virus (HIV) infection. HIV infection and its associated diseases may cause extraordinary itching. One memorable itching patient had no known risk factors for HIV, but her husband had undergone coronary artery bypass graft surgery several years earlier during which he became infected, later spreading HIV to the patient.

## Examination

- Careful skin examination should be performed for signs of skin diseases including distribution of lesions, lesional morphology, primary and secondary lesions
- Patients need a complete cutaneous examination, and need to understand the importance of looking elsewhere for diagnostic clues
- Examine for excoriations and lichenification

    Secondary lesions on the upper midback suggest that a skin disease is responsible, whereas sparing is associated with systemic causes of itching

- Examine mucous membranes as needed
- Testing for dermatographism may help in urticarial diseases
- Make a special effort to look for evidence of scabies and other infestation
- Occasionally, investigation of mental status, mood, hallucinations, personality disorders, and similar may be required
- Although rarely necessary, the clinician should consider performing a complete physical examination or refer the patient to another physician willing to do so
- When the differential diagnosis includes systemic diseases and internal malignancy, patients should be evaluated properly
- Patients with pruritus of unknown origin usually should be considered to have an underlying disorder

## Laboratory investigation

This rarely yields useful information, as the clinical examination usually produces the correct diagnosis. However, in the setting of generalized itching of unknown etiology, evaluation to exclude internal disease may be indicated (see chapter 4: Systemic causes of itching) including:

- Testing for hematologic disorders

    Complete blood count with differential

    Erythrocyte sedimentation rate

    Serum protein electrophoresis

- Liver transaminases, creatinine, blood urea nitrogen, glucose or glycosylated hemoglobin
- Thyroid function tests (thyroid stimulating hormone, T4)
- Chest X-ray
- Skin biopsy, possibly including direct immunofluorescence

    Biopsies may lead to the diagnosis of 'prebullous' bullous pemphigoid, dermatitis herpetiformis and other inflammatory dermatoses

■ Further investigation may be required depending on the situation including

HIV screening

Urine for 5-hydroxyindoleacetic acid (5HIAA) and mast cell metabolites

Serum iron and ferritin

Stool studies for ova and parasites and occult blood

## Further investigation

When all else fails, consider re-evaluation of any indicated historical, examination or laboratory data in 6–12 months. In the interim, empiric treatment and the passage of time often brings resolution of the itching. Clinicians should not hesitate to use therapeutic trials of antipruritic approaches as a diagnostic aid.

## Further reading

1. Kantor GR, Lookingbill DP. Generalized pruritus and systemic disease. *J Am Acad Dermatol* 1983;9: 375–82

2. Kantor GR. Evaluation and treatment of generalized pruritus. *Clev Clin J Med* 1990;57:521–6

3. Kantor GR. Pruritus and systemic disease. *Curr Concepts Skin Dis* 1991;12:17–21

4. Kantor GR. Diagnostic evaluation of the patient with generalized pruritus. In Bernhard J, ed. *Itch: Mechanisms and Management of Pruritus*. New York: McGraw Hill, 1994:337–46

5. Kantor GR. Investigation of the elderly patient with pruritus. *J Ger Dermatol* 1995;3:1–7

6. Kantor GR, Bernhard JD. Investigation of the pruritic patient in daily practice. *Sem Dermatol* 1995;14: 290–6

7. Klecz RJ, Schwartz RA. Pruritus. *Am Fam Phys* 1992; 45:2681–6

8. Lober CW. Should the patient with generalized pruritus be evaluated for malignancy. *J Am Acad Dermatol* 1988;19:350–2

9. Lyell A. The itching patient, a review of causes of pruritus. *Scott Med J* 1972;17:334-8

10. O'Donnell BF, Alton B, Carney D, *et al.* Generalized pruritus: when to investigate further. *J Am Acad Dermatol* 1993;28:117

11. Rajka G. Investigation of patients suffering from generalized pruritus, with special reference to systemic disease. *Acta Derm Venereol* 1966;46:190–4

12. Sarno AM, Bernhard JD. Drug-induced pruritus without a rash. In Bernhard J, ed. *Itch: Mechanisms and Management of Pruritus*. New York: McGraw Hill, 1994:329–35

13. Sher TH. Clinical evaluation of generalized pruritus. *Comp Ther* 1992;18:14–9

# Systemic causes of itching 4

Systemic conditions occasionally cause itching and can be summarized by the mnemonic BLINKED: B= blood disease, bugs; L= liver disease; I= infection, immunologic or autoimmune disease; N= neoplastic disease, neuropsychiatric diseases; K= kidney disease; E= endocrinologic disease; D= drugs

This chapter treats all neurological and psychiatric diseases as systemic diseases and includes pregnancy and the menopause which can also contribute to itching

Published estimates of the prevalence of systemic diseases in patients with generalized itching range from 10 to 50%[1-4]. However, these estimates are likely to be at least ten-fold higher than is expected in community practice due to investigator bias.

In a study of 44 cases of generalized pruritus, Kantor and Lookingbill[4] compared itching patients to age- and sex-matched patients with psoriasis. There was no difference in the prevalence of systemic diseases.

If the clinician believes that a systemic evaluation is required, tests to consider may include a complete blood count with differential, multi-chemistry panel (including creatinine, liver transaminases, albumin and protein), thyroid studies, and chest radiograph.

Although infections may be a systemic disease, these are addressed in chapter 5: Infections, infestations, bites and stings.

## Endocrine diseases

### Autoimmune progesterone or estrogen dermatitis

Autoimmune progesterone dermatitis includes itching, urticaria, papulovesicular eruptions, and bullous erythema multiforme[5-7]. It consists of a recurrent eruption, primarily on the extremities after receiving oral estrogen/progesterone replacement for the treatment of climacteric symptoms.

- Recurrence of the eruption 5 to 10 days prior to the menses with spontaneous resolution following menses is typically present
- Intradermal skin testing to progesterone sensitivity may confirm the diagnosis
- Treatment with conjugated estrogens often results in remission

Autoimmune estrogen dermatitis was reported in a recent study[8].

- Women exhibiting severe premenstrual exacerbations of papulovesicular eruptions, urticaria, eczema, or generalized pruritus were tested by intradermal skin tests and proved to have an unrecognized sensitivity to estrogen
- Most had a positive delayed tuberculin-type skin test or an urticarial reaction to intradermal estrogens
- Antiestrogen therapy with tamoxifen or elimination of oral estrogen therapy may be helpful

### Diabetes mellitus

Generalized itching is not more common in diabetic patients than in the generalized population. However, vulvar itching may be much more common in diabetic women (rates approach 20%) than in normal women controls (6%) and is associated with poor diabetes control[9].

■ Screening for diabetes in patients with generalized itching may not be cost-effective, but such screening in vulvar disease patients may prove diagnostic

## Perimenopausal itching

Episodic itching is an occasional finding in perimenopausal women. Other stigmata of the menopause state such as hot flashes may be present[10].

■ Hormone replacement therapy with ethinyl estradiol is usually sufficient to control pruritus due to this cause

## Thyroid disease

Severe generalized itching may be the presenting symptom in hyperthyroidism, particularly in the setting of thyroid storm. Excoriations, lichenification, and dermatitis may be present[11,12].

■ Readily diagnosed by history of weight loss, heat intolerance, other symptoms and screening laboratory studies

Hypothyroidism may be a cause of localized or generalized itching.

■ Typical changes include xerotic, scaling skin that may be easily irritated (Figure 1)
■ Asteatotic dermatitis may be more common
■ Readily diagnosed by history of weight gain, cool intolerance, lethargy and screening laboratory studies

# Hematologic diseases

Hematologic diseases, especially the malignant conditions, are associated with significant itching.

## Hypereosinophilic syndrome

Hypereosinophilic syndrome is a rare disorder typically affecting middle-aged males which must be distinguished from eosinophil leukemia[13–15].

■ Itchy red papules, nodules and urticarial wheals may develop
■ Concurrent polycythemia and mastocytosis have been reported
■ Cardiac and neurologic abnormalities are associated
■ Aquagenic pruritus has also been reported

Because eosinophilia may be found in a large number of other dermatologic conditions, other hypereosinophilic conditions such as infectious diseases must be ruled out. Treatment may be difficult, and systemic steroids and chemotherapeutic agents may be required.

## Iron deficiency

Although iron deficiency is often listed as a cause of itching, the association between iron deficiency and itching is far from proven, and rigorous controlled trials have not been performed[16–21].

Iron deficiency may be a sign of polycythemia vera, numerous other cancers, and other systemic conditions which themselves cause itching. Until further evidence emerges, the association of iron deficiency with itching must be considered as secondary to other factors or diseases.

## Job's syndrome

This is a rare hyper-IgE syndrome in which red hair and cold abscesses are found[22].

■ Chronic atopic dermatitis may be associated in early childhood
■ Abnormal neutrophil chemotaxis function allows frequent bacterial and candidal infections of the skin, sinuses and respiratory tract
■ Serum levels of IgE are often elevated to ten times normal (>2000 IU/ml)

## Paraproteinemia (Myelomatosis)

Pruritus may be the original presenting complaint, although the mechanism is unknown[23].

## Polycythemia vera

### Clinical features and pathophysiology

Between 30–50% of untreated patients develop an invisible, severe, prickly and distressing discomfort within minutes of water contact, which can last 15–60 minutes[24].

- Platelet aggregation has been suggested as a possible mechanism and source of pruritogenic factors including histamine
- Mast cell degranulation and mediator-release by mast cells is not likely to be responsible for water-induced pruritus[25]
- Water-induced itching may precede development of polycythemia vera by years, thus this diagnosis must be suspected in all patients with water-induced itching

### Treatment

- Topical corticosteroid and systemic antihistaminic agents are occasionally helpful
- Ultraviolet (UV) B irradiation may help
- Aspirin has been reported effective[26]
- In an open trial, cimetidine (900 mg daily) helped the majority of patients[27]
- Intramuscular interferon-α suppresses the increased hematopoiesis, and the majority of patients with intractable pruritus obtain relief[28,29]

    One-third of patients treated with interferon may not be able to tolerate the side-effects

For other hematologic conditions, see malignancy below.

## Liver diseases

Virtually any liver disease may contribute to itching (Table 1).

- Serum screening may demonstrate abnormalities in the following non-specific tests: alkaline phosphatase, total and direct bilirubin, cholesterol, aspartate aminotransferase (AST, SGOT), alanine aminotransferase (ALT, SGPT), γ-glutamyltranspeptidase (GGT), and fasting cholesterol
- More specific tests, i.e. invasive cholangiography, may be required for definitive diagnosis
- Drugs including chlorpromazine, contraceptive pills and testosterone can induce cholestasis[30–33]
- Itching has also been mentioned as a presenting feature of the arteriohepatic syndrome in children[34]

### Pathogenesis

- The exact mechanism of itching in liver disease remains unclear, but it seems to be related to cholestasis
- Bile salts do not appear to be the sole itch mediators
- Histaminergic pathways may be involved
- Impaired excretion of large, centrally-acting, endogenous opioid peptides may contribute to pruritus[31,32,35]

### Treatment

- Resins such as cholestyramine or colestipol are often effective and can be considered the first line of therapy[36,37]

    These are best taken before and after eating breakfast

- Antihistamines may be beneficial, but failure is frequent

    Since the observed efficacy may be related to sedation, choosing a centrally acting agent, such as diphenhydramine or hydroxyzine, may be a reasonable choice

- Phenobarbital may temporarily improve itching, but its effects are not generally sustained longer than several weeks

**Table 4.1** Liver diseases presenting with itching

| Disease | Diagnostic tests | Expected test result |
|---|---|---|
| Biliary atresia | Cholangiogram | Abnormal biliary structure |
| Carcinoma of pancreatic head or bile ducts[38] | Cholangiogram | Stricture |
| | CT or MRI scan | Mass lesion |
| Choledocholithiasis | Cholangiogram | Filling defects |
| Cholestasis of pregnancy[30,32] | Bilirubin | Elevated |
| | Transaminases | Elevated |
| Chronic pancreatitis | Serum amylase and lipase | Elevated |
| | Cholangiogram | Obstruction |
| Drug-induced hepatitis/ cholestasis | Drug withdrawal | Prompt improvement |
| Hemochromatosis[39,40] | Iron studies | Excess iron |
| | Liver biopsy | Demonstration of iron and damage |
| Hepatitis B and C[41] | Hepatitis serology | Positive |
| Primary biliary cirrhosis[42] | Antimitochondrial antibody | Positive |
| | Elevated immunoglobulins | Elevated IgM |
| | Liver biopsy | Bile duct destruction |
| Primary sclerosing cholangitis | Cholangiogram | Strictures |

Table adapted from reference 43

- Flumecinol 600 mg, a hepatic enzyme inducer, was safe at the above doses, and short-term treatment with 300mg daily significantly ameliorated itching in primary biliary cirrhosis[44]
- Rifampicin, which inhibits the uptake of bile acids by hepatocytes and is an antimicrobial agent, has been used to treat pruritus at 300 to 450 mg twice daily[45,46]

    Prolonged administration in primary biliary cirrhosis does not seem to exacerbate liver disease

- Ondansetron, a specific serotonin type 3 receptor antagonist, relieves itching in cholestatis within 30–60 minutes[47,48]
- Ursodeoxycholic acid and methotrexate have an advantage in not only relieving pruritus but also potentially retarding disease progression in primary biliary sclerosis, although this remains to be proved[49,50]

    Ursodeoxycholic acid 600 mg/day may affect itch intensity after 6 months or more of use

- Epomediol is an anticholestatic agent that has been shown to ameliorate itching in patients with intrahepatic cholestasis of pregnancy[51]
- Subhypnotic injected doses (15 mg) of propofol relieve pruritus associated with liver disease[52–54]
- Primary biliary cirrhosis (cholestatic pruritus) responds to one or two continuous (24-hour) intravenous infusions of naloxone[55] (0.2 mg/kg/min)
- Plasma perfusion in four patients through the ion resin BR–350 was found to be an effective, safe and expensive treatment for

symptomatic relief of intractable pruritus in cholestatic liver disease[56]

- A number of patients treated with the teratogenic agent thalidomide reported an improvement in itch[57]
- Itching in patients with cholestasis due to pancreatic carcinoma may achieve itch palliation and jaundice relief with surgical insertion of a stent[38]
- Phototherapy improves cholestatic pruritus and primary biliary cirrhosis, probably by its ability to enhance excretion of bile acids and other possible pruritogens into urine[58]

## Malignancy

Virtually any malignancy can cause itching as a paraneoplastic disorder (see Box 4.1). In cancer patients there is little evidence that histamine participates in itch mediation.

- Burtin and colleagues[70] found a decreased skin response in cancer patients to histamine injection, as the presence of a tumor may mimic the effects of general administration of histamine $H_1$ antagonists on the skin response to histamine

Some neoplasms are more frequently associated with pruritus, e.g. lymphoma. Itching in cancer patients may be due to an idiopathic paraneoplastic mechanism, physical obstruction (e.g. obstruction of bile ducts), a pruritic malignant skin infiltrate, or alternatively a primary skin disease[59,71].

- The etiology of paraneoplastic itching is poorly understood[72]. Although there is no doubt paraneoplastic itching can occur, no reliable epidemiologic study has ever demonstrated increased rates of malignant disease in itching patients compared with a control population

Failure of generalized itching to respond to conventional therapy or persistent unexplained

---

> **Box 4.1** Malignancies associated with itching (from reference 59)
>
> Breast carcinoma[60]
> Carcinoid syndrome[61]
> Cutaneous T-cell lymphoma
> Hodgkin's disease[62,63]
> Gastrointestinal tract cancers:
>     tongue, stomach and colon[64]
> Kaposi sarcoma[65] (Figure 2)
> Leukemia[66]
> Lung cancer[67,68]
> Malignant mastocytoma
> Multiple myeloma
> Non-Hodgkin lymphomas[63]
> Polycythemia rubra vera[69]
> Prostatic carcinoma
> Thyroid carcinoma
> Uterine carcinoma

---

itching should warrant evaluation for underlying malignant disorders[73–77]. Examples of itching in malignancy are listed below.

### Lymphoma

- Hodgkin's disease has an itch prevalence of 10–30%[62,63,78,79]

  Gobbi and colleagues[80,81] reported that severe pruritus in Hodgkin's disease predicts a poor prognosis

  Return of itching following successful treatment should be regarded as evidence of tumor recurrence

- Non-Hodgkin's lymphoma may cause itching less frequently (2%)
- Cutaneous T-cell lymphoma (see chapter 9: Other itching conditions),
- Peripheral T-cell lymphoma, and other cutaneous lymphomas are notoriously pruritic

## Other malignant conditions

- Leukemia: less than 5% experience itching, but malignant infiltrates may itch
- Polycythemia rubra vera: itch prevalence of 30–50% (see Hematologic diseases, above)
- Carcinoid syndrome: itching may be a component, but flushing and other associated signs are much more frequent
- Central nervous system tumors (see Neuropsychiatric diseases, below)
- Aquagenic pruritus has been reported in association with the following malignant and non-malignant neoplastic diseases

    Acute lymphoblastic leukemia[82]

    Cervical squamous cell carcinoma[83]

    Hypereosinophilic syndrome[84]

    Juvenile xanthogranuloma[85]

    Myelodysplastic syndrome[83]

    Polycythemia rubra vera[86]

## Treatment

Many patients with paraneoplastic itching have incurable malignant disease. In this group of patients, non-specific antipruritic treatment should be considered.

- Hydration of the skin surface may relieve itching
- A simple, effective therapeutic approach is to apply emollients (lotions, creams and ointments) on dry skin twice daily
- Emollients with camphor and menthol, phenol or pramoxine, may provide safe relief from pruritus
- Age-old remedies including cool compresses and shake lotions (e.g. calamine) may be helpful
- Baths with colloidal oatmeal, therapeutic salts, or milk-oil baths may provide short-term relief
- Occasionally, topical corticosteroids may be useful adjunctive agents

For tumor-induced physical obstruction, consider organ-specific therapy.

- Pancreatic or other gastrointestinal carcinoma-induced cholestasis: operative stent placement, rifampicin, and ursodeoxycholic acid (see Liver diseases, above)
- Urinary obstruction: catheter placement may relieve renal-pruritus

# Neuropsychiatric diseases

Abnormalities of the nervous system may contribute to itching or cause itching.

Psychogenic pruritus and self-excoriation are diagnoses of exclusion, e.g. patients with the itch of primary biliary cirrhosis may only have excoriations visible.

Psychiatric diseases, especially depression, modulate itch perception. Occasionally patients with longstanding, intractable itching may develop depressive symptoms as the result of their itching; the depression does not always cause itching.

## Pathogenesis

There is no topic which is likely to be more complex and multifactorial.

- Itch mediators including histamine, endogenous opioids and neuropeptides may be affected by neuropsychiatric diseases
- Focal neurologic disease may directly stimulate peripheral or central itch pathways
- Personality disorders, affective disorders, and psychoses may precipitate or enhance itching and complaints of itching

## Focal central nervous system diseases

The approach to focal central nervous system disease depends upon the diagnosis and feasibility and availability of therapy. Focal neurologic disease may create the perception of itch as reported in the following conditions.

- Brain tumors: in a study of 77 patients with brain tumors[87], 13 complained of itching with six of these complaining of nostril itch
- Brainstem glioma: episodic, unilateral facial itching was reported in two children with neurofibromatosis with brainstem glioma[88]
- Cerebrovascular accident: patients with unilateral pruritus after a stroke have been described[89–91]

  Relief has been reported with carbamazepine or amitriptyline

- Cervical spinal cord compression may cause reversible itching and burning in the lower extremities[92]
- Degenerative joint disease in the spine has been linked to dermatomal itching[93]
- Guillain-Barré syndrome has been reported to present with intractable itching[94]
- Multiple sclerosis[95–98]: paroxysmal attacks of several minutes of intense itching that start and end abruptly and recur several times a day; controlled effectively by carbamazepine
- Intramedullary vascular malformation[99]: segmental pruritus of the T2 dermatome was described as due to an intramedullary vascular malformation
- Intramedullary neoplasm and syringomyelia: a patient with dermatomal pruritus and rash was attributed to a cervicothoracic syrinx and a thoracic spinal cord tumor[100]
- Neurofibromatosis may induce itching within a segmental distribution or generalized itching[101,102]
- Nocardia brain abscess has been associated with unilateral itching[103]
- Tabes may give rise to segmental pruritus

## Psychiatric conditions and itching

### Psychogenic itching

If itching is associated with significant psychopathology, such as anxiety, depression, or schizophrenia, and is temporally associated with the onset of the itching, it can be called psychogenic itching. Because patients with psychiatric disease are not immune from developing skin diseases or itching from systemic diseases (e.g. hepatic or renal disease), psychogenic itching is a diagnosis of exclusion.

### Clinical features

Prior history of neuropsychiatric disease may be extremely helpful. Obtaining a complete medication history on patients may provide clues to this diagnosis that may not be found from direct questioning of the patient.

- No primary lesions are ever seen, but secondary lesions are often present
- Secondary lesions range from lichenification to excoriations

  Excoriations usually spare the upper back where patients find it difficult to reach

  Insight into excoriations: patients who acknowledge that they have significant itching and cannot stop their scratching behavior seem to be quite different from those who state that they never scratch, yet have actively bleeding excoriations

### Neurotic excoriations

Neurotic excoriations is not a specific neuropsychiatric disease, but rather a symptom of a wide range of psychiatric disorders, for example major depression.

Sufferers with this disorder are driven to pick, scratch, rub, or otherwise abuse their skin to produce the lesions. Even minor irritation of the skin give rise to an exaggerated response. Virtually everyone with an insect bite may be driven to scratch or rub at the site; what distinguishes these patients from others is that they cannot seem to stop scratching and digging[104,105]. Even following cessation of symptoms from an original insult or skin irregularity, they persist in deriving some satisfaction from continuing their skin-destructive behavior.

Many patients also experience impairment in social or occupational functioning.

- To emphasize the importance of this condition, one study shows that as many as one-third of neurotic excoriation patients may contemplate suicide[106]
- Critically, these patients lack delusions of infection or infestation

Excoriations are often relatively deep, and may be punctate or linear (Figures 3, 4). In long-standing disease, scarring is frequently found. Active lesions and scars are typically found on relatively accessible skin, including the arms, legs, neck, face and upper torso[107].

Obsessive–compulsive disorder is a frequent cause of this disorder[108], and these same patients may suffer from other obsessive–compulsive behaviors.

- Obsessive–compulsive disorder is an anxiety disorder characterized by intrusive uncontrollable thoughts and mounting anxiety, that, in this case, is relieved by picking or otherwise abusing the skin
- These thoughts make no sense to patients and often occur when patients are inactive or at night
- Precipitating psychosocial stressors may initiate the behavior in some patients

### Delusions of parasitosis

To understand this disorder, one must understand some definitions as summarized by Koo and Gambla[109].

- A delusion is a false belief that cannot be corrected by argument or persuasion and may or may not be founded logically

  Consider as an example a patient with itchy, irritant contact dermatitis who misinterprets the symptoms from the dermatitis as an infection with subcutaneous worms

- By contrast, an hallucination is a perception not founded in objective reality

  Consider as an example a patient who has no itching, but hallucinates that itching is occurring

- Since itching has no objective findings, delineating differences between delusions and hallucinations is not always straightforward

Schizophrenia is a disease in which patients have delusions, but also other symptoms including loss of interpersonal skills, deficits of mental functioning, and hallucinations.

- Schizophrenic patients with delusions of parasitosis may be at risk for suicide, so a cautious approach to these patients is indicated

Monosymptomatic hypochondriacal psychosis is a delusional ideation that revolves around one particular hypochondriacal concern. Sufferers are most commonly middle-aged women, but no age or gender is immune from this disorder[109].

- Patients with this disorder may appear normal and rational in virtually every other way
- Hypochondriacs may feel itching or crawling sensations of the skin and may misinterpret these as parasitosis, but this is not usually delusional

  Unlike delusions of parasitosis, 'illusions of parasitosis' result from actual environmental stimuli that are incorrectly attributed to insects or other small organisms biting or infesting the person, their home, or their working environment

  The occasional patient will have actual arthropods responsible for their condition and careful examination should help identify true infestation as a possibility

In hypochondriacs, logic, reason and appropriate symptomatic treatment generally improve the condition. Patients with true delusions will not respond to discussion or reason.

- Patients often bring in shreds of tissue, crusts, skin and other debris as 'proof' of their parasitosis

  Because it would be a serious problem to miss true parasitosis, it is critical to carefully examine patients for evidence of true parasitosis and to microscopically examine any materials that patients bring for evaluation

- As further 'proof' patients may involve their friends and relatives in this delusion

  A patient recently evaluated by the author not only brought in her 'worms' in a medicine bottle, but she arrived with a testimony from her mother who had also 'observed' the parasites: the 'worms', however, consisted of sebum expressed from follicular orifices (Figure 5)

Delusional patients show no primary signs, but secondary signs are frequently present.

- Patients may have multiple excoriations and factitial ulcerations from their attempts to remove the 'parasites' with their fingernails or other instruments (Figure 6)
- Eczematous changes may be present from patients' attempts to remove the 'parasites' with topical alcohol, gasoline, permethrin, antibacterial or antifungal agents, and scores of medically recognized agents or home remedies
- Patients may also be at risk of suicide

  A patient with symptoms of itching, burning, and stinging of the skin believed he was being devoured by 'yellow bacteria': within one hour of consultation he was admitted to a locked psychiatric facility for seriously threatening suicide

## Other itching disorders and psychiatric diseases

Localized, generalized or epidemic itching may be a sign of psychiatric disease.

- Chronic itching hand dermatitis may be seen in those with handwashing rituals due to obsessive–compulsive disorder[110]

- Anogenital itching can be a sign of obsessive–compulsive disorder, erotic fantasies, sexual dysfunction, guilt and shame[104,111]
- Generalized itching can be a sign of a delusional state, including delusions of parasitosis, foreign bodies and poisoning
- Poison ivy dermatitis has been reported to cause secondary mania[112]
- 'Telepathic pruritus'[113]

  There is a reported case of a paranoid schizophrenic man with the delusion that two other men used mental telepathy to make him itch

- Community hysteria has been reported to induce community-wide itching at an elementary school

  The author also knows of instances of pseudoscabies hysteria in his son's nursery school

### General approach to psychiatric treatment

The first step is to make a correct diagnosis and not to ignore other contributory causes of itching. Psychiatric disease may only be a component of the patient's clinical picture rather than the entire explanation. The itch–scratch cycle may create itching in any given patient, and proper topical, systemic, and physical dermatologic treatment aimed at arresting the itch sensations may be a vital component of therapy.

Do not hesitate to recommend formal evaluation by your psychiatric colleagues, some patients will actually be relieved. Professional counselling may be an important replacement or a vital adjunct to pharmacologic therapy in virtually all psychiatric conditions[104,107,114,115].

### Pharmacologic therapy

#### Anxiety disorders

- Alprazolam may be beneficial for patients with itching and anxiety for short periods; longer duration therapy may necessitate weaning

- Similarly, buspirone, a non-addictive agent, may require weeks to achieve effect
- Some depressed patients may present with symptoms of anxiety, and antidepressant therapy, especially doxepin, may be useful

### Delusional disorders

Neuroleptic medications are the treatment of choice, however, since patients by definition have a delusion, introducing a neuroleptic agent may be challenging to accomplish, and will have to be carefully done.

- Patients may be unwilling to see psychiatrists and other mental health professionals
- A strategy that may work is to explain the role of 'stress' in exacerbating the symptoms of the disease, then use the neuroleptic agent to treat the 'stress'

The neuroleptic agents pimozide[116] and haloperidol may be helpful. Prior to prescribing the clinician must be familiar with side-effects.

### Depression

- Remember that maximal efficacy may require weeks with any single agent
- If a primary dermatologic disease is complicated by depression, consider antidepressants, including doxepin or amitriptyline (25–150 mg/day), both of which have potent antihistaminic activity as well as neuropsychiatric efficacy

    These agents have frequent side-effects

- For depression with secondary itching (no primary dermatologic disease), antidepressants including sertraline, fluoxetine, and paroxetine have fewer side-effects than tricyclic agents

### Obsessive–compulsive disorder

- Clomipramine may be beneficial but this agent has frequent side-effects
- Fluoxetine may also be beneficial

## Pharmacologic causes of itching

Essentially any drug may cause an adverse reaction in the skin which can be associated with itching[117].

- In double-blind, placebo-controlled trials, placebo causes itching in up to 5% of cases, so caution should be exercised in assigning itching causation to any individual agent

The most common itching reactions are morbilliform and urticarial reactions and any therapeutic agent can cause a morbilliform reaction. This section will not describe these intensely itchy reaction patterns, as entire texts are devoted to the subject.

- Litt and Pawlak cite 340 drugs that may cause itching[118]
- It has been hypothesized by Bernhard[119] that subclinical sensitivity to any drug may cause itching
- Management consists of identification and elimination of the offending agent, and use of topical and systemic antipruritic agents[120]

Itching may also occur without evident skin lesions being present through a variety of mechanisms[117,121,122].

- Hepatotoxicity (rarely observed without other associated hepatitis symptoms)
    Chloroform
    Valproic acid

- Cholestasis
    Azathioprine
    Oral contraceptives and other estrogenic agents
    Erythromycin estolate
    Chlorpromazine
    Penicillamine
    Promazine
    Sulfadiazine
    Testosterone and other anabolic steroids
    Tolbutamide

- Photoreactions
  Psoralen photochemotherapy with 8 methoxypsoralen

- Neurologic mechanisms[123]
  Butorphanol
  Codeine
  Cocaine
  Fentanyl
  Morphine
  Tramadol

- Dry skin and increased scaliness
  Beta-blockers
  Busulfan
  Clofibrate
  Nafoxidine
  Niacin
  Retinoids such as acitretin, etretinate, and
  isotretinoin
  Tamoxifen

- Idiopathic mechanisms[124–127]
  Antimalarial agents including amodiaquine,
  chloroquine, halofantrine, and hydroxy-
  chloroquine
  Clonidine
  Gold salts
  Lithium

Systemic drugs have also been uncommonly reported to cause localized itching.

- Anafranil may cause genital itching
- Dexamethasone may cause genital itching[128,129]
- Dobutamine may cause scalp itching[130]
- Enalapril may cause vulvo-vaginal itching[131]
- Foscarnet may cause anal itching
- Iodoquinol may cause anal itching
- Meperidine can cause mild facial itching in 10% of treated patients
- Quinidine was reported to cause localized itching[132]
- Spinal opiate analgesia with various agents can cause facial itching[133]

- Transmucosal fentanyl citrate caused nose itching in 65% and body itching in 10% of treated patients[134]

# Pregnancy

Irritation, rashes and other skin changes are common in pregnancy. Pregnant women acquire all of the same itchy diseases non-pregnant patients acquire[135] (atopic dermatitis, scabies, psoriasis, etc.).

- Whenever possible, consider a therapeutic ladder such as: topical emollients, oatmeal and emollient bath additives, topical corticosteroid agents, and antihistamines diphenhydramine, hydroxyzine, or dexchlorpheniramine, and mequitazine (from the third month)[135]
- Although not a specific antipruritic agent, benzodiazepines such as oxazepam have been recommended as a secondary treatment

## Polymorphic eruption of pregnancy

Synonyms[136,137]: pruritic urticarial papules and plaques of pregnancy[138,139] (PUPP); toxemic rash of pregnancy; late-onset prurigo of pregnancy; early-onset prurigo of pregnancy; prurigo gestationis; prurigo annularis; erythema multiforme gestationis; prurigo gestationis of Besnier, and papular dermatitis of pregnancy of Spangler.

### Pathogenesis

- Antiepidermal cell surface antibodies have been identified in a patient with PUPP[139]
- Leakage of circulating small immune complexes through dilated upper dermal vessels has been reported but not confirmed[140]

### Clinical features

An intensely pruritic eruption most common in primigravidas beginning in the third trimester of pregnancy, with an incidence of 1:120 to 1:240 pregnancies[141,142]. It presents as red urticarial papules and plaques that begin on the abdominal striae and spread to involve the thighs and occasionally the buttocks and arms (Figure 7). Increased maternal weight gain[143,144] and increased neonatal birth weight have been implicated in one study and refuted in another[145].

- There is no associated increase in fetal morbidity or mortality
- There is a case report[146] of a neonate born with polymorphic eruption of pregnancy similar to the mother's eruption

Itching usually subsides rapidly or within several weeks after childbirth. Treatment is supportive with reassurance, topical emollients, topical (or rarely systemic) corticosteroid agents, and phototherapy.

### Herpes gestationis (pemphigoid gestationis)

#### Pathogenesis

This is an autoimmune disease with circulating IgG autoantibodies with complement-fixing capacity that bind to a structural protein of the hemidesmosome – complement is consistently demonstrated bound to the basement membrane zone (BMZ).

Associations exist with major histocompatability complex class I and II antigens suggesting an immunogenetic predisposition may be relevant. Circulating IgM anti-BMZ antibodies may be found without the skin eruption.

#### Clinical features

May present in any pregnancy from the first to the third trimesters and can be more severe in subsequent gestations. Incidence of 1:7000 to 1:55000 pregnancies. The initial presentation of urticarial papules and plaques typically progress to blisters within days to weeks (Figure 8).

- There is a controversial increase in fetal prematurity, morbidity and mortality

#### Treatment

- Topical corticosteroid and antihistamine agents are generally not effective
- Systemic corticosteroid agents at 0.5–1 mg/kg/day may be required to initially control the disease, with lower maintenance doses

### Pruritic folliculitis of pregnancy

A disseminated, red, follicular papular eruption, which may be a form of hormonally induced acne[147]. (May be a variant of polymorphic eruption of pregnancy; see above.)

### Intrahepatic cholestasis of pregnancy (pruritus gravidarum)

#### Pathogenesis

Estrogens may profoundly affect liver metabolism in a subset of pregnant patients. This condition may also occur as a premenstrual syndrome in non-pregnant women[148].

#### Clinical features

The condition begins in the third trimester and may be localized to the abdomen or widespread. There is an incidence of up to 1:100 pregnancies[149–151].

- The patient complains of itching without evident skin change except secondary excoriations
- There is a reported possible increased risk of fetal distress
- Elevated post-prandial bile acids, alkaline phosphatase and transaminases may be seen
- Impaired vitamin K absorption may predispose to bleeding diathesis
- Itching usually subsides rapidly or within several weeks of childbirth
- It can recur with subsequent pregnancies and with the use of oral contraceptive pills –

recurrent attacks increase the risk of cholelithiasis

### Treatment

- Topical corticosteroid and antihistamine agents are generally not effective
- Cholestyramine may help eliminate bile acids and pruritogens, or ursodeoxycholic acid may improve itching, serum concentrations of bile salts, and transaminase levels[152]
- Epomediol may also ameliorate itching in intrahepatic cholestasis of pregnancy[153]

## Renal diseases

Itching is a significant problem for up to 60% of patients undergoing long-term hemodialysis. In patients with end-stage renal disease[154], itching is usually generalized and can be so severe and intractable that sleep deprivation and contemplation of suicide can result[155,156].

- Localized itching such as nose itching has also been reported in this population
- Itching severity usually reaches its peak when patients have been without treatment for 2 days and is at its nadir the day of dialysis
- Screening for renal disease in patients with generalized itching is worthwhile

### Pathogenesis

In patients with chronic renal failure and itching the following are abnormal:

- Histamine is elevated in the blood of uremic patients and hemodialysis does not reduce plasma histamine concentrations; intracutaneous histamine reactions are stronger in patients with uremic itching[157,158]

  Dermal mast cell counts are increased in uremia[159]

  Whereas tolerance to chronically elevated histamine should occur over time thereby decreasing histamine-mediated itching, itching actually increases as the duration of dialysis increases

  Intravenous histamine administration is not known to cause itching

- Substance P, which functions in the transmission of pain and itch sensations, is increased in uremia[160]
- Parathyroid hormone may be increased or normal in itching uremic patients, and this is not associated with abnormal calcium and phosphorus metabolism

  When parathyroid hormone is injected it is not itself pruritogenic

- Skin nerve terminal numbers have been reported as increased and decreased in uremia[161,162]

Patients with chronic renal failure and itching do not have abnormal calcium or phosphorus metabolism; cutaneous neuronal markers and neuropeptides; dermo-epidermal barrier; or water content in the affected skin[163,164].

### Treatment

- Renal transplantation is the most effective and difficult therapeutic intervention
- Topical corticosteroid agents and oral antihistamines are generally not effective[165]
- Ultraviolet B phototherapy is the treatment of choice in moderate to severe uremic pruritus

  Despite this statement, it is clear that a number of patients do not respond well to this modality

Other treatments have been reported to be effective:

- Azelastin, an antiallergic drug, alleviates itching in some patients[166]
- Capsaicin 0.025% cream depletes substance P in peripheral sensory neurons, and

- most who can tolerate therapy report marked relief or complete resolution of itching[167]
- Erythropoietin therapy lowers plasma histamine concentrations in patients with uremia and has been reported to result in marked improvement of pruritus[168]
- Lidocaine administered intravenously, oral charcoal, and nicergoline are not as efficacious, but have some demonstrated efficacy
- Neurotropin lowers the level of substance P and appears to be effective in itch relief
- Nutritional adjustment and higher dialysis efficacy may reduce the prevalence and degree of pruritus in hemodialyzed patients[169]
- Sauna baths at 75 °C have been reported to help[170]
- Thalidomide, a teratogenic agent, is generally effective in itching unresponsive to available therapy[171]
- Activated charcoal has been reported to help[172]

## Sundry systemic conditions that itch

- Amyloidosis in the form of familial primary cutaneous amyloidosis has been reported to be associated with severe itching beginning in childhood[173]

    Primary cutaneous amyloidosis is uncommon in Europeans

    A British family was described in which an extremely rare variant was inherited as an autosomal dominant itching disorder

- Angina pectoris may present as nasal bridge itching[174,175]

    One patient had itching upon walking or sexual intercourse which was relieved by rest, The process was associated with severe atherosclerotic heart disease as was proved when the itching was relieved by coronary-artery bypass surgery

- Angiolymphoid hyperplasia with eosinophilia may occur anywhere on the body, and represents an unusual, itchy, benign neoplasm[176]
- Aniline intoxication resulting from ingestion of rape oil denatured with aniline can cause fever, itch, adenopathy, hepatomegaly, and varied exanthems[177]
- Prodromal itching may occur in childhood asthma[178]

    In a prospective study of 79 children with asthma, 26 had prodromal itching 1–30 mins before the asthma attack, and 17 had prodromal itching during the early part of the attack; the itching lasted up to 30 mins

- Crohn's disease has been reported to be associated with palatal itching, in association with red, burning gingiva[179]
- Dumping syndrome postprandial itching occurred in a postgastrectomy patient, which was relieved by pectin administration[180]
- Eosinophilic cellulitis (Well's Syndrome): any single or multiple sites may be involved with itchy, red plaques occasionally associated with fever; biopsy specimens reveal diagnostic features[181]
- Focal dermal hypoplasia (Goltz syndrome): patients may have generalized xerosis and itching[182]
- Graft versus host disease

    Affects 25–50% of patients who live longer than 100 days after bone marrow transplantation

    Skin involvement occurs in 80–90% of those with other graft vs. host disease[183]

    Clinically, itching morbilliform eruptions, scaling and ichthyosis, or even sclerodermoid appearances, may be present[184] (Figure 9)

    Treatment is generally by means of immunosuppressive agents

- Infections: see chapter 5: Infections, infestations, bites and stings

- Juvenile rheumatoid arthritis can cause a rash which may be quite itching[185,186] (Figure 10)
- Lupus erythematosus, especially chronic cutaneous disease, is pruritic in advancing disease (Figure 11)
- Porphyria cutanea tarda may cause itching and this has been reported to reflect the severity of the disease[187]
- Progressive systemic sclerosis: although uncommon, itching may be severe in advancing areas and therapeutically refractory to all measures[188]
- Sarcoidosis rarely presents with itching[189–191]
- Sjogren's syndrome with its associated dry skin can cause severe, recalcitrant itching[192,193]
- Starvation-associated itching: eating disorder-induced starvation was reported associated with itching[194]

# References

1. Gilchrest BA. Pruritus: pathogenesis, therapy, and significance in systemic disease states. *Arch Int Med* 1982;142:101–5

2. Moore P. Patients presenting with pruritus. *Practitioner* 1995;239:58–61

3. Rajka G. Investigation of patients suffering from generalized pruritus, with special references to systemic diseases. *Acta Derm Venereol* 1966;46:190–4

4. Kantor GR, Lookingbill DP. Generalized pruritus and systemic disease. *J Am Acad Dermatol* 1983;9: 375–82

5. Bolaji II, O'Dwyer EM. Post-menopausal cyclic eruptions: autoimmune progesterone dermatitis. *Eur J Obstet Gynecol Reprod Biol* 1992;47:169–71

6. Hart R. Autoimmune progesterone dermatitis. *Arch Dermatol* 1977;113:426–30

7. Stephens CJ, Wojnarowska FT, Wilkinson JD. Autoimmune progesterone dermatitis responding to tamoxifen. *Br J Dermatol* 1989;121:135–7

8. Shelley WB, Shelley ED, Talanin NY, *et al.* Estrogen dermatitis. *J Am Acad Dermatol* 1995;32:25–31

9. Neilly JB, Martin A, Simpson N, *et al.* Pruritus in diabetes mellitus: investigation of prevalence and correlation with diabetes control. *Diabetes Care* 1986;9: 273–5

10. Greaves MW. Pruritus. In Champion RH, Burton JL, Ebling FJG, eds. *Textbook of Dermatology*, 5th edn. Oxford: Blackwell Scientific Press, 1992: 527–35

11. Barnes HM, Sarkany I, Calnan CD. Pruritus and thyrotoxicosis. *Trans St Johns Hosp Dermatol Soc* 1974;60:59–62

12. Tormey WP, Chambers JP. Pruritus as the presenting symptom in hyperthyroidism. *Br J Clinical Practice* 1994;48:224

13. Chusid MJ, Dale DC, West BC, *et al.* The hypereosinophilic syndrome. *Medicine* 1975;54:1–27

14. Kazmierowski JA, Chusid MJ, Parillo JE, *et al.* Dermatologic manifestations of the hypereosinophilic syndrome. *Arch Dermatol* 1978;114: 531–5

15. Newton JA, Singh AK, Greaves MW, *et al.* Aquagenic pruritus associated with the idiopathic hypereosinophilic syndrome. *Br J Dermatol* 1990;122: 103–6

16. Lewiecki EM, Rahman F. Pruritus. A manifestation of iron deficiency. *J Am Med Assoc* 1976;236: 2319–20

17. Rector WG Jr, Fortuin NJ, Conley CL. Non-hematologic effects of chronic iron deficiency. A study of patients with polycythemia vera treated solely with venesections. *Medicine* 1982;61:382–9

18. Salem HH, Van der Weyden MB, Young IF, *et al.* Pruritus and severe iron deficiency in polycythaemia vera. *Br Med J Clin Res Ed* 1982;285:91–2

19. Staubli M. Pruritus – a little known iron-deficiency symptom. *Schweizer Med Wochen J Suisse Med* 1981; 111:1394–8

20. Tucker WF, Briggs C, Challoner T. Absence of pruritus in iron deficiency following venesection. *Clin Exp Dermatol* 1984;9:186–9

21. Valsecchi R, Cainelli T. Generalized pruritus: a manifestation of iron deficiency. *Arch Dermatol* 1983; 119:630

22. Hill HR, Ochs HD, Quie PG, *et al.* Defect in neutrophil granulocyte chemotaxis in Job's syndrome of recurrent 'cold' abscesses. *Lancet* 1974;2:617–19

23. Zelicovici Z, Lahav M, Cahane P. Pruritus as a presentation of myelomatosis. *Br Med J* 1977;2:1154

24. Archer CB, Camp RDR, Greaves MW. Polycythaemia vera can present with aquagenic pruritus. *Lancet* 1988;1:1451

25. Buchanan JG, Ameratunga RV, Hawkins RC. Polycythemia vera and water-induced pruritus: evidence against mast cell involvement. *Pathology* 1994; 26:43–5

26. Fjellner B, Hägermark ÖA. Pruritus in polycythaemia vera. Treatment with aspirin and possibility of platelet involvement. *Acta Derm Venereol* 1979; 59:505–12

27. Weick JK, Donovan PB, Najean Y, *et al.* The use of cimetidine for the treatment of pruritus in polycythemia vera. *Arch Int Med* 1982;142:241–2

28. Finelli C, Gugliotta L, Gamberi B, *et al.* Relief of intractable pruritus in polycythemia vera with recombinant interferon alfa. *Am J Hematol* 1993;43:316–8

29. Muller EW, de Wolf JT, Egger R, *et al.* Long-term treatment with interferon-alpha 2b for severe pruritus in patients with polycythaemia vera. *Br J Haematol* 1995;89:313–8

30. Khandelwal M, Malet PF. Pruritus associated with cholestasis. A review of pathogenesis and management. *Digestive Dis Sci* 1994;39:1–8

31. Bergasa NV, Jones EA. The pruritus of cholestasis. *Sem Liver Disease* 1993;13:319–27

32. Bergasa NV. The pruritus of cholestasis. *Sem Dermatol* 1995;14:302–12

33. Aldersley MA, O'Grady JG. Hepatic disorders. Features and appropriate management. *Drugs* 1995; 49:83–102

34. Ryatt KS, Cotterill JA, Littlewood JM. Generalized pruritus in a baby as a presenting feature of the arteriohepatic dysplasia syndrome. *Clin Exp Dermatol* 1983;8:657–61

35. Bergasa NV, Talbot TL, Alling DW, *et al.* The pruritus of cholestasis: potential pathogenic and therapeutic implications of opioids. *Gastroenterology* 1995; 108:1582–8

36. Datta DV, Sherlock S. Cholestyramine for long term relief of the pruritus complicating intrahepatic cholestasis. *Gastroenterology* 1966;50:323–32

37. Gillespie DA, Vickers CR. Pruritus and cholestasis: therapeutic options. *J Gastroenterol Hepatol* 1993;8: 168–73

38. Ballinger AB, McHugh M, Catnach SM, *et al.* Symptom relief and quality of life after stenting for malignant bile duct obstruction. *Gut* 1994;35: 467–70

39. Hamilton DV, Gould DJ. Generalized pruritus as a presentation of idiopathic haemochromatosis. *Br J Dermatol* 1985;112:629

40. Nestler JE. Hemochromatosis and pruritus. *Ann Int Med* 1983;98:1026

41. Fisher DA, Wright TL. Pruritus as a symptom of hepatitis C. *J Am Acad Dermatol* 1994;30:629–32

42. Spivey JR, Jorgensen RA, Gores GJ, *et al.* Methionine-enkephalin concentrations correlate with stage of disease but not pruritus in patients with primary biliary cirrhosis. *Am J Gastroenterol* 1994;89: 2028–32

43. Ghent CN. Cholestatic pruritus. In Bernhard JD, ed. *Itch: Mechanism and Management of Pruritus.* New York: McGraw-Hill, 1994:229–42

44. Turner IB, Rawlins MD, Wood P, *et al.* Flumecinol for the treatment of pruritus associated with primary biliary cirrhosis. *Aliment Pharmacol Ther* 1994;8: 337–42

45. Podesta A, Lopez P, Terg R, *et al.* Treatment of pruritus of primary biliary cirrhosis with rifampin. *Digestive Dis Sci* 1991;36:216–20

46. Gregorio GV, Ball CS, Mowat AP, *et al.* Effect of rifampicin in the treatment of pruritus in hepatic cholestasis. *Arch Dis Child* 1993;69:141–3

47. Raderer M, Muller C, Scheithauer W. Ondansetron for pruritus due to cholestasis. *New Engl J Med* 1994; 330:1540

48. Schoworer H, Hartmann H, Ramadori G. Relief of cholestatic pruritus by a novel class of drugs; 5-hydroxytryptamine type 3 (5-HT3) receptor antagonists: effectiveness of ondansetron. *Pain* 1995;61: 33–7

49. Floreani A, Zappala F, Mazzetto M, *et al.* Different response to ursodeoxycholic acid in primary biliary cirrhosis according to severity of disease. *Digestive Dis Sci* 1994;39:9–14

50. Matsuzaki Y, Doy M, Tanaka N, *et al.* Biochemical and histological changes after more than four years of treatment of ursodeoxycholic acid in primary biliary cirrhosis. *J Clin Gastroenterol* 1994;18:36–41

51. Molina C. Epomediol ameliorates pruritus in patients with intrahepatic cholestasis of pregnancy. *J Hepatol* 1992;16:241–2

52. Borgeat A, Wilder-Smith OH, Mentha G. Subhypnotic doses of propofol relieve pruritus associated with liver disease. *Gastroenterology* 1993;104:244–7

53. Borgeat A, Savioz D, Mentha G, *et al*. Intractable cholestatic pruritus after liver transplantation – management with propofol. *Transplantation* 1994; 58:727–9

54. Gonzalez MC, Iglesias J, Tiribelli C, *et al*. Subhypnotic doses of propofol relieve pruritus associated with liver disease. *Gastroenterology* 1993;104: 244–7

55. Hoofnagle JH, Jones EA. A controlled trial of naloxone infusions for the pruritus of chronic cholestasis. *Gastroenterology* 1992;102:544–9

56. Alarabi AA, Wikstrom B, Loof L, *et al*. Treatment of pruritus in cholestatic jaundice by bilirubin- and bile acid-adsorbing resin column plasma perfusion. *Scan J Gastroenterol* 1992;27:223–6

57. McCormick PA, Scott F, Epstein O, *et al*. Thalidomide as therapy for primary biliary cirrhosis: a double-blind placebo controlled pilot study. *J Hepatol* 1994;21:496–9

58. Rosenthal E, Diamond E, Benderly A, *et al*. Cholestatic pruritus: effect of phototherapy on pruritus and excretion of bile acids in urine. *Acta Paediatrica* 1994;83:888–91

59. Fleischer AB, Jr, Michaels JR. Pruritus in cancer patients. *J Geriat Dermatology* 1995;3:172–81

60. Twycross RG. Pruritus and pain in en cuirass breast cancer. *Lancet* 1981;2:696

61. Mengel CE. Cutaneous manifestations of the malignant carcinoid syndrome: severe pruritus and orange blotches. *Ann Int Med* 1963;58:989–93

62. Alexander LL. Pruritus and Hodgkin's disease. *J Am Med Assoc* 1979;241:2598–9

63. Bluefarb SM. *Cutaneous Manifestations of Malignant Lymphomas*. Springfield: Charles C. Thomas, 1959

64. Shoenfeld Y, Weinburger A, Ben-Bassat M, *et al*. Generalized pruritus in metastatic adenocarcinoma of the stomach. *Dermatologica* 1977;155:122–4

65. Lotz R, Rosler HP, Zapf S, *et al*. Radiotherapy in HIV positive patients. *Fortschritte Med* 1990;108:35–9

66. Bonvalet D, Foldes C, Civatte J. Cutaneous manifestations in chronic lymphocytic leukemia. *J Dermatol Surg Oncol* 1984;10:278–82

67. Beeaff DE. Pruritus as a sign of systemic disease, report of metastatic small cell carcinoma. *Arizona Med* 1980;37:831–3

68. Thomas S, Harrington CI. Intractable pruritus as the presenting symptom of carcinoma of the bronchus: a case report and review of the literature. *Clin Exp Dermatol* 1983;8:459–61

69. de Wolf JT, Hendriks DW, Egger RC, *et al*. Alpha-interferon for intractable pruritus in polycythemia rubra vera. *Lancet* 1991:337:241

70. Burtin C, Noirot C, Giroux C, *et al*. Decreased skin response to intradermal histamine in cancer patients. *J Allergy Clin Immunol* 1986;78:83–9

71. Storck H. Cutaneous paraneoplastic syndromes. *Medizinische Klinik* 1976;71:356–72

72. Curth HO. A spectrum of organ systems that respond to the presence of cancer. How and why the skin reacts. *Ann New York Acad Sci* 1974;230:435–42

73. Rosenberg FW. Cutaneous manifestations of internal malignancy. *Cutis* 1977;20:227–34

74. Cormia FE. Pruritus, an uncommon but important symptom of systemic carcinoma. *Arch Dermatol* 1965;92:36–9

75. De Conno F, Ventafridda V, Saita L. Skin problems in advanced and terminal cancer patients. *J Pain Symptom Management* 1991;6:247–56

76. Higgins EM, du Vivier AW. Cutaneous manifestations of malignant disease. *Br J Hosp Med* 1992;48: 552–4, 558–61

77. Lober CW. Pruritus and malignancy. *Clin Dermatol* 1993;11:125–8

78. Czarnecki DB, Downes NP, O'Brien T. Pruritic specific cutaneous infiltrates in leukemia and lymphoma. *Arch Dermatol* 1982;118:119–21

79. Degos R, Civatte J, Blanchet P, *et al*. Prurit, seule manifestation pendant 5 ans d'une maladie de Hodgkin. *Ann Med Interne* 1973;124:235–8

80. Gobbi PG, Attardo-Parrinello G, Lattanzio G, *et al*. Severe pruritus should be a B-symptom in Hodgkin's disease. *Cancer* 1983;51:1934–6

81. Gobbi PG, Cavalli C, Gendarini A, *et al*. Reevaluation of prognostic significance of symptoms in Hodgkin's disease. *Cancer* 1985;56:2874–80

82. Ratnanal RC, Burrows NP, Marcus RE, *et al*. Aquagenic pruritus and acute lymphoblastic leukemia. *Br J Dermatol* 1993; 129:346–9

83. Ferguson JE, August PJ, Guy AJ. Aquagenic pruritus associated with metastatic squamous cell carcinoma of the cervix. *Clin Exp Dermatol* 1994; 19:257–8

84. Newton JA, Singh AK, Greaves MW, *et al*. Aquagenic pruritus associated with the hypereosinophilic syndrome. *Br J Dermatol* 1990;122:103–6

85. Handfield-Jones SE, Hills RJ, Ive FA, *et al.* Aquagenic pruritus associated with juvenile xanthogranuloma. *Clin Exp Dermatol* 1993;18:253–5

86. Abdel-Naser MB, Gollnick H, Orfanos CE. Aquagenic pruritus as a presenting symptom of polycythemia vera. *Dermatology* 1993;187:130–3

87. Adreev VC, Petkov I. Skin manifestations associated with tumours of the brain. *Br J Dermatol* 1975;92: 675–8

88. Summers CG, MacDonald JT. Paroxysmal facial itch: a presenting sign of childhood brainstem glioma. *J Child Neurol* 1988;3:189–92

89. King CA, Huff J, Jorizzo JL. Unilateral neurogenic pruritus: paroxysmal itching associated with central nervous system lesions. *Ann Int Med* 1982;97:222–3

90. Shapiro PE, Braun CW. Unilateral pruritus after a stroke. *Arch Dermatol* 1987;123:1527–30

91. Massey EW. Unilateral neurogenic pruritus following stroke. *Stroke* 1984;15:901–3

92. Ulicny TL, Dastur KJ, Gray GH Jr. CT demonstration of cervical spinal cord compression – cause of reversible itching and burning in the lower extremities. *J Computed Tomography* 1982;6:57–60

93. Grob JJ, Bonerandi JJ. Dermatomal pruritus of the upper limb: a manifestation of nerve root compression due to degenerative spine disease? *J Dermatol* 1987;14:512–3

94. Sampson RN. Hypnotherapy in a case of pruritus and Guillain-Barré syndrome. *Am J Clin Hypnosis* 1990;32:168–73

95. Musaph H. Psychogenic pruritus. *Dermatologica* 1967;135:126–30

96. Yamamoto M, Yabuki S, Hayabara T, *et al.* Paroxysmal itching in multiple sclerosis: a report of three cases. *J Neurol Neurosurg Psychiatry* 1981;44: 19–22

97. Osterman PO. Paroxysmal itching in multiple sclerosis. *Br J Dermatol* 1976;95:555–8

98. Koeppel MC, Bramont C, Ceccaldi M, *et al.* Paroxysmal pruritus and multiple sclerosis. *Br J Dermatol* 1993;129:597–8

99. Vuadens P, Regli F, Dolivo M, *et al.* Segmental pruritus and intramedullary vascular malformation. *Schweizer Archiv Neurol Psychiatrie* 1994;145:13–6

100. Kinsella LJ. Carney-Godley K. Feldmann E. Lichen simplex chronicus as the initial manifestation of intramedullary neoplasm and syringomyelia. *Neurosurgery* 1992;30:418–21

101. Riccardi VM. Pathophysiology of neurofibromatosis. *J Am Acad Dermatol* 1980;3:157–66

102. McFadden JP, Logan R, Griffiths WAD. Segmental neurofibromatosis and pruritus. *Clin Exp Dermatol* 1988;112:265–8

103. Sullivan MJ, Drake ME Jr. Unilateral pruritus and Nocardia brain abscess. *Neurology* 1984;34:828–9

104. Koblenzer CS. *Psychocutaneous disease.* Orlando, Fl: Grune and Stratton, 1987

105. Laihinen A. Psychosomatic aspects in dermatoses. *Ann Clin Res* 1987;19:147–9

106. Phillips KA, Taub SL. Skin picking as a symptom of body dysmorphic disorder. *Psychopharmacol Bul* 1995;31:279–88

107. Fried RG. Evaluation and treatment of "psychogenic" pruritus and self-excoriation. *J Am Acad Dermatol* 1995;32:532–3

108. Koo JY. Treating compulsive behaviors in dermatology. *Western J Med* 1991;155:523

109. Koo J, Gambla C. Delusions of parasitosis and other forms of monosymptomatic hypochondriasis. *Dermatol Clin* 1996;14:429–38

110. Hatch ML, Paradis C, Friedman S, *et al.* Obsessive–compulsive disorder in patients with chronic pruritic conditions: case studies and discussion. *J Am Acad Dermatol* 1992;26:549–51

111. Espin Montanez J, Iranzo Prieto V. A case of anal pruritus of psychic origin. *Actas Luso-Espanolas Neurologia Psiquiatria* 1969;28:184–91

112. D'Mello DA, MacAuley L. Poison ivy dermatitis and secondary mania. *J Nervous Mental Dis* 1994;182: 116–7

113. Bernhard JD, Gardner MR. Nonrashes. 6. Telepathic pruritus. *Cutis* 1990;45:59

114. Gupta MA, Gupta AK, Haberman HF, *et al.* The self-inflicted dermatoses: a critical review. *Gen Hosp Psychiat* 1987;9:45–52

115. Fruensgaard K. Psychotherapeutic strategy and neurotic excoriations. *Int J Dermatol* 1991;30:198–203

116. Damiani JT, Flowers FP, Pierce DK. Pimozide in delusions of parasitosis. *J Am Acad Dermatol* 1990; 22:312–3

117. Sarno AM, Bernhard JD. Drug–induced pruritus without a rash. In *Itch: Mechanisms and Management of Pruritus.* New York: McGraw Hill, 1994:329–335

118. Litt JZ, Pawlak WA Jr. *Drug Eruption Reference Manual,* 5th edn. Cleveland: Wal-Zac Enterprises, 1996

119. Bernhard JD. Clinical aspects of pruritus. In Fitzpatrick TB, Eisen AZ, Wolff K, *et al.* eds. *Dermatology in General Medicine,* 3rd edn. New York: McGraw Hill, 1987:78–90

120. Kantor GR. Diagnostic evaluation of the patient with generalized pruritus. In *Itch. Mechanisms and Management of Pruritus.* New York: McGraw Hill, 1994:337–46

121. Mehta M (ed). *PDR Guide to Drug Interactions, Side Effects, Indications.* Montvale: Medical Economics Data, 1992

122. Bork K. *Cutaneous Side Effects of Drugs.* Philadelphia: WB Saunders, 1988:313–6

123. Manschreck TC. The treatment of cocaine abuse. *Psychiatric Quart* 1993;64:183–97

124. Brasseur P, Agnamey P, Ekobo AS, *et al.* Sensitivity of Plasmodium falciparum to amodiaquine and chloroquine in central Africa: a comparative study in vivo and in vitro. *Trans Roy Soc Trop Med Hygiene* 1995;89:528–30

125. Mnyika KS, Kihamia CM. Chloroquine-induced pruritus: its impact on chloroquine utilization in malaria control in Dar es Salaam. *J Trop Med Hygiene* 1991;94:27–31

126. Fain O, Frilay Y, Sitbon M, *et al.* Pruritus caused by hydroxychloroquine. *Rev Med Interne* 1994;15:433

127. Ezeamuzie IC, Igbigbi PS, Ambakederemo AW, *et al.* Halofantrine-induced pruritus amongst subjects who itch to chloroquine. *J Trop Med Hygiene* 1991; 94:184–8

128. Zaglama NE, Rosenblum SI, Sartiano GP, *et al.* Single, high-dose intravenous dexamethasone as an antiemetic in cancer chemotherapy. *Oncology* 1986; 43:27–32

129. Klygis LM. Dexamethasone-induced perineal irritation in head injury. *Am J Emerg Med* 1992;10:268

130. McCauley CS, Blumenthal MS. Dobutamine and pruritus of the scalp. *Ann Int Med* 1986;105:966

131. Heckerling PS. Enalapril and vulvovaginal pruritis. *Ann Int Med* 1990;112:217–222

132. Holt RJ. Uncharacteristic cutaneous reactions induced by quinidine. *Drug Intell Clin Pharm* 1982;16: 615–6

133. Fischer HB, Scott PV. Spinal opiate analgesia and facial pruritus. *Anaesthesia* 1982;37:777–8

134. Goldstein-Dresner MC, Davis PJ, Kretchman E, *et al.* Double-blind comparison of oral transmucosal fentanyl citrate with oral meperidine, diazepam, and atropine as preanesthetic medication in children with congenital heart disease. *Anesthesiology* 1991;74: 28–33

135. Anonymous. Strategy of treatment of pruritus during pregnancy. The Drugs and Pregnancy Study Group. *Ann Pharmacotherapy* 1994;28:17–20

136. Holmes RC, Black MM. The specific dermatoses of pregnancy: a reappraisal with special emphasis on a proposed simplified clinical classification. *Clin Exp Dermatol* 1982;7:65–73

137. Holmes RC, Black MM. The specific dermatoses of pregnancy. *J Am Acad Dermatol* 1983;8:405–12

138. Alcalay J, Wolf JE. Pruritic urticarial papules and plaques of pregnancy: the enigma and the confusion. *J Am Acad Dermatol* 1988;19:1115–16

139. Trattner A, Ingber A, Sandbank M. Antiepidermal cell surface antibodies in a patient with pruritic urticarial papules and plaques of pregnancy. *J Am Acad Dermatol* 1991;24:306–8

140. Kasp-Grochowska E, Beck J, Holmes RC, *et al.* The role of circulating immune complexes in the aetiology of polymorphic eruption of pregnancy. *Arch Dermatol Res* 1984;276:71–3

141. Lawley TJ, Hertz KC, Wade TR, *et al.* Pruritic urticarial papules and plaques of pregnancy. *J Am Med Assoc* 1979;241:1696–9

142. Roger D, Vaillant L, Fignon A, *et al.* Specific pruritic diseases of pregnancy. A prospective study of 3192 pregnant women. *Arch Dermatol* 1994;130:734–9

143. Pauwels C, Bucaille-Fleury L, Recanati G. Pruritic urticarial papules and plaques of pregnancy: relationship to maternal weight gain and twin or triplet pregnancies. *Arch Dermatol* 1994;130:801–2

144. Cohen LM, Capeless EL, Krusinski PA, *et al.* Pruritic urticarial papules and plaques of pregnancy and its relationship to maternal–fetal weight gain and twin pregnancy. *Arch Dermatol* 1989;125:1534–6

145. Roger D, Vaillant L, Lorette G. Pruritic urticarial papules and plaques of pregnancy are not related to maternal or fetal weight gain. *Arch Dermatol* 1990; 126:1517

146. Uhlin SR. Pruritic urticarial papules and plaques of pregnancy. Involvement in mother and infant. *Arch Dermatol* 1981;117:238–9

147. Borradori L, Saurat JH. Specific dermatoses of pregnancy. Toward a comprehensive view? *Arch Dermatol* 1994;130:778–80

148. Dahl MG. Premenstrual pruritus due to recurrent cholestasis. *Trans St Johns Hosp Dermatol Soc* 1970; 56:11–3

149. Furhoff WR. Itching in pregnancy. A 15-year follow-up study. *Acta Med Scand* 1974;196:403–10

150. Fisk NM, Bye WB, Storey GNB. Maternal features of obstetric cholelithiasis: 20 years experience at King George V Hospital. *Aust NZ J Obstet Gynaecol* 1988; 28:172–6

151. Waine C. Beware of itching during late pregnancy. *Practitioner* 1995;239:97–100

152. Palma J, Reyes H, Ribalta J, *et al.* Effects of ursodeoxycholic acid in patients with intrahepatic cholestasis of pregnancy. *Hepatology* 1992;15: 1043–7

153. Molina C. Epomediol ameliorates pruritus in patients with intrahepatic cholestasis of pregnancy. *J Hepatol* 1992;16:241–2

154. Shoop KL. Pruritus in end stage renal disease. *Anna J* 1994;21:147–53

155. Ståhle-Bäckdahl M. Pruritus in hemodialysis patients. *Skin Pharmacol* 1992;5:14–20

156. Ståhle-Bäckdahl M. Uremic pruritus. *Sem Dermatol* 1995;14:297–301

157. Francos GC, Kauh YC, Gittlen SD. Elevated plasma histamine in chronic uremia. Effects of ketotifen on pruritus. *Int J Dermatol* 1991;30:884–9

158. Stockenhuber F, Kurz RW, Sertl K, *et al.* Increased plasma histamine levels in uraemic pruritus. *Clinical Sci* 1990;79:477–82

159. Leong SO, Tan CC, Lye WC, *et al.* Dermal mast cell density and pruritus in end-stage renal failure. *Ann Acad Med Singapore* 1994;23:327–9

160. Kaku H, Fujita Y, Yago H, *et al.* Study on pruritus in hemodialysis patients and the antipruritic effect of neurotropin. plasma levels of substance P, somatostatin, IgE, PTH and histamine. *Nippon Jinzo Gakkai Shi* 1990;32:319–26

161. Fantini F, Baraldi A, Sevignani C, *et al.* Cutaneous innervation in chronic renal failure patients. An immunohistochemical study. *Acta Derm Venereol* 1992; 72:102–5

162. Szepietowski J, Thepen T, van Vloten WA, *et al.* Tyrosine hydroxylase immunoreactive fibres in the skin of hemodialysed patients. *Acta Derm Venereol* 1994;74:75

163. Yosipovitch G, Tur E, Morduchowicz G, *et al.* Skin surface pH, moisture, and pruritus in haemodialysis patients. *Nephrol Dial Transplant* 1993;8:1129–32

164. Tan JK, Haberman HF, Coldman AJ. Identifying effective treatments for uremic pruritus. *J Am Acad Dermatol* 1991;25:811–8

165. Ostlere LS, Taylor C, Baillod R, *et al.* Relationship between pruritus, transepidermal water loss, and biochemical markers of renal itch in haemodialysis patients. *Nephrol Dial Transplant* 1994;9:1302–4

166. Matsui C, Ida M, Hamada M, *et al.* Effects of azelastin on pruritus and plasma histamine levels in hemodialysis patients. *Int J Dermatol* 1994;33:868–71

167. Breneman DL, Cardone JS, Blumsack RF, *et al.* Topical capsaicin for treatment of hemodialysis-related pruritus. *J Am Acad Dermatol* 1992;26:91–4

168. De Marchi S, Cecchin E, Villalta D, *et al.* Relief of pruritus and decreases in plasma histamine concentrations during erythropoietin therapy in patients with uremia. *New Engl J Med* 1992;326:969–74

169. Hiroshige K, Kabashima N, Takasugi M, *et al.* Optimal dialysis improves uremic pruritus *Am J Kidney Dis* 1995;25:413–9

170. Snyder D, Merrill JP. Sauna baths in the treatment of chronic renal failure. *Trans Am Soc Artif Intern Organs* 1966;12:188–92

171. Silva SR, Viana PC, Lugon NV, *et al.* Thalidomide for the treatment of uremic pruritus: a crossover randomized double-blind trial. *Nephron* 1994;67: 270–3

172. Pederson JA, Matter BJ, Czerwinski AW, *et al.* Relief of idiopathic generalized pruritus in dialysis patients treated with activated oral charcoal. *Ann Int Med* 1980;93:446–8

173. Newton JA, Jagjivan A, Bhogal B, *et al.* Familial primary cutaneous amyloidosis. *Br J Dermatol* 1985; 112:201–8

174. Puddu V. A case of acute myocardial infarction with an atypical symptomatology: cutaneous itching. *Am Heart J* 1971;82:431

175. Reichstein RP, Stein WG. Nasal pruritus as atypical angina? *New Engl J Med* 1983;309:667

176. Vallis RC, Davies DG. Angiolymphoid hyperplasia of the head and neck. *J Laryngol Otol* 1988;102: 100–1

177. Casado de Frias E, Andujar PH, Oliete F, *et al.* Intoxication caused by ingestion of rape oil denatured with aniline. *Am J Dis Child* 1983;137:988–91

178. David TJ. Wybrew M. Hennessen U. Prodromal itching in childhood asthma. *Lancet* 1984;2:154–5

179. Gargiulo AV, Ladone JA, Toto PD, Logiudice J. Crohn's disease: early detection by gingival biopsy. *Periodontal Case Reports* 1989;11:20–2

180. Harries AD, Tredee R, Heatley, *et al.* Pruritus as a manifestation of the dumping syndrome. *Br J Dermatol* 1982;107:707–9

181. Aberer W, Konrad K, Wolff K. Wells' syndrome is a distinctive disease entity and not a histological diagnosis. *J Am Acad Dermatol* 1988;18:105–14

182. Temple IK, MacDowall, Baraitser M, *et al*. Focal dermal hypoplasia (Goltz syndrome). *J Med Genet* 1990; 27:180–7

183. Parker C. Skin lesions in transplant patients. *Dermatol Clin* 1990;8:313–25

184. Wick MR, Moore SB, Gastineau DA, *et al*. Immunologic, clinical, and pathologic aspects of human graft-versus-host disease. *Mayo Clin Proc* 1983;58:603–12

185. Schaller J, Wedgwood RJ. Pruritis associated with the rash of juvenile rheumatoid arthritis. *Pediatrics* 1970; 45:296–8

186. Henry K. Adult Still's disease presenting with fever and a pruritic rash. *Minn Med* 1986;69:525–6

187. Bonnetblanc JM, Dutheil MJ, Bernard P. Pruritus and tardive cutaneous porphyria. *Annales Dermatol Venereol* 1986;113:133–6

188. Claman HNL. Mast cell changes in a case of rapidly progressive scleroderma – ultrastructural analysis. *J Invest Dermatol* 1989;92:290–5

189. Goldberg A, Lang A, Mekori YA. Prolonged generalized pruritus associated with selective elevation of IgA as the presenting symptoms of sarcoidosis. *Ann Allergy Asthma Immunol* 1995;74:387–9

190. Burke M, Hallak A, Almog C. Sarcoidosis presenting with acute pleurisy, hemoptysis, pruritus and eosinophilia. *Respiration* 1987;51:248–51

191. Powell RF, Smith EB. Pruritic cutaneous sarcoidosis. *Arch Dermatol* 1976;112:1465–6

192. Feuerman EJ. Sjögren's syndrome presenting as recalcitrant generalized pruritus. Some remarks about its relation to collagen diseases and the connection of rheumatoid arthritis with the Sicca syndrome. *Dermatologica* 1968;137:74–86

193. Aso K. Senile dry skin type Sjögren's syndrome. *Int J Dermatol* 1994;33:351–5

194. Gupta MA, Gupta AK, Voorhees JJ. Starvation-associated pruritus: a clinical feature of eating disorders. *J Am Acad Dermatol* 1992;27:118–20

# Infections, infestations, bites and stings 5

This chapter will highlight some of the more common and curious itchy phenomena driven by other organisms, and will skip some of the more uncommon dermatoses caused by infections and infestations. This chapter is not meant to be a comprehensive list of infections, infestations, bites and stings

## Bacterial infections

### Folliculitis

This is superficial inflammation and/or infection of hair follicles, which presents as erythematous pustules at hair follicles (Figure 5.1; Figure 12). Predisposing factors include friction and exposure to occlusive oils.

- Gram-positive organisms are the most common cause of folliculitis[1]
- Other causes include gram-negative bacteria, *Pseudomonas, Candida* and *Pityrosporum*
- Treatment: topical antibiotics such as mupirocin, erythromycin and clindamycin, or systemic antibiotics in widespread disease
- Recurrent folliculitis may suggest the staphylococcal carrier state; thus treatment with the combination of either intranasal mupirocin twice daily or rifampin (300 mg twice daily) combined with appropriate systemic antistaphyloccocal antibiotics for 14 to 30 days
- If folliculitis is severe and there are frequent recurrences, systemic retinoid therapy (isotretinoin 1.0 mg/kg/day for 15–20 weeks) is usually highly effective

### Impetigo

- Superficial infection most commonly caused by group A streptococci or Staphylococcus aureus
- Most common in young children[2], but may occur at any age
- Appearance is usually crusted erosions, but blisters may be present
- May be highly contagious and contacts may have unrecognized disease
- Rare association of glomerulonephritis with streptococcal impetigo
- Treatment with topical mupirocin for limited disease is efficacious[3], but extensive disease may require a 7 to 10 day course of erythromycin, cephalexin, oxacillin, or azithromycin

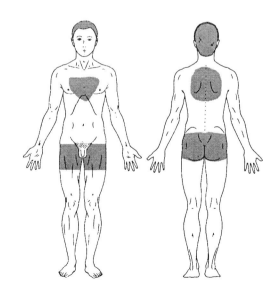

**Figure 5.1** Areas typically affected by folliculitis

**Intertriginous dermatitis (Intertrigo)**

Moist areas of the body, particularly the axillae, groin, inframammary folds, and toe web spaces can develop an inflammatory bacterial condition not related to candidiasis or tinea[4].

- In one study of toe web spaces[5] 41% of those thought to have tinea pedis had a gram-negative bacillus present, and this presence was related to symptoms of itching/soreness and cracking/fissuring

The typical appearance involves erythema, mild scaling, and maceration (Figure 13). Treatment involves keeping the skin dry with excellent hygiene and the use of powders, soaks with aluminum acetate, and topical antibiotic agents or topical azole antifungal agents.

**Leprosy (Hansen's disease)**

A bacterial infection with *Mycobacterium leprae* which has manifold clinical presentations ranging from anesthetic patches or plaques to widespread infiltrative plaques. Neurologic damage may induce itching[6].

- Thorough discussion of this disease of worldwide distribution is beyond the scope of this text

**Syphilis**

Although not commonly regarded as an itchy disease, one-third of patients with secondary syphilis complain of itching. The itchy rash begins at 2 to 3 months following initial infection with *Treponema pallidum*[7,8].

- Examination reveals a widespread rash consisting of small, scaly, round to oval, erythematous macules and papules (Figure 14)
- Palms and soles may bear 'copper pennies' and mucous membranes may have distinct white patches to condyloma lata

- Diagnosis rests upon clinical suspicion, serologic testing; although diagnostic, darkfield examination is becoming rare
- Rarely, luetic biliary disease may cause itching[9]
- Treatment includes benzathine penicillin and contact tracing; testing for the human immunodeficiency virus guides appropriate care

**Cat scratch disease**

- Cat scratch disease is usually a benign, self-limited illness characterized by regional lymphadenopathy and constitutional symptoms
- Cases of cat scratch disease have been seen with skin manifestations that included erythema nodosum, erythema multiforme, erythema marginatum, and non-specific maculopapular, petechial, and morbilliform rashes[10]

  A case of cat scratch disease has been reported in which the patient's principal symptom was an itchy rash

# Fungal infections

**Tineas**

Pathophysiology

Most of the infectious agents of the dermatophytoses are classified in three genera, *Epidermophyton*, *Microsporum* and *Trichophyton*. On the basis of primary habitat, the organisms may be grouped as geophilic (soil associated), zoophilic (animal associated), and anthropophilic (human associated). Although infection with any organism can cause itch, zoophilic and geophilic species are more likely to be inflammatory and itchy[11,12].

- 'Barn itch' in rural workers is due to *Trichophyton verrucosum* infection from animals[13]

- *Trichophyton rubrum* is the most common cause worldwide of tinea pedis, nail infection, tinea cruris, and tinea corporis
- Although the incidence of tinea capitis is declining in developed nations, tinea pedis and onychomycosis are becoming more common
- The increased use of athletic shoes both by men and women and communal bathing could be contributing factors

The dermatophytes have the ability to invade keratinized tissue (skin, hair, and nails) but are usually restricted to the non-living cornified layer of the epidermis because of their inability to penetrate viable tissue of an immunocompetent host. However, invasion does elicit a host response ranging from mild to severe (Figure 15).

- Acid proteinases, elastase, keratinases, and other proteinases reportedly act as virulence factors
- The development of cell-mediated immunity correlated with delayed hypersensitivity and an inflammatory response is associated with clinical cure, whereas the lack of, or a defective, cell-mediated immunity predisposes the host to chronic or recurrent dermatophyte infection[14]

### Clinical presentation

Inflammatory tineas and other superficial fungi may be strikingly itchy. However, many tineas are not itchy because the organisms cause little host response. Even if immunity does develop, certain dermatophytes such as *Trichophyton rubrum* produce substances that diminish the immune response.

- Clinically, the typical appearance of most dermatophyte infections is a scaling ring on any part of the body (Figure 5.2)
- A wide variety of other morphologies exist including scaling patches, plaques, hyperpigmented patches and plaques, and bullous lesions

Tinea infections are named according to the body location affected: feet, tinea pedis; body, tinea cruris; groin, tinea cruris; hand, tinea manus; face, tinea facei; body, tinea corporis; scalp, tinea capitis; and nails, tinea unguium.

- At times, the immune response to tinea infections may be extensive, including boggy, inflamed, draining kerion reactions in the scalp
- Autoeczematization or generalized itchy dermatophytid reactions may occur

### Treatment

Topical treatment with topical antifungal agents (i.e. azoles such as ketoconazole or sulconazole, allyl amines such as terbinafine or naftifine, and others) is indicated for limited body surface areas and when the infection does not involve the nails or hair. Systemic treatment is required when the eruption is extensive or involves hair or nails[15].

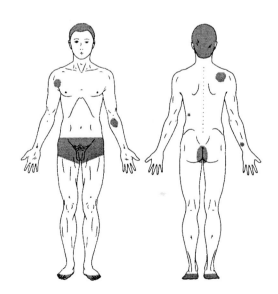

**Figure 5.2** Areas typically affected by tinea

- Griseofulvin has limited activity and numerous side-effects and is losing its place as a useful therapeutic agent

  Griseofulvin has weak affinity for keratin

  Griseofulvin is still a drug of choice for the treatment of tinea capitis in children

- Itraconazole and terbinafine are the best systemic agents with high and specific activity against dermatophytes and strong affinity for keratin

  Terbinafine is an allylamine and has been found to be effective and safe in brief therapy of dermatophyte infections[16]

  Itraconazole is a broad-spectrum triazole which has also been found to be effective and safe in brief therapy of dermatophyte infections[17]

  Fluconazole belongs to the class of azoles and has primarily been studied in candidiasis[18]

For extreme inflammation associated with kerion formation or dermatophytid reaction, a brief burst of a systemic corticosteroid agent for 1 to 2 weeks may be a useful adjunct in therapy.

## Pityrosporum folliculitis

Pityrosporum folliculitis typical affects men and women in their second and third decade. Patients present with itching follicular papules and pustules localized to the upper trunk or upper arms. Direct microscopy reveals round yeast cells and sometimes even hyphae[19]. Treatment is directed at decreasing yeast counts.

- Topical treatments daily until clear may be helpful, and these include selenium sulfide 2.5% lotion or azole antifungal creams
- Systemic agents including brief courses of terbinafine or itraconazole for 1 to 2 weeks may clear the condition

## Viral infections

### Acquired immunodeficiency syndrome (AIDS)

Itching is an occasional initial presentation in AIDS. Common causes include eosinophilic folliculitis, seborrheic dermatitis, drug eruptions, acquired ichthyosis, pruritic papular eruption of AIDS, and scabies[20,21]. However, all itchy conditions can affect this population.

- As many as half of all itching AIDS patients may never have specific causative nor categoric diagnoses identified

Some of the identified itchy conditions are as follows.

### Eosinophilic pustular folliculitis

Widespread eruption of follicular pustules and papules. Most commonly found on the face and trunk, but may present on the extremities. This condition is so itchy that excoriations and prurigo nodules are the most common finding[22].

- Generally resistant to oral antihistamine and topical steroid therapy
- Ultraviolet (UV) B phototherapy may be effective in many patients[23]
- Systemic isotretinoin in doses of 1 mg/kg per day may also be effective
- Other reported treatments have included antihistamines such as cetirizine, antifungal agents such as itraconazole, and antibiotics such as metronidazole

### Seborrheic dermatitis

Typical appearance is of papules, patches and plaques with striking, greasy scale. Often this is an extensive eruption on the upper, central face which may also involve the upper trunk and extremities[24].

- As in non-AIDS patients, pathogenesis may be due to overgrowth and/or abnormal response to the yeast *Pityrosporum ovale*

- Treatment with topical corticosteroid agents (e.g. hydrocortisone, desonide or aclometasone) and antifungal creams (e.g. clotrimazole or ketoconazole) may be helpful
- Systemic antifungal agents such as ketoconazole, itraconazole, and fluconazole may be required

### Drug eruptions

Drug eruptions, especially morbilliform (maculopapular) eruptions may be more common in the human immunodeficiency virus (HIV)-infected population.

- Agents especially likely to cause drug eruptions include trimethoprim–sulfamethoxazole and other antibiotics, as well as phenytoin[25]

The typical appearance is discrete truncal macules and papules that coalesce, then generalize, usually lasting a few days to a few weeks. Systemic antihistamines and topical corticosteroid agents can help the symptoms, but do not make the eruption disappear sooner. Although generally helpful in this condition, systemic corticosteroid agents are usually avoided in order to prevent further immunosuppression.

### Insect bite reactions

Insect bite reactions may be markedly more inflammatory and itchy in the HIV-infected population, especially prior to the onset of severe immunosuppression. Erythematous macules, papules, nodules and excoriations in a typical distribution for bites may be more evident than the patient's historical reaction pattern.

### Pruritic papular eruption

The pruritic papular eruption of AIDS is characterized by generalized, itchy, skin-colored papules and nodules. Chronic lesions are excoriated and hyperpigmented[26–29].

- The condition typically waxes and wanes, and is generally resistant to oral antihistamine and topical steroid therapy
- UVB and PUVA phototherapy has been a successful treatment in many patients, and is considered quite safe[30,31]

### Scabies

Due to the immunocompromized status of AIDS patients, infestations with the mite, *Sarcoptes scabiei* tend to be more florid. Typical scabies may be present and erythematous macules and papules in the web spaces, gluteal cleft, and genitalia may be seen in this population. More commonly, the appearance is crusted (Norwegian) scabies with hyperkeratotic patches and plaques in a generalized distribution[20].

- Note the hyperkeratotic debris under fingernails is teeming with mites
- Therapy for scabies should be more thorough than in non-immunocompromized patients since these patients are more likely to host numerous mites
- An emerging therapy is systemic ivermectin, but in immunocompromized patients this also may require repeated courses for cure
- See also discussion below regarding scabies

### Acquired ichthyosis

Early in the history of HIV disease, patients with severe acquired ichthyoses were identified. This exceptionally dry, cracked skin is most commonly seen on the extremities, but can be generalized[32].

- Itching probably results from irritants and allergens breaking through the compromized cutaneous barrier
- Therapy is aimed at restoring this barrier by using topical emollients and minimizing use of both soap and hot water

### Staphylococcal skin infections

These infections may be asymptomatic, or their predominant symptom may be itching.

- Treatment with antistaphylococcal agents with or without rifampin may be helpful

### Kaposi sarcoma

Kaposi sarcoma, particularly tumors of this condition, may be complicated by itching[33].

### Herpes simplex

Itching in genital herpes infection is likely to be more problematic in women than in men. First-episode genital herpes patients have local pain and itching 98% of the time. Treatment with antiviral agents decreases morbidity[34,35].

- Oral or intravenous acyclovir treatment produces quicker healing, less pain and decreased itching[36]
- Oral valacyclovir and oral famciclovir are significantly more bioavailable than acyclovir and thus are significantly more effective; moreover they may be used two to three times daily rather than the five times daily required of acyclovir

### Herpes zoster

This is caused by infection with *Herpesvirus varicellae* (the varicella-zoster virus). Although the most common symptom is a burning or lancinating pain, itching may also occur either acutely or as part of post-herpetic neuralgia. Treatment with antiviral agents clearly decreases morbidity.

- Oral or intravenous acyclovir treatment produces quicker defervescence, faster healing, and fewer skin lesions
- Oral valacyclovir and oral famciclovir are more bioavailable than acyclovir and thus are significantly more effective; moreover they may be used three times daily rather than the five times daily required of acyclovir[37]

### Varicella (chicken pox)

This is caused by infection with *Herpesvirus varicellae* (the varicella-zoster virus). Infection with associated prodrome is followed within two to three weeks by crops of itchy erythematous macules with delicate vesicles (dew drop on a rose petal), followed by crusting and resolution[38] (Figure 16).

- With impaired immune function, e.g. lymphomas, HIV, etc., this otherwise bothersome itchy problem may occasionally prove fatal
- Varicella or zoster in the first trimester of pregnancy has potential to cause teratogenesis including central nervous system, eye, and extremity defects[39]

### Treatment

- Non-specific antipruritic measures including shake lotions (e.g. calamine), oral antihistamines and colloidal oatmeal baths may be particularly helpful
- If bacterial infections arise on the skin or are suspected internally, systemic antibiotic treatment benefits patients
- Treatment with antiviral agents clearly decreases morbidity
- Oral or intravenous acyclovir treatment produces quicker defervescence, faster healing, and fewer skin lesions[40]
- Although not conclusive, oral valacyclovir and oral famciclovir are more bioavailable than acyclovir and thus are significantly more effective; moreover they may be used three times daily rather than the five times daily required of acyclovir
- Zoster immune globulin injection may benefit the extremely immunocompromized

## Miscellaneous viral exanthems

- A wide variety of non-varicella viral exanthems may occur in childhood and can present as itchy rashes
- Echoviruses, parvoviruses, Coxsackie viruses and myriads of others produce transient but impressive eruptions that are often asymptomatic

   Some virus exanthems have exotic names identifying their itching components, such as papular-purpuric 'gloves and socks' syndrome, caused by parvovirus B19 and other viruses[41]

   Others, like Dengue fever may present with itching, as well as nausea, vomiting, myalgia[42]

- If itching is a major component, then supportive measures including shake lotions (e.g. calamine), sedating oral antihistamines at bedtime, and colloidal oatmeal baths may be used

## Parasitic diseases

Virtually any parasitic pathogen can cause generalized itching or chronic urticaria. Eosinophilia on complete blood count may be a helpful diagnostic clue[43].

- Filarial worm infection can cause intense itching

   In a study[44] in Lagos, Nigeria, of 268 patients with generalized itching without obvious skin diseases, filariasis was responsible in 57%

- Although not generally found in the developed world, onchocerciasis is one of the most common causes of severe itching in Africa[45]

   In rural, at-risk communities in Nigeria, up to 22% of the population may be infected with Onchocerca volvulus; other communities may have infection rates varying from 1–46%[46,47]

- Onchocerciasis has an incubation period of months and has numerous cutaneous findings from widespread excoriations to onchocercomas. Onchocercal blindness is the main long-term risk

Other parasitic infections of note include:

- Giardia: this protozoan may cause urticaria and itching without skin lesions[48–50]

   Look for a history of drinking or swimming in unpurified water and recurrent, foul-smelling diarrhea

- *Ancyclostoma*: the hookworm (*A. braziliense, A. duodenale,* and related organisms such as *Necator americanus*) may cause urticaria, but are famous for causing cutaneous larva migrans

   Cutaneous larva migrans is an intensely itchy eruption caused by cutaneous penetration of worms[51]

   Skin contact with tropical sandy beaches and other sandy, warm and moist regions sets the stage for cutaneous penetration

   Clinically, single or multiple serpiginous, erythematous, possibly vesicular elevated tracts are seen which can advance several cm per day (Figure 17)

   Treatment with 10% thiabendazole suspension four times daily until 2 days after the last tract clears is helpful[52,53]

- Ascaris may cause urticaria; look for history of weight loss
- Malaria may present with itching and constitutional symptoms[54]

   More commonly the antimalarial drugs with which people are treated induce intense itching

- *Schistosoma* may cause itching, urticaria associated with abdominal discomfort and constitutional symptoms
- *Entamoeba histolytica* may also contribute to itching[55]

- *Strongyloides* may cause urticaria but more commonly causes larva currens or cutaneous larva migrans[56,57,58]

    Larva currens is a migratory, serpentine, urticarial eruption produced when a worm burrows through the skin. The advancement can be as much as 10 cm per hour

- *Gnathostoma* may cause many symptoms including cutaneous larva migrans, but below is an outstanding clinical example[59]

    A Laotian woman was reported to have had two weeks of pruritus associated with fleeting erythematous patches on her abdomen and a peripheral eosinophilia

    She withdrew a Gnathostoma spinigerum from the skin of her abdomen

- *Trichinella* may cause a maculopapular eruption or urticaria associated with myalgia, periorbital edema, and constitutional symptoms
- *Trypanosoma* may cause intense itching one or more years following infection[60]
- *Trichuris* (whipworm) infection may cause skin itching in association with symptoms that mimic those of inflammatory bowel disease[57,61,62]

### *Enterobius vermicularis*

The pinworm is one of the most common intestinal parasites in humans. Enterobius eggs have been found in a 10 000-year-old human coprolite.

- In a survey of 206 families in a shanty town in a water-poor area of Lima, Peru, pinworm infection was found most commonly in children of primary school age[63]

    42% of primary school age children were infected

    Even when successfully cured, 52% of children under 5-years-old became reinfected within 6 months of treatment

### Life-cycle

Fecal–oral transmission is the route of infection. The adult worms reside and mate in the area of the cecum and ascending colon. Then females migrate to lay their ova in the perianal area.

- Perianal itching is the cardinal symptom of pinworm infestation, and scratching behavior helps to reinfect hosts and hand contact spreads eggs to others[64]
- Vaginal itching may also be present, and, on at least one occasion, live adult worms of *Enterobius vermicularis* were found in the high vagina[65]

### Diagnosis

Intense anal itching is often accompanied by dermatitic changes, excoriations and secondary infection suggest the diagnosis. Collection of pinworms or ova from the perianal area on to cellophane or other clear plastic tape, application of the tape to a microscopic slide followed by potassium hydroxide, and microscopic examination permits diagnosis (Figure 18).

- The eggs appear more rounded on one side than the other, measure 50–60 μm by 20–30 μm, and are usually found in abundance, as each female lays 11 000 eggs

### Treatment

- Meticulous personal hygiene is essential to prevent spread of the parasites by the fecal-oral route
- Treatment with oral mebendazole is indicated for the entire family

## Infestations

### Pediculosis

### Epidemiology

Pediculosis is a common cause of itching, especially in children and sexually active young adults. Transmission occurs by direct contact with an infested person or indirectly by contact with clothing, personal grooming articles, bedding, or upholstered furniture containing viable nits or lice[66].

- In general, girls have longer hair and are more likely to share grooming implements than boys, hence higher infection rates of head lice are often seen among girls

Extreme examples of head louse infestation have been recorded.

- In a study of school children in Yunlin County, Taiwan[67], an overall infestation rate of 40% was found, varying by school from 59% to 7%

    The rate of infestations was highest among school children of grade 2 (45%) and lowest in grade 3 (35%)

    The rate of infestations of girls (65%) was much higher than that of boys (9%)

    The average number of head lice in each infested girl was 5.7

- When newly arrived Ethiopian immigrants in Israel were screened for ectoparasitic insects and mites, 65.1% were found to be infested with *Pediculus humanus capitis*[68]
- In a report from Israel[69], 15–20% of 5000 school children were infested with lice and another 25–30% had signs of previous lice infestations
- In 1994 it was estimated that pediculosis affects 6–12 million people in the USA[70]
- In Nigeria, a survey of 6882 primary school children living in Ilorin[71], revealed that 3.7% of the children were infested with *Pediculus humanus capitis*

    Girls had a higher infestation rate (5.6%) than boys (2.1%)

### Pathophysiology

Three organisms cause pediculosis: *Pediculus humanus capitis* (head louse: Figure 19),

*Pediculus humanus corporis* (body louse) and *Pthirus pubis* (pubic louse: Figure 20)[72].

- The pubic louse can live in the scalp hair, but prefers short hair areas such as the pubic region, body hair, the axillae, eyebrows, and eyelashes
- Pubic lice are often spread by sexual contact, and are highly contagious with a single contact

### Clinical appearance

Pediculosis can be caused by distinctly different organisms, but they produce equivalent disorders, with itching, bites, and nits on the hairs. Diagnosis is made on the basis of finding nits, silvery-white eggs, firmly attached to the hair shaft concentrated on the crown, behind the ears, and at the nape of the neck[73,74].

- Nits have a distinct clinical appearance that protrude from the hair shaft at an acute angle (Figure 21)
- Hair casts can be confused with nits, yet represent noninfectious keratin deposits[75]

    Hair casts are small cylindrical structures, encircling individual scalp hairs but easily movable along the involved hair shafts

Lice infestation may be asymptomatic, or accompanied by itching, lymphadenopathy, erythema, excoriation, bite reaction, impetigo, blepharitis, conjunctivitis, and crusting.

- Pediculid is an itchy, generalized 'id' reaction associated with pediculosis
- Papular autoeczematization and bullous eruptions have been reported[76,77]

- Pediculosis should not be confused with other parasitic infestations, such as *Liposcelis mendax*[78]

### Treatment

Treatment of body louse infestation is mainly a matter of cleanliness; washing the patient, and their clothing, combs, brushes, hats, and other accoutrements is essential. Treatment is usually affected with topical crotamiton, malathion, permethrin, lindane, ivermectin and other insecticides[79–82].

- The pediculicide is worked into the affected hair-bearing region and left for 5–15 minutes before being washed out
- An exception to this is malathion which requires time to absorb into the keratin[83]
- Removal of adherent nits can be accomplished by soaking the hair in a 1:1 solution of water and vinegar for 30 minutes and combing out
- Treatment of all potential familial contacts is critical, as is treatment of essentially anything inanimate the affected body areas have contacted[84]
- Resistance to all insecticides is becoming more prevalent[85–87]
- Although it has been used by millions of people worldwide with little difficulty, severe reactions to lindane therapy may occur when increased skin absorption of lindane occurs

    Lindane should be used with precautions to avoid excess skin penetration and should not be used to treat infants, young children, or pregnant or lactating women[88,89]

- Single treatment with pediculocides can produce failure rates as high as 40%, so re-treatment in 7–10 days is necessary

## Scabies

### Epidemiology

Caused by *Sarcoptes scabiei var. hominis*, 'the itch' may be man's most widespread arthropod infestation. Scabies most commonly infests children and adolescents, but it can easily infest all ages. The organism is spread through close personal or intimate contact, but may occasionally be spread through casual contact.

Although traditionally passed from person to person, *Sarcoptes scabiei* may infest other animals, and this infestation can spread to man.

- Three types of host relations and, accordingly, forms of sarcoptosis are suggested at the infection from an alien host: pseudo-sarcoptosis, temporary self-curable and typical lingering sarcoptosis[90]
- Symptoms of animal scabies are more localized than traditional scabies, and clinically present as erythematous papules or pustules where animal contact has occurred[91,92]
- If animal scabies are suspected, treatment of the affected animal is necessary
- When acquired from other animals, the variety of *Sarcoptes scabiei* is often different

    Camels - S. Scabiei var. cameli
    Cats - Notoedres cati[93]
    Cows - S. Scabiei var. bovis[94]
    Dogs - S. Scabiei var. canis
    Goats - S. Scabiei var. caprae
    Pigs - S. Scabiei var. suis[95]
    Sheep - S. scabiei var. ovis
    Water buffaloes - S. Scabiei var. bubalis[96]

- Other animal hosts of *S. Scabiei* include the Arabian oryx, barbary sheep, elands, ferrets, mountain gazelles and Nubian ibexes[97,98]
- Mites survive for 24–36 h at room conditions and fomites may spread the contagion or reinfect patients
- In one study of infested patients[99], *S. scabiei* was found in dust samples from 44% of infested patients' homes, and live mites, at the time the dust samples were analyzed, were present in 64% of these homes

    Live mites were recovered most often from bedroom floors or overstuffed chairs and couches; only a small number of mites were recovered from beds, or other furniture

    Mites were found less commonly in nursing homes

## Scabies facts

- Copulation occurs in a small burrow excavated by the female[66]

  After copulation, the fertilized female enlarges the burrow and begins egg-laying

- Gradual skin penetration occurs from production of a lytic secretion as well as action of the legs

  Females crawl 2–3 mm each day, depositing eggs and feces (scybala)

  Approximately 40–50 eggs are laid by each mite and larvae emerge from the eggs after 3–4 days

  Larvae go to the skin surface where they dig short burrows in which they transform into nymphs

- The average number of adult female mites on an individual suffering from the common form of scabies is about 12, but in crusted scabies there can be hundreds to thousands of mites present

- The mite fertility index is determined by the number of eggs in the mite burrow and is highest from September to December and much lower in January to July[100]

## Pathophysiology

A cell-mediated immune response occurs at the bite site. Humoral immunity is also implicated in the pathogenesis, including immunologic reactions mediated by antibodies of IgG, IgM, and, especially, IgE[101]. Infection leads to elevated levels of tumor necrosis factor-alpha, a protein produced mainly by macrophages during inflammatory processes[102,103].

- Immunologic reactions may not eliminate mites from the skin surface, but may induce scratching, a crude but potentially effective way of forcibly removing mites from the skin surface

## Clinical symptoms

- Itching is worse at night and begins 3 to 4 weeks after the infection is acquired

- Immediate and delayed-type hypersensitivity are involved

- Often members of the patient's immediate or extended family itch

- Since infestation does not produce immunity to repel subsequent re-infestation, second infestations may be accompanied by immediate symptoms

## Clinical appearance

The pathognomonic lesions of scabies are burrows, which are usually 0.5–1.5 mm wide and 5–15 mm long, slightly raised, scaling, meandering lines (Figure 22).

- The distal end of the burrow harboring the mite may have a tiny vesicle[104]

- Burrows may be numerous, but are detected in only 40% of patients

- Secondary features may frequently confuse the clinical picture

  Eczematous changes are common

  Secondary infection such as impetigo may also be severe and extensive

  Numerous excoriations may suggest neurotic excoriations

- In infants the palms, soles, ankles, wrists, face, scalp and trunk are commonly involved[105]

  Palm and sole vesicles, vesiculopustules and bullae may be seen

- In children and young adults lesions may be found on the wrists, the sides of the fingers, the finger web-spaces, the feet and ankles

  The gluteal cleft may be involved, but patients rarely forward the history of itching in this location

- In men, the penis and scrotum may have highly inflammatory papules and nodules (Figure 23)

- Due to the immunocompromized status of the elderly, neonates, and the immunosuppressed, infestations with scabies tend to be more florid
- Cases of crusted scabies have been reported in the following clinical situations

  AIDS[106]

  Bone marrow transplant[107]

  Chronic graft-versus-host disease[108]

  Diabetes[109]

  Elderly[110]

  Malignant tumors including adult T-cell leukemia[111]

  Individuals with learning disabilities and physical debilitation[112]

  Neonates and infants treated with corticosteroids[113]

  Selective IgA deficiency[114]

- Crusted (or Norwegian) scabies is characterized by hyperkeratotic, psoriasiform lesions of the hands, nails, trunk, feet, ears, and scalp which can harbor hundreds or thousands of mites[115,116]

  Note the subungual debris contains numerous mites

  Crusted scabies can spread in epidemic fashion

*Unusual clinical variants*
- Localized bullous scabies mimicking bullous pemphigoid is described[117,118]
- Pseudo T-cell lymphoma due to scabies in a patient with Hodgkin's disease[119]
- Vesicular scabies in an elderly patient receiving high-dose prednisone therapy[120]
- An infant with biopsy-proven scabies developed nodular lesions with atypical histiocytes and Langerhans cell features[121]

  Within six months after treatment all skin lesions gradually disappeared

*Adverse consequences of scabies*
- Persisting recurrent itching papules may persist for months to years following cure[122]
- Scabid: an unusual id reaction to scabies[123]

- Sepsis, including fatal sepsis, is associated and is most common with Norwegian scabies in patients with acquired immunodeficiency syndrome[124,125]
- Acute hematogenic osteomyelitis after impetiginized scabies has been reported[126]
- Acute glomerulonephritis has been temporally associated with scabies[127,128]
- Angioimmunoblastic lymphadenopathy has been reported[129]
- Generalized urticaria may be a consequence of scabies[130]

## Diagnosis

Most commonly, the initial diagnosis is made by clinical suspicion based on the patient's history and physical examination. Definitive diagnosis is made by finding microscopic evidence of infestation including mites, eggs or scybala. Techniques vary for scabies examination, but the single most critical factor is the choice of the body site[131].

- Examining the tiny dark dot at the end of typical burrows gives the highest microscopic yield of mites (Figure 24)
- Random body sites rarely demonstrate mites or their products
- The skin is gently scraped with a scalpel and the material placed in a drop of 10% potassium hydroxide or mineral oil on a microscope slide[132]
- The Burrow Ink Test may also help identify scabies infection
- Fluorescence-microscopic techniques seem more sensitive than other approaches, but are time-consuming and require expensive equipment[133]

## Treatment

*General guidelines*

Therapy for scabies should be more thorough in immunocompromised patients since these patients are more likely to host numerous mites. Whatever agent is chosen, the entire family should be treated once, and, given failure rates, re-treatment in one week is reasonable.

- Treatment failures can occur with children having more than one household of contacts; i.e. when divorced parents have separate homes or where children are cared for by grandparents
- Sensitivity to these issues helps eradicate the infestation from the family unit
- Careful instruction in proper application can enhance chances of cure
- Failure due to organism resistance is a growing problem for all scabicides

*Scabicides*

- Benzyl benzoate (10–20%) emulsion is highly effective in the treatment of scabies[134]

    Eczematous eruptions may frequently occur with benzyl benzoate

- Crotamiton (10%) is an effective scabicide and appears to be safe in children[135,136]
- Lindane (1% gamma benzene hexachloride) is also highly effective and is less irritating and more elegant than permethrin[137]

    Lindane has been associated with neurotoxic reactions, especially seizures, and has caused death when used excessively or ingested

    The use of lindane is problematic in infants, young children, pregnant or lactating women, and patients with AIDS

    Two hours after a single topical application of lindane, an HIV infected man experienced a new-onset generalized seizure, possibly due to intrinsic lowered seizure threshold[88]

- Monosulfiram (25%) solution diluted in two parts water may be applied[138]

    Multiple repeated applications are required for cure

- Permethrin (5%) cream is an agent of choice and is highly effective[137]

    Permethrin is a mild irritant and can cause stinging and burning

- Sulfur precipitate (5–10%) in petrolatum or other base is an inexpensive, effective treatment[139,140]

    Sulfur ointment application is the antithesis of elegant

- Malathion (0.5%) in aqueous base can be an effective scabicide if left on the skin for 24 hours
- Ivermectin systemically (200 μg/kg body mass) as a single oral dose is an emerging treatment[141,142]

    Repeated courses are required in the immunocompromized

    Ivermectin may also be applied topically, but like other treatments two applications are required[143]

## Bites and itchy stings

### Epidemiology

It has been estimated that there are one billion insects on Earth for every human, thus bites and stings are universal human experiences. Clearly, since these itchy disorders are dependent upon the life-cycles of the insects themselves, bites and stings tend to be episodic.

### Pathophysiology

Strict differentiation between infestation and arthropod bites is somewhat arbitrary, whereas stinging seems more clearly defined. Infesting arthropods often bite for sustenance. Since stings are not typically itchy, they will not be emphasized in this text.

An insect bite may produce direct effects of the toxin injected (generally non-immunologic), or components of the toxin may promote lymphocyte and monocyte infiltration as a delayed-type hypersensitivity response, and local cell proliferation as a more general response to the local damage and inflammatory stimulus[144].

- When bitten initially by most arthropods, aside from symptoms from the physical skin damage, no reaction usually occurs
- Only after repetitive exposure does one begin to develop hypersensitivity, manifest by a typical bite
- With prolonged exposure an immediate weal reaction occurs, to be followed by the delayed papular reaction
- Immunologic tolerance may occur with resultant lack of reaction

In studies of mosquito bites (from which one may generalize to other bites):

- Bite reactions were found to consist of both an immediate and a delayed reaction
- The eruption and time course of the immediate whealing reaction are consistent with type I hypersensitivity
- The eruption and time course of the delayed reaction were consistent with cutaneous eosinophil and basophil hypersensitivity

  Delayed mosquito-bite papules seem to be cutaneous late-phase reactions mediated by eosinophils or they could also represent type IV lymphocyte-mediated immune reactions

- Positive rates of immediate reaction increased from early childhood to adolescence and decreased with age from adulthood[145]
- The appearance and intensity of the delayed reaction decreased with age
- Five stages of reactivity have been described[146]

  Stage 1 – No reaction
  Stage 2 – Delayed reaction only
  Stage 3 – Immediate and delayed reaction
  Stage 4 – Immediate reaction only
  Stage 5 – No reaction

## Clinical appearance

Itchy bites and stings can produce myriads of morphologic appearances (Figures 25, 26).

- Erythematous macules, papules, and wheals

  Crusted or ecchymotic macules, papules, and wheals may appear from excoriation

  Dermatitis and impetigo may also arise secondarily from scratching

- Papulovesicles, vesiculopustules, and bullae
- Bites and stings in hypersensitive individuals may also produce systemic symptoms

  Urticaria, Arthus-like reactions and angioedema may result

  These reactions may be severe and life threatening[147]

## Treatment

Whenever possible, avoiding the bite is critical. Topical corticosteroids and anesthetics applied to the affected area are often effective in relieving itching.

For many arthropods, the most effective treatments are preventative, including donning protective clothing, use of repellents, and avoidance of locations at-risk[148,149].

### Repellents

- Citronella, an oil extracted from a grass, has a strong scent and is a marginally effective repellent
- N,N-diethylmetatoluanide (DEET) is the most effective insect repellant
- Insect repellents can be absorbed transcutaneously

  There are few reports of adverse reactions involving repeated use of DEET, most often on young children

  Some toxicology handbooks recommend that if insect repellents with DEET are used on young children, the concentrations must be below 15%

- Dimethylphthalate is a widely used repellent

- Persons known to be hypersensitive (e.g. angioedema) to insect bites and stings should carry an epinephrine injection kit to use as a first aid measure

## Non-scabieitic mites

Non-scabieitic mites prefer to dine on the blood of animal hosts, but when their favorite meal is unavailable, they bite humans. People who handle animals are most likely to be affected, but virtually anyone is subject to being bitten since we all live within reach of birds, rats, mice and other animals. Often, these bites are mysterious and require some degree of historical investigation to discern.

There are too many types of mites to comprehensively cover in this section and the interested reader is referred to more complete references[150]. Some of the important genera are listed below.

*Cheyletiella*
- Cheyletiella, a non-burrowing species of mite, may be found in dogs (*C. yasguri*), cats (*C. blakei*), rabbits (*C. parasitovorax*), and other animals, and can cause severe itching[151]
- A common veterinary term for this condition is 'walking dandruff'[152]
- A wide variety of clinical signs may be seen, but most commonly erythematous papules are found in areas that have been in contact with the infested animal or animal's favorite sites[153,154]
- Antiscabietic treatment of the affected patient does not result in cure
- Treatment of affected animals usually results in clearance

*Demodex*
- *Demodex folliculorum* is a normal inhabitant of the skin and is a worm-like mite that infests hair follicles above the level of sebaceous glands in various mammals

Demodicosis can be shared between a boy and his dog[155]
- When excessive numbers of mites are present, intense irritation and itching, somewhat resembling scabies, may appear
- As in the case of scabies infestation, HIV infection may create more severe itching and signs such as folliculitis[156]
- Treatment of the patient (and rarely the dog) with topical permethrin, mercuric oxide, or metronidazole helps[157,158]

*Eutromicula*
- Trombiculid mites cause 'chigger' bites, intensely itchy spots which usually arise from walking or working in long grasses or fields.
- Larvae on grasses attach to a susceptible human or non-human host, insert a sword-like appendage into the skin and form a stylostome from salivary secretions into the lower epidermis
- Enzymes digest the skin and digestate and serum are withdrawn through the stylostome over the next 2–3 days
- Mites then drop off to complete their life cycle
- *E. alfreddugusi* is the most common 'chigger' mite in the United States, but related mites include *Neotromicula autumnalis* in Europe and *Acomatacarus australensis* in Asia, Australia and Pacific islands
- Trombiculid mites can cause epidemic outbreaks of mite dermatitis
- The best protection arises from the use of protective clothing and insect repellent

*Pyemotes*
- *Pyemotes ventricosus* is found in wood and may affect those who work with timber
- *Pyemotes tritici* lives in grain, and reports of *Pyemotes ventricosus* as the grain itch mite may in fact be misidentification of species

- Grain itch mites have caused several large epidemics of dermatitis during the 19th and 20th centuries
- Varicelliform or chigger-bite-like dermatitis is typically seen, but constitutional symptoms are reported

*Dermanyssus*

- *Dermanyssus gallinae* and bird mites, usually affect those in the poultry business, but can affect anyone living or working within the vicinity of infested birds and their nests
- Medical sleuths can take pride in uncovering mysterious bites, such as pigeon mite (*Dermanyssus gallinae*) infestation involving two patients, two nurses, and one physician in a hospital[159–161]

  The first patient developed a diffuse, itchy erythematous maculopapular rash on his trunk and extremities

  Dermanyssus gallinae was identified on the patient and his bedding

  A second patient complained of scalp itching, and also had mites present on her pillow and bed linen

  The intern taking care of both patients, and two nurses who had contact with these patients, had mite infestation

  Pigeons roosting on the air conditioners and near the doors connecting the patients' rooms to a sunporch were the source of the mites

*Ornithonyssus*

- Chronic itching can also be caused by other bird mites, *Ornithonyssus sylviarum* and *O. bursa*[162]
- *O. baconi*, the tropical rat mite, can cause bites, dermatitis and urticaria[163]

### Miscellaneous other mite dermatitides

For a full description see Blankenship[150].

- *Acarus siro* causes 'Baker's itch' and lives in stored products such as cheese

- *Glycyphagus domesticus* causes 'Grocer's itch' and lives in hay, animal and other food
- *Rhizoglyphus parasiticus* and *R. hyacinthi* cause 'Coolie itch' and live in onions, plant bulbs and tea
- *Carpoglyphus lactis* causes 'dried fruit itch' and lives in dried fruit, feathers and skin

### Fleas

Fleas are small, reddish-brown, wingless insects with a laterally compressed body and a pronounced third pair of legs adapted to leaping. While more than 2000 species and subspecies of flea are known, only nine have significant medical and veterinary importance, and only six involve man. However these six may be vectors of bacteria, viruses, rickettsiae and intestinal parasites[164].

- *Pulex irritans*, the human flea still exists, may cause intense itching, and may spread in an epidemic fashion
- *Ctenocephalides felis* and *C.canis*, the cat and dog fleas, are nearly universal and may cause few symptoms on the infested animal[165]
- Eggs drop easily from pet hosts to be widely distributed throughout the home
- *Ceratophyllus gallinae*, the bird flea, can cause mystery itching[166]

  An epidemic of flea bite dermatitis occurred in a Singapore warehouse which had been colonized by wild Myna birds infested with the flea Ceratophyllus gallinae

Clinically, like other bites, a flea bite shows first as a hemorrhagic punctum, accompanied by itching, and leads to an erythema with or without central wheal.

- Human flea bites range from small red welts to severe rash and itching; they are usually found only on wrists, ankles and legs

  They may occur as multiple, grouped bites (breakfast, lunch and dinner)

■ Animal flea bites are often found from the mid-calf down or where the patient has had contact with flea-infested clothing or bedding[167]

Treatment is supportive, but eliminating the fleas from the environment by washing infested clothing, bedding, and other suspected infested items is crucial. If spread from animals, treatment of the animal and its environment is key.

## Beetles

*Paederus fuscipes* dermatitis is a self-healing itching, blistering irritant contact dermatitis caused by a small insect. This beetle does not bite or sting, but accidental brushing against or crushing the beetle over the skin provokes the release of its coelomic fluid which contains paederin, a potent vesicant agent[168,169].

■ The lesions usually resembles the accidental dropping of a caustic or hot liquid
■ The uncommon association of acute dermatitis with minimal or no complaints, which would be noteworthy in the case of chemical or thermal burns, facilitates diagnosis

Carpet beetle dermatitis may cause recurrent bites[170], and in one case a woolen rug in the patient's bedroom was infested with carpet beetle larvae, *Anthrenus verbasci*.

## Bedbugs

*Cimex lectularius* and *C. hemipterus* live in household furniture and flooring and are nocturnal feeders. Because these insects are starvation-resistant, they may survive for months of no feeding in an empty house, before feasting on new inhabitants.

■ Bites can be asymptomatic to fiercely itchy bullae, and appear in the morning following feeding

## Lepidopterans

Lepidopterism is the term used to describe the aggregate adverse medical effects resulting from contact with adult or larval forms of butterflies and moths. Histamine, histamine-releasing substances, kinin activators, and other as yet undefined proteins are responsible for cutaneous, cardiovascular, neurologic, and constitutional signs and symptoms of lepidopterism. Insect venom is injected into the skin through specialized caterpillar hairs when contact occurs with the insect (or vegetation laden with insect debris)[171,172].

■ The offending setae are tapering, hollow microcapillaries which are open at both ends, and serve as microneedles from which irritant substances may be liberated when penetrating into the skin
■ The resulting inflammatory reactions are attributable to combined mechanical and toxic effects
■ Clinically, irritation may be noted immediately after contact or may be delayed for days
■ Mild cases of lepidopterism will resolve spontaneously; systemic corticosteroids may aid in the treatment of more serious cases
■ Lepidopterism may occur in epidemic fashion[173,174]

## Mosquitoes

Mosquitoes are mankind's most common itch-inducing insect; there are few people who have not experienced this arthropod assault.

■ The flight speed of some West African mosquitoes has been estimated as high as 120cm/s[175]

Hypersensitivity to mosquito venom is highly variable between individuals, and with tolerance may change over the course of one season in an individual[176].

- Severe Arthus-type reactions may occur, with bloody bullae formation, chills, and fever several hours after the mosquito bite
- Exaggerated insect bite reactions are seen in patients with HIV infection and chronic lymphocytic leukemia
- Systemic anaphylaxis from mosquito bites has also been reported[177]
- Potent topical corticosteroid and anesthetic agents may mitigate the symptoms
- In mosquito-sensitive subjects, prophylactically administered cetirizine is an effective drug against both immediate and delayed mosquito-bite symptoms[178,179]

### Sandflies

These insects belong to the genera *Phlebotomus* and *Lutzomyia*. A particularly unpleasant, phlebotomine, itching condition is known as harara or urticaria multiformis endemica in the Middle Eastern countries[180].

- Clinically, one sees urticarial papules, vesicles, vesiculopustules, and bullae on exposed skin which may be complicated by secondary infection

## Marine bites and stings

### Swimmer's itch

This phenomenon typically occurs in the summer within 30–90 minutes of immersion into cercaria-infested fresh water or saltwater[181]. After 6–12 hours there is intensely pruritic macular eruption and in a few cases secondary skin infection may also develop.

- The distribution of this disorder ranges from the fresh water lakes of Montana, USA[182] to the rice paddy fields of Thailand[135,183]
- Numerous cercarial species that use snails as their host are implicated in this disease[184], including *Trichobiharzia ocellata*, *T. szidati*, *Diplostomum spathaceum* and *Schistosoma spindale*
- Cercariae are able to invade human skin and cause dermatitis in human volunteers after repeated exposure[185,186]
- To identify cercaria-infested water test fresh waterfowl fecal material for the presence of miracidia, and snails for the presence of cercariae

> In an amazing study, swimmer's itch-producing cercariae were verified by placing several species on the arms of human volunteers and waiting for a reaction

A different type of swimmer's itch, found in Hawaii, is caused by a toxic strain of the finely filamentous, velvety, dark olive-green or black algae *Microcolus Lyngbyaceus*[187].

- This is also recognized by the name 'stinging seaweed' dermatitis

### Seabather's eruption

Seabather's eruption is an erythematous macular or papular dermatitis, with or without urticarial eruption, that develops in individuals who have been swimming in the ocean. It is a highly itchy eruption under swimwear and occurs sporadically in Florida, the Caribbean[188], and as far north as New York and Bermuda[189].

The disease is caused by several species of Cnidaria larvae, including *Linuche unguiculata* (thimble jellyfish) and *Edwardsiella lineata* (sea anemone). Applying larvae to the skin of healthy subjects produced a dermatitis indistinguishable from seabather's eruption. Systemic hypersensitivity symptoms may occur but are unlikely. Children are more likely than adults to have systemic symptoms.

- The average duration of the eruption and itching was reported as 12.5 days and recurrences may occur[190]
- It resolves spontaneously within 2 weeks

Symptomatic treatment is the mainstay of therapy for this self-limited rash, but is often ineffective.

## Other marine assaults

Cnidarians such as jellyfish[191] and sea anemones may sting man, inducing burning and intense itching[192].

- Portuguese man-of-war stings can cause intense itching (Figure 27)

  These organisms contain cnidoblasts which contain a nemotocyst which injects venom when the cell touches prey[193]

Treatment of the linear, erythematous and vesicular eruption is symptomatic with topical corticosteroid agents

Sea urchin (Echinoderm) spines which are imbedded in the skin can cause foreign body granulomas which are usually asymptomatic, but may itch[194,195]. They arise as a delayed reaction a few months after the initial injury by sea-urchin spines[195]. Spontaneous resolution may occur.

- Many injuries such as those from sea urchins can be avoided by wearing shoes when walking in shallow water or tide pools

## References

1. Feingold DS. Staphyloccocal and streptoccocal pyodermas. *Semin Dermatol* 1993;12:331–5
2. Shrimer DL, Schwartz RA, Jammiger CK. Impetigo. *Cutis* 1995;56:30–2
3. Bork K, Brauers J, Kresken M. Efficacy and safety of 2% mupirocin ointment in the treatment of primary and secondary skin infections – an open multicentre trial. *Br J Clin Pract* 1989;43:284–8
4. Guitart J, Woodley DT. Intertrigo: a practical approach. *Comp Ther* 1994;20:402–9
5. Noble WC, Hope YM, Midgley G, *et al.* Toewebs as a source of gram–negative bacilli. *J Hosp Infect* 1986; 8:248–56
6. Browne SG. Some less common neurological findings in leprosy. *J Neurol Sciences* 1965;2:253–61
7. Cole GW, Amon RB, Russell PS. Secondary syphilis presenting as a pruritic dermatosis. *Arch Dermatol* 1977;113:489–90
8. El Shiemy, S, Farid M, Saliam TH, *et al.* Clinical study on syphilis in Abu Dhabi with special stress on the unusual presentation of the disease. *Int J Dermatol* 1984;23:120–2
9. Sarkani I. Pruritus and cholestatic jaundice due to secondary syphilis. *Proc Roy Soc Med* 1973;66:237–8
10. Daye S, McHenry JA, Roscelli JD. Pruritic rash associated with cat scratch disease. *Pediatrics* 1988;81:559–61
11. Weitzman I, Summerbell RC. The dermatophytes. *Clin Microbiol Rev* 1995;8:240–59
12. Aly R. Ecology and epidemiology of dermatophyte infections. *J Am Acad Dermatol* 1994;31:S21–5
13. Schwartz ME. Barn itch. *Am Fam Phys* 1983;27:149–53
14. Dahl MV. Suppression of immunity and inflammation by products produced by dermatophytes. *J Am Acad Dermatol* 1993;28:S19–S23
15. Degreef HJ, DeDoncker PR. Current therapy of dermatophytosis. *J Am Acad Dermatol* 1994;31:S25–30
16. Balfour JA, Faulds D. Terbinafine. A review of its pharmacodynamic and pharmacokinetic properties, and therapeutic potential in superficial mycoses. *Drugs* 1992;43:259–84
17. Van Cutsem J. Itraconazole and therapy of fungal infections. *Curr Prob Dermatol* 1996;24:194–202
18. Montero-Gei F, Perera A. Therapy with fluconazole for tinea corporis, tinea cruris and tinea pedis. *Clin Inf Dis* 1992;14 (Suppl 1):577–81
19. Back O, Faergemann J, Hornqvist R. Pityrosporum folliculitis: a common disease of the young and middle-aged. *J Am Acad Dermatol* 1985;12:56–61
20. Penneys NS. *Skin Manifestations of AIDS.* London: Dunitz, 1990
21. Hoover WD Jr, Lang PG. Pruritus in HIV infection. *J Am Acad Dermatol* 1991;24:1020–1
22. Buchness MR, Sanchez M. HIV-associated pruritus. *Clinics Dermatol* 1991;9:111–4

23. Buchness MR, Lim HW, Hatcher VA, *et al.* Ultraviolet B phototherapy of eosinophilic pustular follicultits in patients with the acquired immunodeficiency syndrome. *N Engl J Med* 1988;318:1183–8

24. Ford GP, Farr PM, Ive FA, *et al.* The response of seborrheic dermatitis to ketoconazole. *Br J Dermatol* 1984;111:603–7

25. Gordin FN, Simon GL, Wofsy CD, *et al.* Adverse reactions to trimethoprim-sulfamethoxazole in patients with the acquired immunodeficiency syndrome. *Ann Int Med* 1984;100:495

26. Bason MM, Berger TG, Nesbitt LT Jr. Pruritic papular eruption of HIV-disease. *Int J Dermatol* 1993;32:784–9

27. Hevia O, Jimenez-Acosta F, Ceballos PI, *et al.* Pruritic papular eruption of the acquired immunodeficiency syndrome: a clinicopathologic study. *J Am Acad Dermatol* 1991;24:231–5

28. Ishii N, Nishiyama T, Sugita Y, *et al.* Pruritic papular eruption of the acquired immunodeficiency syndrome. *Acta Derm Venereol* 1994;74:219–20

29. Liautaud B, Pape JW, DeHovitz JA et al. Pruritic skin lesions. A common initial presentation of acquired immunodeficiency syndrome. *Arch Dermatol* 1989;125:629–32

30. Pardo RJ, Bogaert MA, Penneys NS, *et al.* UVB phototherapy of the pruritic papular eruption of the acquired immunodeficiency syndrome. *J Am Acad Dermatol* 1992;26:423–8

31. Meola T, Soter NA, Ostreicher R, *et al.* The safety of UVB phototherapy in patients with HIV infection. *J Am Acad Dermatol* 1993;29:216–20

32. Bremmer S. Acquired ichthyosis in AIDS. *Cutis* 1987;39:421–3

33. Lotz R, Rosler HP, Zapf S, *et al.* Radiotherapy in HIV positive patients. *Fortschritte Med* 1990;108:35–9

34. Corey L, Adams HG, Brown ZA, *et al.* Genital herpes simplex virus infections: clinical manifestations, course, and complications. *Ann Int Med* 1983;98:958–72

35. Weller TH. Varicella and zoster II. *N Engl J Med* 1983;309:1434–40

36. Huff JC. Antiviral treatment in chickenpox and herpes zoster. *J Am Acad Dermatol* 1988;18:204–6

37. Pereira FA. Herpes simplex: evolving concepts. *J. Am Acad Dermatol* 1996;35:503–20

38. Arvin AM. Varicella zoster virus: overview and clinical manifestations. *Semin Dermatol* 1996;15:4–7

39. Waterson AP. Virus infections (other than rubella) during pregnancy. *Br Med J* 1979;3:564–6

40. Balfour HH Jr, Kelly JM, Suarez CS *et al.* Acyclovir treatment of varicella in otherwise healthy children. *J Pediatrics* 1990;116:633–9

41. Feldmann R, Harms M, Saurat JH. Papular-purpuric 'gloves and socks' syndrome: not only parvovirus B19. *Dermatology* 1994;188:85–7

42. Hwang KP, Su SC, Chiang CH. Clinical observations of dengue fever among children. *Kaohsiung J Med Sci* 1989;5:50–7

43. Rozenman D, Kremer M, Zuckerman F. Onchocerciasis in Israel. *Arch Dermatol* 1984;120:505–7

44. Olumide YM, Oresanya F. Generalized pruritus as a presenting symptom in Nigeria. *Intern J Dermatol* 1987;26:171–3

45. De Sole G. Criterion for inclusion in onchocerciasis control programmes based on ivermectin distribution. *Trans Roy Soc Trop Med Hyg* 1995;89:224–5

46. Anosike JC, Onwuliri CO. Studies on filariasis in Bauchi State, Nigeria. 1. Endemicity of human onchocerciasis in Ningi Local Government Area. *Ann Trop Med Parasitol* 1995;89:31–8

47. Akogun OB, Musa-Hong H, Hellandendu H. Onchocerciasis in Taraba State, Nigeria: intensity, rate of infection and associated symptoms in 14 communities of Bali district. *Applied Parasitol* 1994;35:125–32

48. Hamrick HJ, Moore GW. Giardiasis causing urticaria in a child. *Am J Dis Child* 1983; 137:761–3

49. McKnight JT, Tietze PE. Dermatologic manifestations of giardiasis. *J Am Board Fam Pract* 1992;5:425–8

50. Spaulding HS Jr. Pruritus without urticaria in acute giardiasis. *Ann Allergy* 1990;65:161

51. Lonsdorf G. Larva migrans. *Hautarzt* 1980;31:450–1

52. Battistini F. Treatment of creeping eruption with topical thiabendazole. *Texas Rep Biol Med* 1969;27 (Suppl 2):645

53. Davis CM, Israel RM. Treatment of creeping eruption with topical thiabendazole. *Arch Dermatol* 1968;97:325–6

54. Klingelberger CE. It's not a viral syndrome, it's malaria. *Ann Emerg Med* 1989;18:207–10

55. Ganor S. Entamoeba histolytica: a possible cause of pruritus. *Int J Dermatol* 1981;20:261

56. Yoshimoto CM. Strongyloides infection in Hawaii: an imported case. *Hawaii Med J* 1993;52:59–61, 76

57. Chaudhry AZ, Longworth DL. Cutaneous manifestations of intestinal helminthic infections. *Dermatol Clin* 1989;7:275–90

58. Orecchia G, Pazzaglia A, Scaglia M, *et al.* Larva currens following systemic steroid therapy in a case of strongyloidiasis. *Dermatologica* 1985;171:366–7

59. Kagen CN, Vance JC, Simpson M. Gnathostomiasis. Infestation in an Asian immigrant. *Arch Dermatol* 1984;120:508–10

60. De Queriroz AC. Tumor-like lesion of the brain caused by *Trypanosoma cruzi. Am J Trop Med Hyg* 1973;22:473–6

61. Juckett G: Common intestinal helminths. *Am Fam Phys* 1995;52:2039–48, 2051–2

62. Buslau M, Marsch WC. Papular eruption in helminth infection – a hypersensitivity phenomenon? *Acta Derm Venereol* 1990;70:526–9

63. Gilman RH, Marquis GS, Miranda E. Prevalence and symptoms of *Enterobius vermicularis* infections in a Peruvian shanty town. *Trans Roy Soc Trop Med Hyg* 1991;85:761–4

64. Jones JE. Pinworms. *Am Fam Phys* 1988;38:159–64

65. Deshpande AD. *Enterobius vermicularis* live adult worms in the high vagina. *Postgrad Med J* 1992;68:690–1

66. Burns DA. Diseases caused by arthropods and other noxious animals. In Champion RH, Burton JL, Ebling FJG, eds. *Textbook of Dermatology*, 5th edn. Oxford: Blackwell Scientific Publications, 1992:1265–324

67. Fan PC, Chao D, Lee KM, *et al.* Chemotherapy of head louse (*Pediculus humanus capitis*) infestation with gamma benzene hexachloride (gamma-BHC) among school children in Szu-Hu District, Yunlin County, Central West Taiwan. *Chung Hua i Hsueh Tsa Chih* 1991;48:13–9

68. Mumcuoglu KY, Miller J, Manor O, *et al.* The prevalence of ectoparasites in Ethiopian immigrants. *Israel J Med Sci* 1993;29:371–3

69. Mumcuoglu KY, Miller J, Gofin R, *et al.* Epidemiological studies on head lice infestation in Israel. I. Parasitological examination of children. *Int J Dermatol* 1990;29:502–6

70. Sokoloff F. Identification and management of pediculosis. *Nurse Pract* 1994;19:62–4

71. Ebomoyi EW. Pediculosis capitis among urban school children in Ilorin, Nigeria. *J Nat Med Assoc* 1994;86:861–4

72. Elgart ML: Pediculosis. *Dermatol Clin* 1990;8:219–28

73. Mumcuoglu KY, Klaus S, Kafka D, *et al.* Clinical observations related to head lice infestation. *J Amer Acad Dermatol* 1991;25:248–52

74. Morsy TA, Sarwat MA, Fawzi AF, *et al.* Some clinical features of pediculosis among school children. *J Egyptian Soc Parasitol* 1994;24:121–5

75. Van Staey A, Suys E, Derumeaux L, *et al.* Hair casts. *Dermatologica* 1991;182:124–7

76. Brenner S, Yust I. Bullous eruption in a case of bullous pediculid. *Cutis* 1988;41:281

77. Brenner S, Ophir J, Krakowski A. Pediculid. An unusual -id reaction to pediculosis capitis. *Dermatologica* 1984;168:189–91

78. Burgess I, Coulthard M, Heaney JL. Scalp infestation by *Liposcelis mendax. Br J Dermatol* 1991;125:400–1

79. Brown S, Becher J, Brady W. Treatment of ectoparasitic infections: review of the English language literature, 1982–1992. *Clin Infect Dis* 1995;20(Suppl 1):S104–9

80. Mumcuoglu KY, Miller J. The efficacy of pediculicides in Israel. *Isr J Med Sci* 1991;27:562–5

81. Kalter DC, Sperber J, Rosen T, *et al.* Treatment of pediculosis pubis. Clinical comparison of efficacy and tolerance of 1% lindane shampoo vs. 1% permethrin creme rinse. *Arch Dermatol* 1987;123:1315–9

82. Janniger CK, Kuflik AS. Pediculosis capitis. *Cutis* 1993;51:407–8

83. Chosidow O, Chastang C, Brue C, *et al.* Controlled study of malathion and d-phenothrin lotions for *Pediculus humanus var. capitis*-infested schoolchildren. *Lancet* 1994;344:1724–7

84. Bergus GR. Topical treatments for head lice. *J Fam Pract* 1996;42:21–2

85. Izri MA, Briere C. First cases of resistance of *Pediculus capitis* Linne 1758 to malathion in France. *Presse Med* 1995;24:1444

86. Mumcuoglu KY, Hemingway J, Miller J, *et al.* Permethrin resistance in the head louse *Pediculus capitis* from Israel. *Med Vet Entomol* 1996;9:427–32

87. Mumcuoglu KY, Miller J. The efficacy of pediculicides in Israel. *Israel J Med Sci* 1991;27:562–5

88. Solomon BA, Haut SR, Carr EM, *et al.* Neurotoxic reaction to lindane in an HIV-seropositive patient. An old medication's new problem. *J Fam Pract* 1995;40:291–6

89. Davies JE, Dedhia HV, Morgade C, *et al.* Lindane poisonings. *Arch Dermatol* 1983;119:142–4

90. Sokolova TV, Lange AB. The parasite-host specificity of the itch mite (*Acariformes: Sarcoptidae*) in man and animals (a review of the literature). *Parazitologia* 1992;26:97–104

91. Morsy TA, Bakr ME, Ahmed MM, *et al.* Human scabies acquired from a pet puppy. *J Egypt Soc Parasitol* 1994;24:305–8

92. Hawkins JA, McDonald RK, Woody BJ. *Sarcoptes scabiei* infestation in a cat. *J Am Vet Med Assoc* 1987; 190:1572–3

93. Chakrabarti A. Human notoedric scabies from contact with cats infested with *Notoedres cati. Int J Dermatol* 1986;25:646–8

94. Mumcuoglu Y, Rufli T. Human infestation by *Sarcoptes scabiei var. bovis* (cattle itch mite). *Hautarzt* 1979;30:423–6

95. Chakrabarti A: Pig handler's itch. *Int J Dermatol* 1990;29:205–6

96. Chakrabarti A, Chatterjee A, Chakrabarti K, *et al.* Human scabies from contact with water buffaloes infested with *Sarcoptes scabiei var. bubalis. Ann Trop Med Parasitol* 1981;75:353–7

97. Yeruham I, Rosen S, Hadani A, *et al.* Sarcoptic mange in wild ruminants in zoological gardens in Israel. *J Wildlife Dis* 1996;32:57–61

98. Phillips PH, O'Callaghan MG, Moore E, *et al.* Pedal *Sarcoptes scabiei* infestation in ferrets (*Mustela putorius furo*). *Austr Vet J* 1987;64:289-90

99. Arlian LG, Estes SA, Vyszenski-Moher DL. Prevalence of *Sarcoptes scabiei* in the homes and nursing homes of scabietic patients. *J Am Acad Dermatol* 1988;19:806–11

100. Sokolova TV, Radchenko MI, Lange AB. The seasonality of scabies morbidity and the fertility of the itch mite *Sarcoptes scabiei de Geer* as an index of the activity of a population of the causative agent. *Vestnik Dermatol Venerol* 1989;11:12–5

101. Morsy TA, el Alfy MS, Arafa MA, *et al.* Serum levels of tumour necrosis factor alpha (TNF-alpha) versus immunoglobulins (IgG., IgM., and IgE.) in Egyptian scabietic children. *J Egypt Soc Parasitol* 1995;25:773–86

102. Cabrera R, Agar A, Dahl MV. The immunology of scabies. *Semin Dermatol* 1993;12:15–21

103. Dahl MV. The immunology of scabies. *Ann Allergy* 1983;51:560–6

104. Moore P. Diagnosing and treating scabies. *Practitioner* 1994;238:632–5

105. Haustein UF. Bullous scabies. *Dermatology* 1995; 190:83–4

106. Schlesinger I, Oelrich DM, Tyring SK. Crusted (Norwegian) scabies in patients with AIDS: the range of clinical presentations. *South Med J* 1994;87:352–6

107. Barnes L, McCallister RE, Lucky AW. Crusted (Norwegian) scabies. Occurrence in a child undergoing a bone marrow transplant. *Arch Dermatol* 1987; 123:95–7

108. Magee KL, Hebert AA, Rapini RP. Crusted scabies in a patient with chronic graft-versus-host disease. *J Am Acad Dermatol* 1991;25:889–91

109. Klein LJ, Cole G. Crusted scabies in a diabetic alcoholic. *Int J Dermatol* 1987;26:467–8

110. Paules SJ, Levisohn D, Heffron W. Persistent scabies in nursing home patients. *J Fam Pract* 1993;37:82–6

111. Egawa K, Johno M, Hayashibara T, *et al.* Familial occurrence of crusted (Norwegian) scabies with adult T-cell leukaemia. *Br J Dermatol* 1992;127:57–9

112. Lang E, Humphreys DW, Jaqua-Stewart MJ. Crusted scabies: a case report and review of the literature. *South Dakota J Med* 1989;42:15–7

113. Camassa F, Fania M, Ditano G, *et al.* Neonatal scabies. *Cutis* 1995;56:210–2

114. Shindo K, Kono T, Kitajima J, *et al.* Crusted scabies in acquired selective IgA deficiency. *Acta Derm Venereol* 1991;71:250–1

115. Hubler WR Jr. Epidemic Norwegian scabies. *Arch Dermatol* 1976;112:179–81

116. Wolf R, Krakowski A. Atypical crusted scabies. *J Am Acad Dermatol* 1987;17:434–6

117. Ostlere LS, Harris D, Rustin MH. Scabies associated with a bullous pemphigoid-like eruption. *Br J Dermatol* 1993;128:217–9

118. Slawsky LD, Maroon M, Tyler WB, *et al.* Association of scabies with a bullous pemphigoid-like eruption. *J Am Acad Dermatol* 1996;34:878–9

119. Walton S, Bottomley WW, Wyatt EH, *et al.* Pseudo T-cell lymphoma due to scabies in a patient with Hodgkin's disease. *Br J Dermatol* 1991;124:277–8

120. Dhawan SS, Weitzner JM, Phillips MG, *et al.* Vesicular scabies in an adult. *Cutis* 1989;43:267–8

121. Talanin NY, Smith SS, Shelley ED, *et al.* Cutaneous histiocytosis with Langerhans cell features induced by scabies: a case report. *Ped Dermatol* 1994;11: 327–30

122. Oberste-Lehn H, Baggesen I. Persisting recurrent itching papullae following scabies. *Dermatol Wochenschrift* 1968;154:437–41

123. Brenner S, Wolf R, Landau M. Scabid: an unusual id reaction to scabies. *Int J Dermatol* 1993;32:128–9

124. Glover A, Young L, Goltz AW. Norwegian scabies in acquired immunodeficiency syndrome: report of a case resulting in death from associated sepsis. *J Am Acad Dermatol* 1987;16:396–9

125. Skinner SM, DeVillez RL. Sepsis associated with Norwegian scabies in patients with acquired immunodeficiency syndrome. *Cutis* 1992;50:213–6

126. Gaida G, Tollner U, Krupe H, *et al.* Acute hematogenic osteomyelitis after impetiginized scabies. *Klin Padiat* 1985;197:489–91

127. Anonymous. Epidemic scabies and associated acute glomerulonephritis in Trinidad. *Bull Pan Am Health Org* 1988;22:103–7

128. Takiguchi Y, Kusama K, Nagao S, *et al.* A case of scabies complicated by acute glomerulonephritis. *J Dermatol* 1987;14:163–6

129. Kleiner-Baumgarten A, Shoenfeld Y, Chowers Y, *et al.* Scabies-associated angioimmunoblastic lymphadenopathy. *Acta Haematol* 1986;76:166–8

130. Witkowski JA, Parish LC. Scabies: a cause of generalized urticaria. *Cutis* 1984;33:277–9

131. Palicka P, Malis L, Samsinak K, *et al.* Laboratory diagnosis of scabies. *J Hyg Epidemiol Microbiol Immunol* 1980;24:63–70

132. Brodell RT, Helms SE. Office dermatologic testing: the scabies preparation. *Am Fam Phys* 1991;44:505–8

133. Bhutto AM, Honda M, Kubo Y, *et al.* Introduction of a fluorescence-microscopic technique for the detection of eggs, egg shells, and mites in scabies. *J Dermatol* 1993;20:122–4

134. Haustein UF, Hlawa B. Treatment of scabies with permethrin versus lindane and benzyl benzoate. *Acta Derm Venereol* 1989;69:348–51

135. Kolarova L, Gottwaldova V, Cechova D, *et al.* The occurrence of cercarial dermatitis in Central Bohemia. *Zentralblatt Hyg Umweltmed* 1989;189:1–13

136. Taplin D, Meinking TL, Chen JA, *et al.* Comparison of crotamiton 10% cream (Eurax) and permethrin 5% cream (Elimite) for the treatment of scabies in children. *Ped Dermatol* 1990;7:67–73

137. Schultz MW, Gomez M, Hansen RC, *et al.* Comparative study of 5% permethrin cream and 1% lindane lotion for the treatment of scabies. *Arch Dermatol* 1990;126:167–70

138. Reid HF, Thorne CD. Scabies infection: the effect of intervention by public health education. *Epidemiol Inf* 1990;105:592–602

139. Kenawi MZ, Morsy TA, Abdalla KF, *et al.* Treatment of human scabies by sulfur and permethrin. *J Egypt Soc Parasitol* 1993;23:691–6

140. Avila-Romay A, Alvarez-Franco M, Ruiz-Maldonado R. Therapeutic efficacy, secondary effects, and patient acceptability of 10% sulfur in either pork fat or cold cream for the treatment of scabies. *Ped Dermatol* 1991;8:64–6

141. Kar SK, Mania J, Patnaik S. The use of ivermectin for scabies. *Nat Med J India* 1994;7:15–6

142. Marty P, Gari-Toussaint M, Le Fichoux Y, *et al.* Efficacy of ivermectin in the treatment of an epidemic of sarcoptic scabies. *Ann Trop Med Parasitol* 1994;88:453

143. Youssef MY, Sadaka HA, Eissa MM, *et al.* Topical application of ivermectin for human ectoparasites. *Am J Trop Med Hyg* 1995;53:652–3

144. Burns DA. Diseases caused by arthropoods and other noxious animals. In Champion RH, Burton JL, Ebling FJG, eds. *Textbook of Dermatology*, 5th ed, Oxford: Blackwell Scientific Publications, 1992:1265–324

145. Oka K. Ohtaki N. Clinical observations of mosquito bite reactions in man: a survey of the relationship between age and bite reaction. *J Dermatol* 1989;16:212–9

146. Reunala T, Brummer-Korvenkontio H, Lappalainen P, *et al.* Immunology and treatment of mosquito bites. *Clin Exp Allergy* 1990;20 (Suppl 4):19–24

147. McCormack DR. Salata KF, Hershey JN, *et al.* Mosquito bite anaphylaxis: immunotherapy with whole body extracts. *Ann Allergy Asthma Immunol* 1995;74:39–44

148. Holmes HS. Stings and bites. Tips on coexisting comfortably with the insects. *Postgrad Med* 1990;88:75–8

149. Honig PJ. Arthropod bites, stings, and infestations: their prevention and treatment. *Ped Dermatol* 1986;3:189–97

150. Blankenship ML. Mite dermatitis other than scabies. *Dermatol Clin* 1990;8:265–75

151. Cohen SR. Cheyletiella dermatitis. A mite infestation of rabbit, cat, dog, and man. *Arch Dermatol* 1980;116:435–7

152. Cohen SR. Cheyletiella dermatitis. A mite infestation of rabbit, cat, dog, and man. *Arch Dermatol* 1980;116:435–7

153. Lee BW. Cheyletiella dermatitis: a report of fourteen cases. *Cutis* 1991;47:111–4

154. Shelley ED, Shelley WB, Pula JF, *et al.* The diagnostic challenge of nonburrowing mite bites. *Cheyletiella yasguri. J Am Med Assoc* 1984;251:2690–1

155. Fulk GW, Clifford C. A case report of demodicosis. *J Am Optometric Assoc* 1990;61:637–9

156. de Jaureguiberry JP, Carsuzaa F, Pierre C, *et al.* Demodex folliculitis: a cause of pruritus in human immunodeficiency virus infection. *Annales Med Interne* 1993;144:63–4

157. Mimioglu MM, Sahin I, Alp U. Demodectic mange in a dog in Beytepe University campus. *Mikrobiyoloji Bulteni* 1979;13:401–5

158. Morsy TA, el Okbi MM, el-Said AM, *et al.* Demodex (follicular mite) infesting a boy and his pet dog. *J Egypt Soc Parasitol* 1995;25:509–12

159. Regan AM, Metersky ML, Craven DE. Nosocomial dermatitis and pruritus caused by pigeon mite infestation. *Arch Int Med* 1987;147:2185–7

160. Sexton DJ, Haynes B. Bird-mite infestation in a university hospital. *Lancet* 1975;1:445

161. Vargo JA, Ginsberg MM, Mizrahi M. Human infestation by the pigeon mite: a case report. *Am J Infect Control* 1983;11:24–5

162. Gupta AK, Billings JK, Ellis CN. Chronic pruritus: an uncommon cause. Avian mite dermatitis caused by *Ornithonyssus sylviarum* (Northern fowl mite). *Arch Dermatol* 1988;124:1102–3, 1105–6

163. Fishman HC. Rat mite dermatitis. *Cutis* 1988;42:414–6

164. Jones JE. Fleas. *Am Fam Phys* 1984;29:143–7

165. Keep JM. Hazards of domestic pets. Ringworm and other skin conditions. *Austral Fam Phys* 1977;6:1527–36

166. Chua EC, Goh KT. A flea-borne outbreak of dermatitis. *Ann Acad Med Singapore* 1987;16:648–50

167. Ayelesworth R, Baldridge D. Dermatophagoides scheremetewski and feather pillow dermatitis. *Minn Med* 1983;63:43

168. Borroni G, Brazzelli V, Rosso R, *et al.* Paederus fuscipes dermatitis. A histopathological study. *Am J Dermatopathol* 1991;13:467–74

169. Gelmetti C, Grimalt R. Paederus dermatitis: an easy diagnosable but misdiagnosed eruption. *Eur J Ped* 1993;152:6–8

170. Ahmed AR, Moy R, Barr AR, *et al.* Carpet beetle dermatitis. *J Am Acad Dermatol* 1981;5:428-32

171. Rosen T. Caterpillar dermatitis. *Dermatol Clin* 1990;8:245–52

172. Allen VT, Miller OF III, Tyler WB: Gypsy moth caterpillar dermatitis – revisited. *J Am Acad Dermatol* 1991;24:979–81

173. Jamieson F, Keystone JS, From L, *et al.* Moth-associated dermatitis in Canadian travellers returning from Mexico. *Can Med Assoc J* 1991;145:1119–21

174. Dinehart SM, Archer ME, Wolf JE Jr, *et al.* Caripito itch: dermatitis from contact with Hylesia moths. *J Am Acad Dermatol* 1985;13:743–7

175. Snow WF. Field estimates of the flight speed of some West African mosquitoes. *Ann Trop Med Parasitol* 1980;74:239–42

176. Fan PC, Chang HN. Hypersensitivity to mosquito bite: a case report. *Kaohsiung J Med Sci* 1995;11:420–4

177. Reunala T, Brummer-Korvenkontio H, Palosuo T. Are we really allergic to mosquito bites? *Ann Med* 1994;26:301–6

178. Coulie P, Wery M, Ghys L, *et al.* Pharmacologic modulation by cetirizine-2 HCl of cutaneous reactions and pruritus in man after experimental mosquito bites. *Skin Pharmacol* 1989;2:38–40

179. Reunala T, Brummer-Korvenkontio H, Karppinen A, *et al.* Treatment of mosquito bites with cetirizine. *Clin Exp Allergy* 1993;23:72–5

180. Mumcuoglu Y, Rufli T. Siphonaptera/fleas: *Schweizerische Rundschau Med Prax* 1979;68:1172–82

181. Anonymous. From the Centers for Disease Control. Cercarial dermatitis outbreak at a state park – Delaware, 1991. *J Am Med Assoc* 1992;267:2581–6

182. Loken BR, Spencer CN, Granath WO Jr. Prevalence and transmission of cercariae causing schistosome dermatitis in Flathead Lake, Montana. *J Parasitol* 1995;81:646–9

183. Kullavanijaya P, Wongwaisayawan H. Outbreak of cercarial dermatitis in Thailand *Int J Dermatol* 1993;32:113–5

184. Kolarova L, Horak P, Fajfrlik K. Cercariae of *Trichobilharzia szidati* Neuhaus, 1952 (*Trematoda: Schistosomatidae*): the causative agent of cercarial dermatitis in Bohemia and Moravia. *Folia Parasitologica* 1992;39:399–400

185. McWilliam LJ, Curry A, Rowland PL, *et al.* Spinous injury caused by a sea urchin. *J Clin Pathol* 1991;44:428

186. Mulvihill CA, Burnett JW. Swimmer's itch: a cercarial dermatitis. *Cutis* 1990;46:211–3

187. Sims JK, Brock JA, Fujioka R, *et al.* Vibrio in stinging seaweed: potential infection. *Hawaii Med J* 1993;52: 274–5

188. MacSween RM, Williams HC: Seabather's eruption – a case of Caribbean itch. *Br Med J* 1996;312:957–8

189. Freudenthal AR, Joseph PR. Seabather's eruption. *New Engl J Med* 1993;329:542–4

190. Wong DE, Meinking TL, Rosen LB, *et al.* Seabather's eruption Clinical, histologic, and immunologic features. *J Am Acad Dermatol* 1994;30:399–406

191. Kokelj F, Del Negro P, Montanari G. Jellyfish dermatitis due to *Carybdea marsupialis. Cont Derm* 1992;27:195

192. Soppe GG. Marine envenomations and aquatic dermatology. *Am Fam Phys* 1989;40:97–106

193. Calton GJ, Burnett JW, Vader W. Study of the nematocyst venoms of the sea anemone, *Bolocera tuediae Toxicon* 1978;16:443–51

194. Haneke E, Kolsch I. Sea urchin granulomas. *Hautarzt* 1980;31:159–60

195. Burke WA, Steinbaugh JR, O'Keefe EJ. Delayed hypersensitivity reaction following a sea urchin sting. *Int J Dermatol* 1986;25:649–50

# Common dermatitis diseases (eczemas) 6

Dermatitis means inflammation of the skin, and in a broad sense this encompasses a large number of itchy dermatoses. Itching dermatoses act via different mechanisms and, in general, itch by virtue of the effects of the inflammatory mediators and the inflammatory cells that they attract

For organizational convenience, the discussion in this chapter will be limited to atopic dermatitis (eczema), contact dermatitis, asteatotic dermatitis, stasis dermatitis, photo-dermatitides and 'neurodermatides'. Complete textbooks are to be found on all of the above topics in more depth; this chapter will present highlights only. Other dermatitides, e.g., seborrheic dermatitis, are discussed under other headings such as localized itching

## Atopic dermatitis (atopic eczema)

This is an idiopathic hereditary disorder in which there is an increased reactivity of the skin to irritants and allergens and an association with asthma and allergic rhinitis. Although the fundamental defects remain largely unknown, it can be exacerbated by psychological, climatic, and behavioral factors.

- Itching leads to an itch–scratch cycle; atopic dermatitis has been called the itch that rashes

Because there are no absolute criteria by which all atopic dermatitis patients are identified, and the disease activity varies, and because it is not a deadly disease, epidemiologic measurement has been hampered. The incidence is unknown, but the prevalence has been reported to be as low as 2% and as high as 20%, but a likely range may be 5–10%[1-3].

- In 30–50% of cases there is a personal or family history of atopic dermatitis, allergic rhinitis, or asthma[4]
- If one parent has atopic dermatitis, the risk in a child is 20%; if both parents are sufferers the risk rises to 50%

- Concordance in monozygotic twins is 73–86% compared with 21–23% in dizygotic twins[5]
- The age of onset is between 2 and 6 months in the majority of cases, and onset occurs in the first year of life in 60%

    Onset before the age of 2 months may occur, but patients at this age are unable to scratch effectively, and the typical signs are diminished

    Although not a common event, the disease may start at any age later in life

- Spontaneous remission may occur in childhood, but patients may continue to demonstrate lower itch thresholds throughout life

### Role of infection

Clinical infection is very common in atopic dermatitis, and in some such cases impaired neutrophil chemotaxis has been demonstrated. Patients with atopic dermatitis are predisposed towards developing superinfection with *Staphylococcus* (Kaposi's varicelliform eruption).

- They carry more staphylococci even without any clinical evidence of infection, and this correlates with disease severity[6–9]
- Atopic dermatitis patients often have IgE antistaphylococcal antibodies, but their contribution to pathogenesis is unknown
- Staphylococcal enterotoxin B applied on intact atopic skin induces dermatitis[10]

Herpes simplex infections may also complicate atopic dermatitis, with a widespread confluent herpetic outbreak, eczema herpeticum. The role of other commensal organisms such as *Pityrosporum ovale* is unknown.

## Immunologic aspects

A broad spectrum of immunologic abnormalities exists in atopic dermatitis[11,12]. It can even be considered an immunologic disease itself because the condition can be transferred by marrow cells that circulate in the blood before infiltrating the skin. Patients with atopic dermatitis often have increased serum total IgE and specific IgE antibody to ingested or inhaled antigens.

- About 80% of patients with atopic dermatitis have increased amounts of total IgE and these patients display positive prick-test reactions to vast numbers of allergens[13]

    20% of patients have normal IgE and no prick-test reactions

- IgE concentrations correlate with disease severity
- IgE-mediated allergy may exacerbate the dermatitis by recruiting leukocytes and enhancing cytokine production, rapidly escalating inflammation

    IgE and their associated mast cell reactions may be epiphenomena

Specific T-cell overproduction and activity play a vital role in the generation of inflammation in atopic dermatitis.

- Affected patients overproduce activated T-cells that migrate to the skin by virtue of their cutaneous lymphocyte-associated antigen ligand
- Defects in cytokine regulation are also seen

    There is excessive interleukin-4 and -5 formation by lymphocytes, which could induce the increased immunoglobulin synthesis observed

    Another lymphokine of critical pathologic importance is interferon-γ, which antagonizes actions of interleukin-4, and is secreted in small quantities by T-cells

    Therapeutically, pharmacologic doses of interferon-γ help signs and symptoms of atopic dermatitis

- There are decreased numbers and activity levels of suppressor T-cells[14]
- Langerhans cells are increased in number but are less able to stimulate lymphocytes
- Mononuclear cells are less responsive to prostaglandins E-2 and D-2, but appear to produce more prostaglandin E-2 than normal

    Atopic monocytes also secrete granulocyte-macrophage colony stimulating factor, a cytokine that causes spongiotic inflammation

- Another hypothesis holds that faulty cyclic nucleotide metabolism of inflammatory cells leads to inflammatory hyper-reactivity and resultant immune responses[15]

    Increased phosphodiesterase activity in atopic monocytes may play an important role in regulating atopic dermatitis inflammatory activities[16]

    Pharmacologic inhibition of phosphodiesterase appears to reverse atopic dermatitis inflammatory activities

## Other pathologic features

- Although widely recommended and accepted as dogma, bovine milk avoidance has not been rigorously proven to decrease atopic dermatitis

- Maternal allergen avoidance during pregnancy and lactation is unlikely to provide a major prophylactic role
- House dust mite allergen reactivity varied from 6–85% depending upon the testing method employed[17,18]

> The former figure refers to extract of a single recombinant allergen whereas the latter figure refers to reactivity to a crude extract
>
> In patients with severe disease, prophylactic measures to decrease house dust mite numbers can reduce clinical disease severity[19]

### Xerosis and skin barrier defects

Xerosis or dry skin is a manifestation of chronic atopic dermatitis, where the skin is more easily irritated than well hydrated skin. Decreased amounts of ceramides and other lipids seems associated with increased transepidermal water loss.

- Lipids are an essential feature of the epidermal barrier controlling water loss

Application of hot water and soaps or detergents to the skin decreases the remaining amount of lipid, further exacerbating the condition. Atopic xerosis shows various stratum corneum functional impairments, probably reflecting increased epidermal proliferation due to a low-level ongoing dermatitis[20].

### Clinical features

In childhood atopic dermatitis the affected sites include the antecubital and popliteal fossae, neck, wrists and ankles, trunk, face, periauricular area and scalp[21] (Figure 6.1).

- The trunk is the most common site in both infants and children
- In severe childhood disease, nails may have trachyonychia, with a rough texture of pitting and ridging

In adulthood, the distribution is similar, but particularly common areas include the antecubital and popliteal fossae (Figure 28), nipples (Figure 29) and hands.

In early disease, erythema and fine scaling are present. With additional scratching or rubbing, papules and lichenified plaques appear, often with visible excoriation.

- In those of African ancestry, a follicular papular lichenification pattern is particularly common
- Despite overt clinical signs of linear excoriation and visible scratching behavior, patients or their parents frequently deny scratching
- Vesiculation may occur independently, or may accompany superinfection with staphylococci or herpes simplex (Figure 30)
- Antimicrobial therapy should be initiated whenever infection is suspected

### Diagnostic criteria

Criteria by Hanifin and others exist, but are of little utility outside clinical studies[22–26].

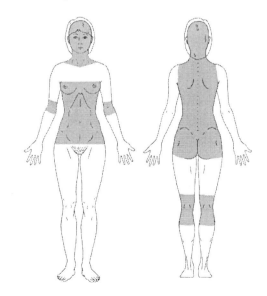

**Figure 6.1** Areas typically affected by atopic dermatitis

- Specialists do not agree on the individual diagnostic signs of atopic dermatitis, but physicians interested in atopic dermatitis agree reasonably well on what constitutes a typical case of atopic dermatitis

## Ophthalmologic abnormalities

- Conjunctival inflammation is a common problem and may represent allergy to pollen or other airborne allergens
- Keratoconus is rarely associated with atopic dermatitis
- Cataracts have been noted to occur, but most of the early reports may have been related to long-term systemic corticosteroid therapy rather than to the disease itself[27,28]

  Cataracts may be posterior capsular or anterior subcapsular zone

In patients with atopic dermatitis, predisposition towards developing other related dermatitides exists, including[29]:

- Allergic contact dermatitis
- Anal itching
- Hand dermatitis
- Juvenile plantar dermatosis
- Lip-lick dermatitis
- Nipple dermatitis
- Nummular dermatitis (primarily of the extremities)
- Pityriasis alba
- Prurigo nodularis
- Vulvar itching

Other manifestations of atopy that occur in one-third to one-half of patients with atopic dermatitis include allergic rhinitis (hay fever) and asthma (reactive airway disease).

## Atopic or atopic-resembling disease as part of other diseases

An eruption resembling atopic dermatitis with or without other atopic disorders and some-times with raised IgE levels may be found in several syndromes. When the disease presents with unusual features, is accompanied by unusual systemic features, or if features of a genetic or immunologic disorder co-exist, clinicians should consider the following conditions in the differential diagnosis[29] (Figure 31):

- Acrodermatitis enteropathica
- Agammaglobulinemia
- Anhidrotic ectodermal defect
- Ataxia telangiectasia
- Cystic fibrosis heterozygote
- Dubowitz syndrome[30]
- Experimental histidine depletion
- Glucagonoma syndrome
- Gluten-sensitive enteropathy
- Hearing loss (genetic)
- Histidinemia
- Hyper-IgE syndrome
- Hurler's syndrome
- Letterer-Siwe syndrome
- Nephrotic syndrome
- Netherton's syndrome
- Phenylketonuria
- Selective IgA deficiency
- Wiskott-Aldrich syndrome

## Prognosis

Spontaneous remission during childhood is well known, but active disease may persist through the first several decades of life. Patients with atopic dermatitis may be more likely to get other dermatitides later in life, and it is probably wise for them to avoid a career with excessive exposure to irritants (for example, beauticians, dishwashers, mechanics).

## Treatment

### Emollients and behavioral changes

Stopping the frequent use of harsh soaps and detergents on the skin is an important part of the therapeutic intervention.

- Mild, non-drying soaps and soap substitutes should be used to reduce the removal of epidermal lipids

The regular use of emollients alone decreases the severity of atopic dermatitis, and when combined with other therapies it is particularly efficacious.

- Emollients may also have a corticosteroid-sparing effect
- Immediately after bathing is an important time to apply emollients to seal water in the hydrated epidermis
- Emollients can also be combined with anti-inflammatory agents such as topical corticosteroids to increase compliance
- Emollients are particularly important to prevent relapse

## Diet

Some studies show that a minority of patients with atopic dermatitis may flare when exposed to individual foods[31-33]. However, studies of long-term food avoidance show no benefit on disease severity of atopic dermatitis[34].

## Miscellaneous measures

- Increasing ambient humidity in dry environments may help xerosis and work to prevent recurrences
- Heat often exacerbates the disease, so keeping the environment cool in winter and summer should be encouraged
- A scrupulously clean environment relatively free of housedust mites may help minimize exacerbations
- Coarse wool clothing may exacerbate the disease and should be avoided, but fine wool may be tolerated[35]
- Education about the appropriate application of emollients and topical therapeutic agents is required; patients frequently apply subtherapeutic quantities

- Treat itching early: application of antipruritic agents prior to erythema and lichenification results in exceptionally rapid response

## Systemic therapy

### Antibiotics

Systemic antibiotics are necessary when infection is present, but may be beneficial for severe exacerbations without obvious infection.

- Antibiotic choice should be aimed at reducing staphylococcal colonization; consider erythromycin, azithromycin, dicloxacillin and cephalexin
- Topical antibiotics may act as a therapeutic adjunct (see discussion below)

### Antihistamines

There is mixed evidence that $H_1$ antihistamines help except by virtue of their sedative action[36-40].

- Bedtime doses of chlorpheniramine, diphenhydramine, hydroxyzine, and trimeprazine may be particularly helpful to diminish the itch–scratch cycle at night
- Of the less sedating antihistamines, cetirizine and loratidine may be more beneficial than astemazole and terfenidine[39,41]

  In addition to antihistaminic effects, cetirizine inhibits inflammatory mediator release and diminishes eosinophil and neutrophil migration[24]

  Loratidine is also likely to have some anti-inflammatory action

### Corticosteroids

Short-term use of prednisone for 7–14 days (0.5–1 mg/kg/day), or the systemic equivalent, may help calm a severe exacerbation.

- Although effective, long-term use cannot usually be justified because of the inevitable and profound side-effects, including osteopenia, cataracts, diabetes, cutaneous atrophy, etc[27].

- When these agents are used, a plan to discontinue therapy as soon as possible should be made explicit

### Other immunologic agents

Cyclosporin has demonstrated efficacy in severe and treatment-refractory atopic dermatitis.

- Short-term use (5 mg/kg/day) for 4–8 weeks results in rapid improvement in itching and other aspects of clinical disease severity[42]
- Long-term use (>3 months) may be indicated in the exceptional patient unable to be controlled with multiple other modalities
- Although its side-effects may be preferable to long-term corticosteroid agents, cyclosporin may cause profound immunosuppression, nephrotoxicity, hypertension and other severe side-effects

Interferon-γ may also have beneficial effects in severe and treatment-refractory atopic dermatitis.

- In adults, 500 000 units were used for 8 weeks and response was equivalent to conventional therapy
- In another study[43], about half the patients with severe disease improved with 6 weeks of treatment, and half of these showed continued improvement 3 months following treatment cessation
- In a placebo-controlled study of 83 patients, those receiving 50 μg/m² of interferon-γ daily for 12 weeks improved their erythema scores, excoriations and erosions and other signs of active dermatitis

    Although some mild toxicity was observed, it was safe and well-accepted by moderate to severe dermatitis patients

### Miscellaneous agents

- A meta-analysis of controlled trials of evening primrose oil in atopic dermatitis, showed that it clearly improved atopic dermatitis[44]

- Given the high placebo-response rate, it is likely that most activity in herbal remedies is through the placebo effect

    A mixture of ten traditional Chinese herbs, found beneficial in open studies, was tested for 2 months in a double-blind placebo-controlled study on adults[45]. Despite poor palatability, itching and disease severity clearly improved and no side-effects were reported

## Topical therapy

### Corticosteroid agents

Short-term (2–8 weeks) administration of these agents is particularly useful in helping to stop the itch–scratch cycle. The stronger the relative potency, the more likely that the agent will be effective[46].

- With the possible exception of some 'soft molecules' (see chapter 11: Treatment) that dissociate side-effects from efficacy, the stronger the potency the greater the risk of local and systemic untoward effects

Failure of hydrocortisone to clear atopic dermatitis is well known, and despite its safety topical hydrocortisone can suppress the hypothalamic–adrenal–pituitary axis.

- When possible, long-term remissions should be maintained with emollients, not corticosteroid agents
- Patients with chronic atopic dermatitis that continuously use these agents should be monitored for local side-effects
- A useful rule for the clinician is to use the least potent corticosteroid agent that works

### Antibiotics

Topical antimicrobials alone serve little role in the treatment of atopic dermatitis, but combined with corticosteroid agents they can be particularly effective.

- Topical mupirocin and hydrocortisone daily is as effective as hydrocortisone twice daily

- The combination of topical hydrocortisone and fusidic acid is more effective in decreasing itching and disease severity than hydrocortisone or fusidic acid alone

*Immune modulating agents*

Topical tacrolimus in open and controlled trials rapidly improves atopic dermatitis symptoms and severity (see chapter 11: Treatment).

*Miscellaneous topical agents*

Topical doxepin is effective in reducing pruritus in patients with atopic dermatitis[39,47].

## Phototherapy

Ultraviolet (UV) A, UVB, combination UVA and UVB, and psoralen photochemotherapy (PUVA) have been used with beneficial results[48]. Suberthyemogenic doses may initially exacerbate disease, but patients become accustomed to UV.

- As a general clinical guide, the appendix contains the Wake Forest University School of Medicine phototherapy protocols for atopic dermatitis

## Psychological treatment

There are psychosomatic influences in atopic dermatitis.

- In one controlled study using standardized mood and personality scales, atopic patients described themselves as being more anxious, more aroused, more depressed and less energetic, and they showed higher neuroticism scores than control patients

    In this study, not all patients were equally affected, and only one of the subgroups was psychologically disabled

    The psychologically disabled patients showed an earlier age of onset of dermatitis, more somatic complaints and a higher level of familial stress, but less intense itching and scratching

Behavioral therapy and other psychological treatments of the patient or family can lead to long-term improvement in skin disease severity, and these should be considered adjuncts to dermatological treatment[49,50].

- If the patient displays unusual psychiatric symptoms, the clinician should consider referral to a mental health professional for further evaluation

# Irritant and allergic contact dermatitis

Contact dermatitis is a common inflammatory skin disorder resulting from cutaneous exposure to irritating agents and allergens[51,52].

- Irritant contact dermatitis is more common than allergic contact dermatitis

    Irritants comprise a broad number of chemicals and particulate substances ranging from organic solvents and water to fiberglass

    Allergens are diverse and, to some degree, idiosyncratic

- The most important therapeutic strategies revolve around limiting exposure to irritants and allergens

## Clinical features

For both irritant and allergic contact mechanisms, erythema, vesicles, and later scaling are present acutely, changing to erythematous lichenified plaques in the case of chronic contact dermatitis (Figure 32).

- Usually, irritant contact dermatitis has no vesicles, whereas vesicles are a common finding in allergic contact dermatitis

The distribution strongly suggests exogenous origin, with frequent involvement of unclothed areas, especially the forearms and hands.

- Sharp angles, streaks and other unusual findings strongly suggest exogenous influences, and are typical of allergic contact dermatitis (Figure 33)

## Predisposed populations

The medical literature boasts of a number of groups that may be at particularly high risk of contact dermatitis. Those who work with foods, chemicals, hair, or frequently use soaps or detergents are at highest risk[53–55].

Note that many cases of occupational dermatitis are hand dermatitis, and the following list is illustrative, not comprehensive. Occupations in which contact dermatitis may occur include:

- Accordion repairers[56]
- Aquarium industry workers[57]
- Aromatherapists[58,59]
- Canning factory workers[60]
- Car mechanics[61]
- Cashiers[62,63]
- Cement workers
- Dental workers
- Electronics industry employees[64]
- Enamellers and decorators in the ceramics industry[65]
- Farm workers including those raising okra, mushrooms, tulips, lilies, potatoes[66,67]
- Fish processing workers[68]
- Food service workers including bakers, caterers, cooks, waiters[69–71]
- Furniture workers[72]
- Grain elevator workers[73]
- Hairdressers[74,75]
- Healthcare workers including nurses, physicians and pharmacists[76–79]
- Horticulturists and flower shop employees[80,81]
- Housewives[82]
- Insulation workers[83]
- Loggers
- Masseurs[83]
- Metalworkers[84,85]
- Milk testers[86]
- Mushroom growers[87]
- Musicians[89,90]
- Newspaper pressroom workers[91]
- Painters, polishers and varnishers[92]
- Photographic technicians[93]
- Plastic industry workers[94]
- Pottery industry workers[95]
- Rubber workers
- Secretaries[96]
- Slaughterhouse workers[97]
- Soldiers[98]
- Textile workers[99]
- Tree surgeons[100]
- Veterinary surgeons[101]
- Warehouse employees[102]

## Irritant contact dermatitis

Although often not recognized by patients, irritant contact dermatitis is more common than allergic contact dermatitis. It usually occurs slowly with chronic exposure to irritants including detergents, soaps, water, and chemical solvents.

- Irritant contact dermatitis is a multifactorial disease, the onset and modulation of which depend on both endogenous and exogenous factors

  Endogenous factors that may be important: age, race, site, gender and history of atopic dermatitis[103]

- Susceptibility to skin irritation is greater in winter than summer[104]
- Particulate matter is also highly irritating
- Examples include hair, wood and sawdust, and powdered metals
- Fiberglass dermatitis itching is discussed separately below

The mechanism of irritant dermatitis produced by repeated or combined exposure to clinical or subclinical doses of irritants is still poorly understood, but is probably related to disruption of the epidermal barrier function and subsequent inadvertent admission of proinflammatory factors and activation of the dermal inflammatory systems[105].

- Irritants increase the response to an allergen in allergic contact dermatitis[106]

  Experimental adverse response to both allergen and irritant applied at the same time was greater than to either alone

## Clinical appearance

The characteristic appearance is poorly marginated erythema, scaling, and skin fissuring, most commonly on the hands, particularly the fingertips, and distal extremities (Figures 34, 35).

- Areas underneath jewelry or subject to anything occlusive are subject to chronic maceration and irritation
- Transdermal medication patches are particularly subject to irritant dermatitis, but allergic contact dermatitis may occur at the site of the adhesive or drug
- Feelings of skin dryness, itching, and stinging – symptoms of contact dermatitis – may occur in the absence of visible signs of irritation
- Irritant dermatitis from overbathing has also been noted to cause generalized itching[107]

## Treatment

- Avoidance of irritants is key
- Topical corticosteroids are frequently used in the treatment of irritant contact dermatitis and improve healing[108]
- Topical emollients help restore the epidermal barrier, and prevent against further irritation[109]

  Some emollient lotions themselves sting and burn eczematous skin, and choice of emollients may rely upon personal preference

  Some patients prefer greasy ointments such as petrolatum which are fabulous but inelegant products, whereas others prefer vanishing lotions that are elegant but provide little emollient

## Allergic contact dermatitis

Allergic contact dermatitis varies depending upon location, occupations, and avocations. Sensitization to the offending chemical or hapten occurs and then re-exposure induces the characteristic eruption. Not all patients are equally susceptible to sensitization. Susceptibility to allergic contact dermatitis may in part be controlled by genetics[110]. Allergic contact dermatitis may appear on any body surface exposed to allergens (Figure 6.2).

- Contact allergens are small compounds that can penetrate the cornified layers of the skin to reach the dermis[111]
- Small molecules react with endogenous proteins to form complete antigens that the lymphocytes may identify[112]
- T-lymphocytes are activated upon appropriate antigen presentation, and release a broad range of inflammatory mediators including interleukin-1, interleukin-2, γ-interferon, and other modulators

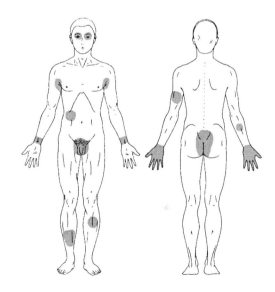

**Figure 6.2** Areas typically affected by allergic contact dermatitis

- T-suppressor cells decrease the capacity to react, and may occur after repeated exposure

Rhus plant dermatitis (poison ivy, oak, and sumac) commonly shows linear vesiculation on exposed skin (Figure 36).

- A common belief without merit is that scratching Rhus dermatitis spreads the eruption
- Within minutes to one hour of exposure, the antigen has soaked into the skin and this occurs hours to days prior to the eruption

Patch testing is a crucial part of management of allergic contact dermatitis. Testing may help identify/confirm the elusive antigen in question.

- To be useful, patch testing requires interpretation, understanding of the limitations of the study, and proper technique
- The innovation of the TRUE Test clearly makes patch testing more standardized and accessible, but may not identify all relevant allergens[113]
- Storrs[114] stated that "furious resolve during investigation coupled with a willingness to be proven wrong and to find the unexpected is most likely to result in a successful outcome for patients with contact dermatitis"
- Contact curiosities: a number of unusual contact dermatitis episodes have been reported, including contact dermatitis due to the following:

  Acupuncture needles[115]
  Condoms (and any other latex object)[76,116]
  Consort contact dermatitis
  Oak moss in a woman's husband's after-shave lotion[117]
  Combined allergy to a partner's seminal fluid and to latex condoms[118]
  Gold[119]
  Incense burning[120]
  Sanitary napkins[121]

Transdermal drug delivery patches[122]
Silver polish contact and photocontact allergy[123]
Stamp pad ink[124]
Tefillin: i.e. ritual Jewish ceremonial wrappings[125]
Tobacco[126]

## Treatment

History and any appropriate testing should be used to determine the irritant or allergen, and avoidance advised. For severe allergic contact dermatitis, brief courses of systemic corticosteroids at 0.5–2 mg/kg/day for 2–3 weeks may be required. Sedating antihistamines at bedtime may help the severely affected patient.

- Caution should be exercised in treating contact dermatitis, since essentially all of the known topical antipruritic agents can themselves cause itching due to allergic contact dermatitis
- Reported cases of sensitization have occurred with the following:

  Benzocaine
  Capsaicin[127,128]
  Corticosteroids (essentially all of the commercially available products)[129–132]
  Crotamiton[133]
  Diphenhydramine
  Doxepin[134,135]
  Eutectic mixture of local anesthetics (EMLA)
  Emollients
  Lidocaine[136,137]
  Menthol[138]
  8-methoxypsoralen (used in PUVA)[139]
  Oatmeal (e.g., used in baths)[140]
  Pramoxine[141]
  Prilocaine[136,142]
  Tar[143]

## Specific contact dermatitis topics

Fiberglass, hand and diaper dermatitis represent three forms of contact dermatitis which require special discussion.

## Fiberglass dermatitis

Fiberglass is widely used for insulation, in roofing materials, in fabrication industries, and as a reinforcement filling material in the electronics industry[144–146]. Fiberglass physical exposure may provoke severe itching in the presence or absence of visible skin changes[147,148].

- Patients are often, but not always, aware of fiberglass exposure
- Handling fiberglass products may induce an irritant contact dermatitis
- Clinically it may resemble scabies, hand dermatitis, folliculitis, petechiae and urticaria; it has also caused generalized pruritus with flexural micropapules[149] (Figure 37)
- Skin stripping and microscopic examination may confirm the presence of glass spicules
- Fiberglass dermatitis may be so severe and difficult to diagnose that, in an extreme case, incarceration for indecent excoriation has occurred[150]

    A 36-year-old man experienced acute, severe, generalized itching which resulted in his scratching being misinterpreted as lewd and indecent behavior

    He was arrested, but released following a history and physical examination which was consistent with fiberglass dermatitis

## Hand and/or foot dermatitis

Hand dermatitis may be relatively asymptomatic, or the itch can be extraordinary.

- In one epidemiologic study[151], the prevalence of hand dermatitis in the general population was 5.2% in men and 10.6% in women

    The prevalence of hand dermatitis among the occupational groups ranged from 2.9% in office workers to approximately 30% in nurses

Hand dermatitis may lead to other forms of dermatitis; susceptibility to irritants at distant sites to hand dermatitis is increased in patients with acute hand dermatitis[152]. A history of childhood atopic dermatitis predisposes towards hand dermatitis, as does being female.

- In a large epidemiologic survey[153], 27% of the individuals who reported childhood atopic dermatitis reported hand dermatitis during the 12 months before the study

Social consequences of hand dermatitis may be trivial or enormous.

- In one study[154], the majority of people with hand dermatitis had consulted physicians and about 20% may take sick leave for their hand dermatitis

    The mean time on sick leave for hand dermatitis was 19 weeks

    Almost 10% changed their occupation because of hand dermatitis, most frequently hairdressers

- In another long-term outcome study[155], one-third of irritant hand dermatitis patients went into remission whereas two-thirds had ongoing disease

    Change of occupation had no significant effect on disease activity

    Hand dermatitis in patients with atopic dermatitis had the most unfavorable long-term prognosis[156]

### *General treatment guidelines*

- Disease with scaling and redness responds to emollients with urea or ammonium lactate with some contributory help from corticosteroids
- For vesicular disease, the use of topical corticosteroids, systemic corticosteroids, systemic antibiotics, tars, and other miscellaneous agents is helpful

    Ultrapotent topical corticosteroids under occlusion may help treatment-refractory disease

- When obvious superinfection is present, use of Burow's solution or potassium permanganate soaks and systemic antibiotics may be helpful
- Whenever occupational limitations allow, decrease exposure to irritants and allergens
- Oral and topical photochemotherapy (PUVA) may help any form of hand dermatitis[157]
- Biofeedback training has been reported as effective for dyshidrosis in a case series[158]
- If the disease does not respond to initial therapy, consider searching for allergens by history and patch testing[159]

*Irritant hand dermatitis*

The clinical appearance includes scaling, mildly erythematous, fissured skin of the finger tips, palms, underneath rings, and dorsal hands (rarely on feet). It is seen most commonly in those who spend a great portion of their time with their hands in irritating chemicals or water.

- Patients with obsessive–compulsive disorder or other neuropsychiatric diseases with compulsive hand washing present tremendous challenges in healing the dermatitic skin[160]

Treatment involves the following:

- Irritant avoidance helps but is often difficult
- If the disease does not respond to initial therapy, consider searching for allergens by history and patch testing[159]
- Restore the normal barrier function with emollients

    These emollients need to be readily accessible, and applied repeatedly during the day

- Topical corticosteroids also help accelerate the healing process, and may be appropriate for one to several months during the healing phase

Low potency corticosteroids have little effect, mid-to high potency agents are more effective

*Dyshidrotic dermatitis (Pompholyx)*

Appears clinically as minute, often non-inflammatory, symmetric, itchy or burning vesicles which begin on the lateral aspects of the fingers and on the palms or soles[161,162] (Figures 38, 39). Hyperhidrosis may exacerbate the disease and may be observed clinically[163,164].

Although neuropsychiatric disease may complicate dyshidrosis (as it may complicate all other itchy dermatoses), there is little evidence to suggest that it is a manifestation of any neurosis, and clinical evidence of such disease is essentially non-existent[160,165].

- Dyshidrotic dermatitis mimics:

    Allergic contact dermatitis due to nickel, Rhus, preservatives, floral shop allergens, etc.[166,167]

    Autoimmune progesterone dermatitis[168]

    Dyshidrotic cutaneous T-cell lymphoma[169,170]

    Dyshidrotic pemphigoid[171,172]

    Linear IgA disease[173]

    Pemphigus vulgaris[174,175]

    Tinea

Treatment involves many of the same approaches employed in irritant hand dermatitis including emollients, potent topical corticosteroids, and avoidance of offending agents[176–179]. Additionally, the use of systemic corticosteroids for brief periods is often required for success.

*Psoriasis*

Psoriasis is not a form of dermatitis, but is considered here as an itchy dermatosis of the palms, which can frequently be mistaken for dermatitides. The appearance is of strikingly erythematous well-circumscribed areas with scaling on the palms and/or soles. The typical changes of psoriasis such as nail pitting and disease elsewhere provide important clues to diagnosis, but may be absent.

Treatment involves the following:

- Use of emollients may help minimize the need for topical corticosteroids
- Potent or ultrapotent topical corticosteroids (occasionally under occlusion[180]) are extremely helpful, but tachyphylaxis occurs
- Alternative antipsoriatic agents including coal tar, calcipotriene, and tazarotene are extremely helpful in long-term management

### Diaper (napkin) dermatitis

Dampness, maceration, fecal enzymes, chemicals, and other irritants in the diaper area lead to diaper dermatitis (Figure 40). Superinfection is occasional, and microbiologic overgrowth may be precipitated by juvenile diabetes, antibiotic therapy, hot weather, and inadequate diaper changing intervals[181].

- In a large sample of Italian infants, the frequency of episodes of diaper dermatitis was 15.2%[182]

  History of atopic dermatitis raised the risk of diaper dermatitis

*Treatment*

Most cases can be cleared with frequent diaper changes, use of super-absorbent disposable diapers (containing gel material in their core), and low-potency topical corticosteroid agents[183,184].

- Contrary to popular belief, disposable diapers may be more gentle and absorbent than cloth diapers, and reduce the incidence and severity of diaper dermatitis[185]
- Occlusive pastes and ointments such as zinc oxide paste may promote healing and are particularly helpful prophylactically

If the eruption lasts for more than 3 days or classic erythematous satellite lesions are present, addition of an antifungal agent such as nystatin powder or a topical azole should help resolve the condition. In secondarily infected diaper dermatitis, bacteria are present in the majority and *Candida* species are present in about half of cases[186].

- Some patients may require topical antibiotics such as mupirocin or fusidic acid, whereas severe disease may need systemic antibiotic agents
- Recalcitrant or clinically atypical eruptions may signify rarer disorders such as psoriasis, Langerhans' cell histiocytosis, or acrodermatitis enteropathica

## Seborrheic dermatitis (dandruff)

Seborrheic dermatitis is not limited to the scalp, but may be found on the forehead, eyebrows, lateral nose, chin, ears, central chest, and intertriginous areas.

- Particularly severe disease is common among patients with HIV-1 disease and Parkinson's disease
- Treatment for all sites is similar, and is discussed in chapter 8: Localized itching

## Asteatotic dermatitis (xerotic dermatitis, eczema Craquelé)

### Predisposing factors

#### Advanced age

The aged epidermis becomes thinner, the corneocytes become less adherent to one another, and there is flattening of the dermoepidermal interface; the dermis becomes atrophic and it is relatively acellular and avascular[187].

- Aged epidermis displays altered drug permeability, increased susceptibility to irritant contact dermatitis, and often severe xerosis[188]
- Barrier integrity and barrier repair are markedly impaired in older individuals compared with younger individuals[189]

This may be attributable to the alteration in lipid composition in the skin of older adults

- One may speculate that older sufferers of atopic dermatitis are more likely to develop this condition

    Note that in young people, atopic xerosis seems to be different and more severe than the xerosis of aging

### Drugs and medical conditions

- Two patients had generalized xerosis and asteatotic dermatitis that developed while they were receiving cimetidine therapy and resolved when cimetidine therapy was discontinued[190]
- Retinoids including vitamin A, isotretinoin, acitretin and etretinate predispose patients towards this phenomenon
- HIV-1 infection seems to predispose patients toward developing asteatotic dermatitis[191–193]

### Behavioral factors

- Excessive bathing and removing the protective lipid layer from the skin with hot water and harsh soaps and detergents is a major factor

    Bathing techniques tolerated by the skin at 22 years of age may not be tolerated at 92 years

- Although seemingly contradictory, inadequate bathing may also predispose patients to develop this condition
- Patients may inadvertently exacerbate their condition by applying irritants, such as alcohol, or allergens, such as neomycin, to their skin

### Clinical appearance

Scaling, roughness, subtle to extreme erythema, and often reticulated cracking on the distal arms and legs is most common (Figure 6.3). With repeated rubbing and use of irritants or

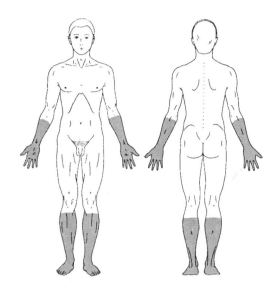

**Figure 6.3** Areas typically affected by asteatotic dermatitis

allergens the process may spread and erythroderma may occur. Nummular dermatitis, with coin-shaped dermatitic patches, is often seen accompanying asteatotic dermatitis[194,195].

### Treatment

Skin cleansing techniques are quite important in prevention and management of asteatotic dermatitis. However, there is no ideal bathing recommendation that encompasses each person at every age in every culture.

- The frequency of bathing and showering should be optimized for the patient
- Bathing water should be kept at the coolest tolerable temperature practical
- Apply an emollient directly on damp skin

    Emollients should be used frequently during the day

    Emollients containing ammonium lactate or urea may be particularly beneficial in this condition

    12% ammonium lactate creams may also help restore the epidermal barrier function

- Room temperatures should be kept low and comfortable and humidity should be kept as high as possible without causing damage
- Encourage minimal use of mild or super-fatted soaps or non-soap cleansers
- Medium potency topical corticosteroid agents are ideal for brief periods to limit the itching

## Stasis dermatitis (gravitational dermatitis, venous eczema)

### Basic pathophysiology

No one knows why stasis dermatitis occurs, but there are morphologic alterations of dermal blood and lymphatic microcirculation that reduce fluid exchange capacity in the blood and lymph vascular systems, leading to tissue necrosis and ulceration[196–198].

- Blood vessels have occluded lumena, and thickening and reduplication of the basement membrane
- Lymphatic vessels show collapsed lumena in the papillary dermis, numerous and complex interdigitations between contiguous endothelial cells and lack of open junctions
- Derangement of the anchoring filaments that normally pull the lymphatic lumen open
- The connective matrix is characterized by fibrosis with formation of dense bundles of collagen and elastic fibers

### Predisposing factors

Allergic contact dermatitis may commonly accompany stasis dermatitis.

- Positive reactions to one or more haptens is found in about 70%[200–207]

  Frequent allergens include bacitracin, balsam of Peru, bronopol, benzoyl peroxide, cetearyl alcohol, epoxy resin, glycols, Lanette E, N and O, lanolin, neomycin, 'para' group, and wool alcohols

  Positive patch reactions following stasis dermatitis may diminish over time, but with 'para' compounds and balsam of Peru a higher degree of persistence is noted

- The poor fluid exchange may restrict clearance of allergens, setting up a reservoir for potential contact allergens
- Furthermore, the density of epidermal Langerhans' cells is increased in areas of stasis
- Corticosteroid hypersensitivity occurs most frequently among patients with stasis dermatitis[207,208]

In a single case report[209], a severe, intensely itchy case of stasis dermatitis associated with low plasma zinc was successfully treated with oral zinc.

- Stasis dermatitis is often a sequela of deep venous thrombosis or varices of the lower limbs.
- It may also be more common in those who stand for extended periods

### Clinical appearance

On the lower extremities, subtle scaling, marked erythema, and hemosiderin brown color are seen, particularly around the ankles.

- Not infrequently, excoriations or other trauma give rise to slowly healing ulcerations
- Secondary infection may also occur, as may autoeczematization or a widespread 'id' reaction

### Treatment

If lower extremity edema is a major component:

- Graduated pressure support hose may be a short-term help in improving the condition, and a long-term adjunct in prophylaxis[210]
- Systemic diuretics may aid in decreasing skin tension, relieving discomfort and improving the condition

■ Leg elevation may be helpful, but strict bedrest should be avoided

Local skin-care measures include using emollients to help restore the skin barrier function.

■ Ointments with little allergenicity such as petrolatum may be ideal

Medium potency topical corticosteroids are extremely important to provide symptomatic relief and to minimize scratching behavior.

■ Ointment vehicles may help reduce the number of topical contactants

If there is secondary infection as a component, the use of Burow's solution (2%) and systemic antibiotics may be helpful.

■ Avoid use of topical antibiotics, especially neomycin

Explore in the patient's history any possibility of topical contact allergy, and eliminate unnecessary contactants.

■ If the condition is refractory to treatment, patch testing is indicated

Ulcers require special care such as the use of hydrocolloid dressings and paste bandages (Unna boot)[211].

## Photodermatitides

A number of distinct photodermatitides exist with different clinical presentations and prognoses. Cutaneous photosensitivity diseases may be idiopathic, produced by endogenous photosensitizers, or associated with exogenous photosensitizers. In general, areas affected include the malar eminences, nose, ears, sides and back of neck (sparing the anterior neck), central upper chest, and posterior forearms and hands.

■ With the exception of photocontact dermatitis, variable areas of exposed or lightly covered skin are usually symmetrically affected, while other areas, often normally uncovered, may be spared

Although this discussion is not comprehensive, separately below will be presented drug phototoxicity, photocontact dermatitis and polymorphic light eruption.

■ Other photodermatitides with itching may include lupus erythematosus, dermatomyositis, chronic actinic dermatitis, photodermatitis of HIV infection, and pellagra[212]
■ Solar urticaria is discussed in chapter 7: Urticarial diseases

### Drug phototoxicity

The action spectra for most phototoxins and photoallergens lie in the UVA range.

### Phototoxic drug eruptions

Common drugs causing phototoxic reactions include diuretics, cardiac agents, antidiabetic agents, psoralens, coal tar, antibiotics, and non-steroidal anti-inflammatory agents.

■ Since the action spectra of most photosensitizers is in the UVA range, sunscreens with effective blockade of UVB do little to prevent phototoxic drug eruptions

### Photoallergic drug eruptions

Common drugs causing photoallergic reactions include topical antimicrobial agents, fragrances, sunscreens, non-steroidal anti-inflammatory agents and psychiatric medications[213].

■ A good chemical UVA sunscreen and most appropriate protective agent for photodermatoses, 4-t-butyl-4'-methoxy-dibenzoylmethane (Parsol 1789), may itself cause photoallergy[214,215]

### Photocontact dermatitis

This is often caused by ingredients in sunscreens and perfumes or plants (phytophotodermatitis). It is similar in appearance to allergic contact dermatitis; discrete and confluent polymorphous patches and linear streaks in photodistributed areas[216,217].

- The condition is usually mild and self-limited but hyperpigmentation may persist
- Failure to recognize phytophotodermatitis in a child may lead to a mistaken diagnosis of child abuse
- Diagnosis is often confirmed by photo-patch testing, and subsequent avoidance of these agents leads to gradual resolution

### Polymorphic light eruption

This is an extraordinarily common dermatosis that affects 5–10% of the population in the spring and summer[218].

- Lesions vary greatly between and within patients, being usually itchy, often grouped, large or small, erythematous or skin-colored papules (Figure 6.3)

  Smooth or irregular, confluent plaques or vesicles and papulovesicles (Figure 41)

  Polymorphic light eruption sine eruption is intense pruritus on sun-exposed skin without visible change resembling polymorphic light eruption

- This condition may be challenging to distinguish from brachioradial pruritus, and it may be the same disorder[219,220]

### Treatment

Reassurance and potent topical corticosteroid agents are helpful, however, severe and recurrent disease may require other measures.

- Prophylactic PUVA and UVB therapy from April to September will decrease itch and rash[221,222]
- Note that phototherapy may trigger the disease, and use of systemic corticosteroid agents may be temporarily required

- Hydroxychloroquine[223] or azathioprine[224] may be effective in select patients

## Lichen simplex chronicus (neurodermatitis circumscripta)

Some clinicians refer to this condition as 'neurodermatitis'. However, this is not as specific as other terms and will not be used further.

Clinically it appears as thick, well-circumscribed plaques which may be hyperpigmented at any site, although favored areas include the neck, anogenital areas, and lower legs. Lesions may be singular or multiple (Figure 42)

### Basic pathophysiology

If rubbed or scratched repeatedly in one spot, for whatever inciting reason, the resultant thick, hyperpigmented, lichenified plaque perpetuates itself, and continues to itch.

- Since the inciting event or events may be diverse, patients with this entity represent a disparate collection of etiologies
- Patients with a history of atopic dermatitis may be at increased risk[225]

Lichen simplex chronicus may be found in perfectly normal, well-adjusted scratching enthusiasts, or it may be seen in those with a great deal of emotional tension[226]. To understand the importance of lichenification and the symptoms which make patients scratch or rub repeatedly, the reader must understand that it takes over 100 000 scratches to make significant lichenification.

- In a classic experiment by Goldblum and Piper[227], four subjects were scratched with a 'scratching machine' for one hour daily until there were visible signs of lichenification on the left side of the back

The weight used on the scratching arm was the maximum that the patient could tolerate without producing burning or excoriations

Lichenification occurred after a minimum of 140 000 scratches, but the mean was 280 000 scratches

- In one psychological study, lichen simplex patients were able to be conditioned to scratch more readily and this scratching behavior is extinguished more slowly than in non-affected individuals[226]
- Lichen simplex curiosities

  A patient was reported with dermatomal lichen simplex chronicus who had a cervicothoracic syrinx and a thoracic spinal cord tumor[228]

  Lithium therapy may have precipitated lichen simplex in one patient; withdrawal resolved the eruption, and rechallenge made it reappear[229]

  The author has seen an unreported case of delusions of parasitosis presenting as facial lichen simplex chronicus·

### Treatment

Treatment of this disorder is challenging, as no single approach works on all patients. Therefore education of patients as to the limitations of treatment can be helpful in their understanding of this meddlesome condition.

### Topical

Whatever therapeutic approach is chosen, patients must use it regularly rather than as needed. Occlusion is highly desirable to keep patients' fingers and fingernails off the plaques and to enhance percutaneous penetration of the agent, and can be readily accomplished with kitchen plastic film.

- Potent or super-potent topical corticosteroids such as halobetasol are often highly effective in improving the condition[230,231]
- Corticosteroid impregnated tape such as

flurandrenolone tape is also easy to use and effective[232]
- Doxepin cream four times daily has been reported as efficacious[233]

### Other approaches

- Intralesional corticosteroid injection has benefit for treatment-resistant plaques
- Sedating antihistaminic agents at bedtime work to help decrease scratching behavior
- In anecdotal experience, one of the most effective treatments is systemic thalidomide (see discussion below) but this is rarely required
- Surgical excision may not be effective, and recurrence of lichen simplex chronicus after surgical excision has been reported[234]

## Prurigo nodularis (Hyde)

As with lichen simplex chronicus, prurigo nodularis is often referred to as 'neurodermatitis'.

### Basic pathophysiology

Virtually anything that itches may create a self-perpetuating itch–scratch cycle. Since the inciting event or events may be diverse, patients with this entity represent a disparate collection of etiologies. Insect bites, including those from household pets[235], may be a common factor in inducing the lesions, but the perpetuation of such lesions is curious.

### Localized cutaneous nerve abnormalities

Hypertrophy of cutaneous papillary dermal nerves is a feature of prurigo nodularis and is suggestive of a chronic peripheral neuropathy[236,237].

- Neuropeptide abnormalities are seen with increased calcitonin gene-related peptide and substance P[238]

Although a number of nerve abnormalities have been identified and are suggestive of a neurocutaneous component in the pathogenesis of prurigo nodularis, it is unknown whether these occur as a consequence of chronic rubbing and picking or whether they are in some way causal[239]. It is noteworthy that all described neurologic abnormalities may not be seen in lesions, arguing against their pathogenic role[240,241].

### Other pathologic abnormalities

- Prurigo nodularis most frequently occurs in connection with a hair follicle[242]
- Merkel cells are present and increased in number in the interfollicular area[243]
- Mast cell numbers are increased and there is evidence of eosinophil degranulation[244]
- Of unknown and unconfirmed significance, about a third of samples in one study[245] were histopathologically positive for acid-fast bacilli and granulomatous changes were present in one sample

### Atopy

The atopic diathesis has been implicated as a contributing factor[246]. One group of investigators found evidence to separate prurigo nodularis into two forms: an atopic and a non-atopic form[247].

- The atopic form is accompanied by cutaneous hypersensitivity to various environmental allergens (a pattern similar to that displayed by atopic dermatitis) and has a younger age of onset
- The non-atopic form has an older age of onset, and does not show any such hypersensitive reactions to environmental allergens

### Contact sensitivity

In exceptional cases, allergic contact dermatitis may play a contributory role. Screening for contact sensitivity with patch testing may occasionally be helpful[248].

### Internal disease associations

Most commonly, patients with prurigo nodularis have disease confined to the skin. This form of itching, like other forms of itching, may be associated with systemic diseases including neuropsychiatric disease[249].

- Essentially any systemic disease that has associated itching may also cause prurigo nodularis, and some of the reported disease associations include the following

  Lymphoma
  Peripheral T-cell lymphoma (Lennert's lymphoma)[250]
  Hodgkin's disease[251,252]
  Gluten sensitive enteropathy[253]
  Human immunodeficiency virus[254,255]
  Uremia[256]
  Depression
  Liver disease
  Although not previously associated with itching disorders, $\alpha$-1 antitrypsin deficiency has been reported to be associated with prurigo nodularis[257]
  Malabsorption[258]

### Prurigo nodularis mimics

Prurigo nodularis-like lesions are also found in other disorders, emphasizing the need for careful evaluation in select patients with uncommon presentations or those in whom treatment is unsuccessful.

- Pemphigoid nodularis[259–261]
- Angiolymphoid hyperplasia with eosinophilia[262,263]
- Multiple cutaneous granular cell tumors[264]

### Clinical appearance

Multiple pea-sized, intensely itchy, well-defined nodules that develop on the skin, particularly on the anterior leg and thigh, but nodules may be located anywhere the fingers or tools may reach[265–267] (Figures 43, 44).

- Lesions are on a background of normal skin
- Signs of excoriation and frank bleeding are frequently seen

## Treatment

### Topical

Whatever therapeutic approach is chosen, patients should use it regularly rather than as needed. Occlusion is highly desirable to keep patients' fingers and fingernails off the nodules and to enhance percutaneous penetration of the agent[268,269].

- Occlusion can be accomplished with plastic self-adhesive bandages
- Potent or super-potent topical corticosteroids such as halobetasol are sometimes effective in improving the condition

  Corticosteroid impregnated tape such as flurandrenolone tape may be helpful

- Topical capsaicin may also have modest efficacy[270]

### Physical

- Cryosurgery

  Cryosurgery alone improves prurigo nodularis but may result in depigmentation[271]

  Cryosurgery combined with intralesional corticosteroids plus lidocaine was reported effective but also may result in depigmentation[272]

- Ultraviolet light[273]

  PUVA may be particularly effective, improving about 90% of patients, but most patients had relapse with need for further treatment[274]

### Systemic

- Retinoid therapy with etretinate may imp-rove select patients[275,276]
- Cyclosporin has also been reported as effective at 3–4.5 mg/kg per day[277]
- Thalidomide may be the most effective agent in prurigo nodularis, but careful monitoring for side-effects and teratogenic considerations are paramount[278,279]

  In one study, four patients were placed into remission with 2–6 months of treatment[280]

  Thalidomide treatment of prurigo nodularis is effective, but may require more than 6 months of therapy

  The most important side-effect, neuropathy, is long standing and possibly irreversible, so monitoring with electromyography and nerve conduction velocity is key[281,282]

- If obsessive–compulsive disorder or other neuropsychiatric diseases are identified, appropriate interventions are required

---

## References

1. Taylor B, Wadsworth J, Wadsworth M, *et al.* Changes in the reported prevalence of childhood eczema since the 1939–45 war. *Lancet* 1984;2:1255–7

2. Thestrup-Pederson K. The incidence and pathophysiology of atopic dermatitis. *J Eur Acad Dermatol Venereol* 1996;7 (Suppl 1):S3–S7

3. Walker RB, Warin RP. The incidence of eczema in early childhood. *Br J Dermatol* 1956;68:1182

4. Pasternak B. The prediction of asthma in infantile eczema: a statistical approach. *J Pediatr* 1965;66:164–5

5. Larsen FS, Holm NV, Henningsen K. Atopic dermatitis. A genetic-epidemiologic study in a population-based twin sample. *J Am Acad Dermatol* 1986;15:487–94

6. Dahl MV. *Staphylococcus aureus* and atopic dermatitis. *Arch Dermatol* 1983;119:840–6

7. Hanifin J, Homburger HA. Staphylococcal colonisation, infection and atopic dermatitis – association not etiology. *J Allergy Clin Immunol* 1986;78:563–6

8. Leyden JJ, Marples RR, Kligman AM. *Staphylococcus aureus* in the lesions of atopic dermatitis. *Br J Dermatol* 1974;90:525–30

9. Noble WC: The role of staphylococci in dermatology. *J Eur Acad Dermatol Venereol* 1996;7 (Suppl 1): S12–S14

10. Strange P, Skov L, Lisby S, *et al*. Staphylococcal enterotoxin B applied on intact normal and intact atopic skin induces dermatitis. *Arch Dermatol* 1996; 132:27–33

11. Hanifin JM. Immunologic aspects of atopic dermatitis. *Dermatol Clin* 1990;8:747–50

12. Leung DYM, Geha RS. Immunoregulatory abnormalities in atopic dermatitis. *Clin Rev Allergy* 1986; 4:67–86

13. Ohman S, Johansson SGO. Allergen-specific IgE in atopic dermatitis. *Acta Derm Venereol* 1974;54: 283–90

14. Braathen LR. T-cell subsets in patients with mild and severe atopic dermatitis. *Acta Derm Venereol* 1985; 114 (Suppl):133–6

15. Hanifin JM. Assembling the puzzle pieces in atopic inflammation. *Arch Dermatol* 1996;132:1230–2

16. Hanifin JM, Chan SC. Monocyte phosphodiesterase abnormalities and dysregulation of lymphocyte function in atopic dermatitis. *J Invest Dermatol* 1995;105 (suppl):84S–88S

17. Gondo A, Saeki N, Tokuda Y. Challenge reactions in atopic dermatitis after percutaneous entry of mite antigen. *Br J Dermatol* 1986;115:485–93

18. Norris PG, Schofield O, Camp RD. A study of the role of house dust mite in atopic dermatitis. *Br J Dermatol* 1988;118:435–40

19. Tan BB, Weald D, Strickland I, *et al*. Double-blind controlled trial of effect of housedust-mite allergen avoidance on atopic dermatitis. *Lancet* 1996;347: 15–18

20. Watanabe M, Tagami H, Horii I, *et al*. Functional analyses of the superficial stratum corneum in atopic xerosis. *Arch Dermatol* 1991;127:1689–92

21. Aoki T, Fukuzumi T, Adachi J, *et al*. Re-evaluation of skin lesion distribution in atopic dermatitis. Analysis of cases 0 to 9 years of age. *Acta Derm Venereol* 1992;176(Suppl):19–23

22. Williams HC, Burney PG, Pembroke AC, *et al*. The UK Working Party's diagnostic criteria for atopic dermatitis. III Independent validation. *Br J Dermatol* 1994;131:406–16

23. Kang KF, Tian RM. Criteria for atopic dermatitis in a Chinese population. *Acta Derm Venereol* 1989;144: 26–7

24. La Rosa M, Ranno C, Musarra I, *et al*. Double-blind study of cetinizine in atopic eczema in children. *Ann Allergy* 1994;73:117–22

25. Rajka G. *Essential Aspects of Atopic Dermatitis*. Berlin: SpringerVerlag, 1989

26. Williams HC, Burney PG, Strachan D, *et al*. The UK Working Party's Diagnostic Criteria for Atopic Dermatitis. II. Observer variation of clinical diagnosis and signs of atopic dermatitis. *Br J Dermatol* 1994;131:397–405

27. Brunsting LA, Reed WB, Bair HL. Occurrence of cataracts and keratoconus with atopic dermatitis. *Arch Dermatol* 1955;72:237–41

28. Schmutz JL, Weber M, Beurey J. Cataracte et dermatologie. *Ann Dermatol Venereol* 1989;116:133–9

29. Champion RH, Parish WE. Atopic dermatitis. In Champion RH, Burton JL, Ebling FJG, eds. *Textbook of Dermatology*, 5th edn. Oxford: Blackwell Scientific, 1992: 589–610

30. Paradisi M, Angelo C, Conti G, *et al*. Dubowitz syndrome with keloidal lesions. *Clin Exp Dermatol* 1994;19:425–7

31. Atherton DJ. Diet and atopic eczema. *Clin Allergy* 1988;18:215–28

32. Benton EC, Barnetson RC. Skin reactions to foods in patients with atopic dermatitis. *Acta Derm Venereol* 1985;114 (Suppl):129–32

33. Sampson HA. Role of immediate food hypersensitivity in the pathogenesis of atopic dermatitis. *J Allergy Clin Immunol* 1983;71:473–80

34. Mabin DC, Sykes AE, David TJ. Controlled trial of a few-foods diet compared with control diet: few-foods diet of no benefit. *Arch Dis Child* 1995;73; 202–7

35. Bendsoe N, Bjornberg A, Asnes H. Itching from wool fibres in atopic dermatitis. *Contact Dermatitis* 1987;17:21–2

36. Hanifin JM. The role of antihistamines in atopic dermatitis. *J Allergy Clin Immunol* 1990;86:666–9

37. Behrendt H, Ring J. Histamine, antihistamines and atopic eczema. *Clin Exp Allergy Suppl* 1990;4:25–30

38. Berth-Jones J, Graham-Brown RA. Failure of terfenadine in relieving the pruritus of atopic dermatitis. *Br J Dermatol* 1989;121:635–7

39. Doherty V, Sylvester DGH, Kennedy CTC, *et al*. Treatment of itching in atopic eczema with antihistamines with a low sedative profile. *Br Med J* 1989;298: 96–7

40. Wahlgren CF, Hägermark Ö, Bergstrom R. The antipruritic effect of a sedative and a non-sedative antihistamine in atopic dermatitis. *Br J Dermatol* 1990; 122:545–51

41. Langeland T, Fagertun HE, Larsen S. Therapeutic effect of loratadine on pruritus in patients with atopic dermatitis. A multi-crossover-designed study. *Allergy* 1994;49:22–6

42. Wahlgren CF, Scheynius A, Hägermark Ö. Antipruritic effect of oral cyclosporin A in atopic dermatitis. *Acta Derm Venereol* 1990;70:323–9

43. Reinhold U, Kukel S, Brzoska J, *et al*. Systemic interferon gamma treatment in severe atopic dermatitis. *J Am Acad Dermatol* 1993;29:58–63

44. Morse PF, Horrobin DF, Manku MS, *et al*. Meta-analysis of placebo-controlled studies of the efficacy of Epogam in the treatment of atopic eczema. Relationship between plasma essential fatty acid changes and clinical response. *Br J Dermatol* 1989; 121:75–90

45. Sheehan MP, Rustin MH, Atherton DJ, *et al*. Efficacy of traditional Chinese herbal therapy in adult atopic dermatitis. *Lancet* 1992;340:13–7

46. Hanifin JM. Pharmacophysiology of atopic dermatitis. *Clin Rev Allergy* 1986;4:43–65

47. Drake LA, Fallon JD, Sober A. Relief of pruritus in patients with atopic dermatitis after treatment with topical doxepin cream. The Doxepin Study Group. *J Am Acad Dermatol* 1994;31:613–6

48. Jekler J, Larko O. UVA solarium versus UVB phototherapy of atopic dermatitis: a paired-comparison study. *Br J Dermatol* 1991;125:569–72

49. Cole WC, Roth HL, Sacks LB. Group psychotherapy as an aid in the medical treatment of eczema. *J Am Acad Dermatol* 1988;18:286–91

50. Melin L, Frederiksen T, Noren P, *et al*. Behavioural treatment of scratching in patients with atopic dermatitis. *Br J Dermatol* 1986;115:467–74

51. Reeves JRT, Maibach HI. *Clinical Dermatology Illustrated. A Regional Approach*. Sydney: Williams & Wilkins and Associates Ltd., 1986

52. Klaus MV, Wieselthier JS. Contact dermatitis. *Am Fam Phys* 1993;48:629–32

53. Goldner R. Work-related irritant contact dermatitis. *Occupat Med* 1994;9:37–44

54. Judd L. A descriptive study of occupational skin disease. *NZ Med J* 1994;107:147–9

55. Goh CL. Common industrial processes and occupational irritants and allergens – an update. *Ann Acad Med Singapore* 1994;23:690–8

56. van Ketel WG, Bruynzeel DP. Occupational dermatitis in an accordion repairer. *Contact Dermatitis* 1992;27:186

57. Tong D. Coral dermatitis in the aquarium industry. *Contact Dermatitis* 1995;33:207–8

58. Selvaag E, Holm JO, Thune P. Allergic contact dermatitis in an aroma therapist with multiple sensitizations to essential oils. *Contact Dermatitis* 1995;33:354–5

59. Schaller M, Korting HC. Allergic airborne contact dermatitis from essential oils used in aromatherapy. *Clin Exp Dermatol* 1995;20:143–5

60. London L, Joubert G, Manjra SI, *et al*. Compensatability and contact dermatitis in the canning industry. *South Af Med J* 1992;81:615–7

61. Meding B, Barregard L, Marcus K. Hand eczema in car mechanics. *Contact Dermatitis* 1994;30:129–34

62. Koch P. Occupational contact dermatitis from colophony and formaldehyde in banknote paper. *Contact Dermatitis* 1995;32:371–2

63. Gollhausen R, Ring J. Allergy to coined money: nickel contact dermatitis in cashiers. *J Am Acad Dermatol* 1991;25:365–9

64. Koh D, Foulds IS, Aw TC. Dermatological hazards in the electronics industry. *Contact Dermatitis* 1990; 22:1–7

65. Motolese A, Truzzi M, Giannini A, *et al*. Contact dermatitis and contact sensitization among enamellers and decorators in the ceramics industry. *Contact Dermatitis* 1993;28:59–62

66. Matsushita T, Aoyama K, Manda F, *et al*. Occupational dermatoses in farmers growing okra (Hibiscus esculentus L.). *Contact Dermatitis* 1989; 21:321–5

67. van Ginkel CJ, Sabapathy NN. Allergic contact dermatitis from the newly introduced fungicide fluazinam. *Contact Dermatitis* 1995;32:160–2

68. Halkier–Sorensen L. Thestrup-Pedersen K. Skin irritancy from fish is related to its postmortem age. *Contact Dermatitis* 1989;21:172–8

69. Acciai MC, Brusi C, Francalanci S, *et al*. Allergic contact dermatitis in caterers. *Contact Dermatitis* 1993; 29:48

70. Dannaker CJ, White IR. Cutaneous allergy to mustard in a salad maker. *Contact Dermatitis* 1987;16: 212–4

71. Tacke J, Schmidt A, Fartasch M, *et al*. Occupational contact dermatitis in bakers, confectioners and cooks. A population-based study. *Contact Dermatitis* 1995;33:112–7

72. Gan SL, Goh CL, Lee CS, *et al*. Occupational dermatosis among sanders in the furniture industry. *Contact Dermatitis* 1987;17:237–40

73. Hogan DJ, Dosman JA, Li KY, *et al*. Questionnaire survey of pruritus and rash in grain elevator workers. *Contact Dermatitis* 1986;14:170–5

74. Holness DL, Nethercott JR. Dermatitis in hairdressers. *Dermatol Clin* 1990;8:119–26

75. van der Walle HB. Dermatitis in hairdressers (II). Management and prevention. *Contact Dermatitis* 1994;30:265–70

76. Weido AJ, Sim TC. The burgeoning problem of latex sensitivity. Surgical gloves are only the beginning. *Postgrad Med* 1995;98:173–4, 179–82, 184

77. Torinuki W. Contact dermatitis to biperiden and photocontact dermatitis to phenothiazines in a pharmacist. *Tohoku J Exp Med* 1995;176:249–52

78. Martins C, Freitas JD, Goncalo M, *et al*. Allergic contact dermatitis from erythromycin. *Contact Dermatitis* 1995;33:360

79. Stingeni L, Lapomarda V, Lisi P. Occupational hand dermatitis in hospital environments. *Contact Dermatitis* 1995;33:172–6

80. Thiboutot DM, Hamory BH, Marks JG Jr. Dermatoses among floral shop workers. *J Am Acad Dermatol* 1990;22:54–8

81. Bruynzeel DP, Tafelkruijer J, Wilks MF. Contact dermatitis due to a new fungicide used in the tulip bulb industry. *Contact Dermatitis* 1995;33:8–11

82. Nava C, Meneghini CL, Sertoli A, *et al*. Contact dermatitis of the hands in housewives: preliminary data of a multicenter study. *Giornale Ital Med Lavoro* 1989;11:109–12

83. Aberer W. Allergy to colophony acquired backstage. *Contact Dermatitis* 1987;16:34–6

84. Goh CL, Gan SL. The incidence of cutting fluid dermatitis among metalworkers in a metal fabrication factory: a prospective study. *Contact Dermatitis* 1994;31:111–5

85. Goh CL, Yuen R. A study of occupational skin disease in the metal industry (1986–1990). *Ann Acad Med Singapore* 1994;23:639–44

86. Herzog J, Dunne J, Aber R, *et al*. Milk tester's dermatitis. *J Am Acad Dermatol* 1988;19:503–8

87. Ueda A, Obama K, Aoyama K, *et al*. Allergic contact dermatitis in shiitake (Lentinus edodes (Berk) Sing) growers. *Contact Dermatitis* 1992;26:228–33

88. Bruhn JN, Soderberg MD. Allergic contact dermatitis caused by mushrooms. A case report and literature review. *Mycopathologia* 1991;115:191–5

89. Buckley DA, Rogers S. 'Fiddler's fingers': violin-string dermatitis. *Contact Dermatitis* 1995;32:46–7

90. Bork K. Allergic contact dermatitis on a violinist's neck from para-phenylenediamine in a chin rest stain. *Contact Dermatitis* 1993;28:250–1

91. Yakes B, Kelsey KT, Seitz T, *et al*. Occupational skin disease in newspaper pressroom workers. *J Occupat Med* 1991;33:711–7

92. Moura C, Dias M, Vale T. Contact dermatitis in painters, polishers and varnishers. *Contact Dermatitis* 1994;31:51–3

93. Rustemeyer T, Frosch PJ. Allergic contact dermatitis from colour developers. *Contact Dermatitis* 1995;32:59–60

94. Tarvainen K, Jolanki R, Forsman-Gronholm L, *et al*. Exposure, skin protection and occupational skin diseases in the glass-fibre-reinforced plastics industry. *Contact Dermatitis* 1993;29:119–27

95. Wilkinson SM, Heagerty AH, English JS. Hand dermatitis in the pottery industry. *Contact Dermatitis* 1992;26:91–4

96. Kanerva L, Estlander T, Jolanki R, *et al*. Contact dermatitis from telefax paper. *Contact Dermatitis* 1992;27:12–5

97. Hansen KS, Petersen HO. Protein contact dermatitis in slaughterhouse workers. *Contact Dermatitis* 1989;21:221–4

98. Wolf R, Movshowitz M, Brenner S. Contact dermatitis in Israeli soldiers. *J Toxicol Envir Health* 1994;43:7–11

99. Hatch KL, Maibach HI. Textile dye dermatitis. *J Am Acad Dermatol* 1995;32:631–9

100. Oliwiecki S, Beck MH, Hausen BM. Occupational allergic contact dermatitis from caffeates in poplar bud resin in a tree surgeon. *Contact Dermatitis* 1992;27:127–8

101. Roger A, Guspi R, Garcia-Patos V, *et al*. Occupational protein contact dermatitis in a veterinary surgeon. *Contact Dermatitis* 1995;32:248–9

102. Ashworth J, Rycroft RJ, Waddy RS, *et al*. Irritant contact dermatitis in warehouse employees. *Occupat Med* 1993;43:32–4

103. Berardesca E, Distante F. The modulation of skin irritation. *Contact Dermatitis* 1994;31:281–7

104. Tupker RA, Coenraads PJ, Fidler V, *et al*. Irritant susceptibility and weal and flare reactions to bioactive agents in atopic dermatitis. II. Influence of season. *Br J Dermatol* 1995;133:365–70

105. Park KB, Eun HC. A study of skin responses to follow-up, rechallenge and combined effects of irritants using non-invasive measurements. *J Dermatol Sci* 1995;10:159–65

106. McLelland J, Shuster S, Matthews JN. 'Irritants' increase the response to an allergen in allergic contact dermatitis. *Arch Dermatol* 1991;127:1016–9

107. Richards W, Church JA. Use of dishwashing liquids for bathing: a cause of generalized pruritis. *Ann Allergy* 1977;39:284

108. Ramsing DW, Agner T. Efficacy of topical corticosteroids on irritant skin reactions. *Contact Dermatitis* 1995;32:293–7

109. Hannuksela A, Kinnunen T. Moisturizers prevent irritant dermatitis. *Acta Derm Venereol* 1992;72:42–4

110. Fisher AA. *Contact Dermatitis,* 3rd edn, Philadelphia: Lea & Febiger, 1986

111. Goh CL. Immunologic mechanism in contact allergy – a review. *Ann Acad Med Singapore* 1988;17:243–6

112. Basketter D, Dooms-Goossens A, Karlberg AT, *et al.* The chemistry of contact allergy: why is a molecule allergenic? *Contact Dermatitis* 1995;32:65–73

113. Lachapelle JM, Bruynzeel DP, Ducombs G, *et al.* European multicenter study of the TRUE Test. *Contact Dermatitis* 1988;19:91–7

114. Storrs FJ. All the things I knew were true about contact dermatitis that aren't. *Cutis* 1993;52:301–6

115. Castelain M, Castelain PY, Ricciardi R. Contact dermatitis to acupuncture needles. *Contact Dermatitis* 1987;16:44

116. Bircher AJ, Hirsbrunner P, L'angauer S. Allergic contact dermatitis of the genitals from rubber additives in condoms. *Contact Dermatitis* 1993;28:125–6

117. Held JL, Ruszkowski AM, Deleo VA. Consort contact dermatitis due to oak moss. *Arch Dermatol* 1988; 124:261–2

118. Fisher AA. Management of "consort dermatitis" due to combined allergy: seminal fluid and latex condoms. *Cutis* 1994;54.66–7

119. Fowler JF Jr. Allergic contact dermatitis to gold. *Arch Dermatol* 1988;124:181–2

120. Hayakawa R, Matsunaga K, Arima Y. Depigmented contact dermatitis due to incense. *Contact Dermatitis* 1987;16:272–4

121. Eason EL, Feldman P. Contact dermatitis associated with the use of Always sanitary napkins. *Can Med Assoc J* 1996;154:1173–6

122. Carmichael AJ, Foulds IS. Allergic contact dermatitis from oestradiol in oestrogen patches. *Contact Dermatitis* 1992;26:194–5

123. Dooms-Goossens A, Debusschere K, Morren M, *et al.* Silver polish: another source of contact dermatitis reactions to thiourea. *Contact Dermatitis* 1988;19: 133–5

124. Fowler JF Jr. Occupational dermatitis from stamp pad ink. *Contact Dermatitis* 1987;16:38

125. Ross B, Brancaccio RR. Allergic contact dermatitis to tefillin. *J Am Acad Dermatol* 1996;34:152–3

126. Pecegueiro M. Airborne contact dermatitis to tobacco. *Contact Dermatitis* 1987;17:50–1

127. Williams SR, Clark RF, Dunford JV. Contact dermatitis associated with capsaicin: Hunan hand syndrome. *Ann Emerg Med* 1995;25:713–5

128. Burnett JW. Capsicum pepper dermatitis. *Cutis* 1989;43:534

129. Dunkel FG, Elsner P, Burg G. Allergic contact dermatitis from prednicarbate. *Contact Dermatitis* 1991; 24:59–60

130. Dunkel FG, Elsner P, Burg G. Contact allergies to topical corticosteroids: 10 cases of contact dermatitis. *Contact Dermatitis* 1991;25:97–103

131. Goh CL. Cross-sensitivity to multiple topical corticosteroids. *Contact Dermatitis* 1989;20:65–7

132. Wilkinson SM, Cartwright PH, English JS. Hydrocortisone: an important cutaneous allergen. *Lancet* 1991;337:761–2

133. Baptista A, Barros MA. Contact dermatitis from crotamiton. *Contact Dermatitis* 1992;27:59

134. Shelley WB, Shelley ED, Talanin NY. Self-potentiating allergic contact dermatitis caused by doxepin hydrochloride cream. *J Am Acad Dermatol* 1996;34: 143–4

135. Taylor JS, Praditsuwan P, Handel D, *et al.* Allergic contact dermatitis from doxepin cream. One-year patch test clinic experience. *Arch Dermatol* 1996; 132:515–8

136. Hardwick N, King CM. Contact allergy to lignocaine with cross-reaction to bupivacaine. *Contact Dermatitis* 1994;30:245–6

137. Handfield-Jones SE, Cronin E. Contact sensitivity to lignocaine. *Clin Exp Dermatol* 1993;18:342–3

138. Wilkinson SM, Beck MH. Allergic contact dermatitis from menthol in peppermint. *Contact Dermatitis* 1994;30:42–3

139. Korffmacher H, Hartwig R, Matthes U, *et al.* Contact allergy to 8-methoxypsoralen. *Contact Dermatitis* 1994;30:283–5

140. Riboldi A, Pigatto PD, Altomare GF, *et al.* Contact allergic dermatitis from oatmeal. *Contact Dermatitis* 1988;18:316–7

141. Cusano F, Luciano S. Contact dermatitis from pramoxine. *Contact Dermatitis* 1993;28:39

142. Thakur BK, Murali MR. EMLA cream-induced allergic contact dermatitis: a role for prilocaine as an immunogen. *J Allergy Clin Immunol* 1995;95:776–8

143. Cusano F, Capozzi M, Errico G. Allergic contact dermatitis from coal tar. *Contact Dermatitis* 1992;27:51–2

144. Bjornberg A, Lowhagen GB, Tengberg JE. Skin reactivity in workers with and without itching from occupational exposure to glass fibres. *Acta Derm Venereol* 1979;59:49–53

145. Koh D, Aw TC, Foulds IS. Fiberglass dermatitis from printed circuit boards. *Am J Indust Med* 1992;21:193–8

146. Sertoli A, Giorgini S, Farli M. Fiberglass dermatitis. *Clin Dermatol* 1992;10:167–74

147. Okano M, Kozuka T, Tanigaki T, *et al.* Fiberglass dermatitis in Japan – report of four cases. *J Dermatol* 1987;14:590–3

148. Wang BJ, Lee JY, Wang RC. Fiberglass dermatitis: report of two cases. *J Formosan Med Assoc* 1993;92:755–8

149. Garcia-Patos V, Pujol RM. Generalized pruritus with flexural micropapules in a 16-month-old girl. Fiberglass dermatitis. *Arch Dermatol* 1994;130:785, 788

150. Weimstein BR, Bernhard JD. Incarceration for excoriation. *Cutis* 1990;46:240

151. Smit HA, Burdorf A, Coenraads PJ. Prevalence of hand dermatitis in different occupations. *Int J Epidemiol* 1993;22:288–93

152. Agner T. Skin susceptibility in uninvolved skin of hand eczema patients and healthy controls. *Br J Dermatol* 1991;125:140–6

153. Meding B, Swanbeck GL. Predictive factors for hand eczema. *Contact Dermatitis* 1990;23:154–61

154. Meding B, Swanbeck G. Consequences of having hand eczema. *Contact Dermatitis* 1990;23:6–14

155. Keczkes K, Bhate SM, Wyatt EH. The outcome of primary irritant hand dermatitis. *Br J Dermatol* 1983;109:665–8

156. Meding B, Swanbeck G. Epidemiology of different types of hand eczema in an industrial city. *Acta Derm Venereol* 1989;69:227–33

157. LeVine MJ, Parrish JA, Fitzpatrick TB. Oral methoxsalen photochemotherapy (PUVA) of dyshidrotic eczema. *Acta Derm Venereol* 1981;61:570–1

158. Koldys KW, Meyer RP. Biofeedback training in the therapy of dyshidrosis. *Cutis* 1979;24:219–21

159. Rietschel RL. Patch testing in occupational hand dermatitis. *Dermatol Clin* 1988;6:43–6

160. Gupta MA, Gupta AK, Haberman HF. Dermatologic signs in anorexia nervosa and bulimia nervosa. *Arch Dermatol* 1987;123:1386–90

161. Crosti C, Lodi A. Pompholyx: a still unresolved kind of eczema. *Dermatology* 1993;186:241–2

162. Plotnick H. Dyshidrosis. *Cutis* 1977;20:373–5

163. Lodi A, Betti R, Chiarelli G, *et al.* Epidemiological, clinical and allergological observations on pompholyx. *Contact Dermatitis* 1992;26:17–21

164. Yokozeki H, Katayama I, Nishioka K, *et al.* The role of metal allergy and local hyperhidrosis in the pathogenesis of pompholyx. *J Dermatol* 1992;19:964–7

165. Hansen O, Kuchler T, Lotz GR, *et al.* My fingers itch, but my hands are bound. An exploratory psychosomatic study of patients with dyshidrosis of the hands (cheiropompholyx). *Zeitschrift Psychosomatische Med Psychoanalyse* 1981;27:275–90

166. Crippa M, Misquith L, Lonati A, *et al.* Dyshidrotic eczema and sensitization to dithiocarbamates in a florist. *Contact Dermatitis* 1990;23.203–4

167. de Groot AC, van Ulsen J, Weyland JW. Peri-anal allergic contact eczema with dyshidrotic eczema of the hands due to the use of Kathon CG moist toilet wipes. *Ned Tijdschrift Geneeskunde* 1991;135:1048–9

168. Anderson RH. Autoimmune progesterone dermatitis. *Cutis* 1984;33:490–1

169. Chan HL, Su IJ, Kuo TT, *et al.* Cutaneous manifestations of adult T cell leukemia/lymphoma. Report of three different forms. *J Am Acad Dermatol* 1985;13:213–9

170. Jakob T, Tiemann M, Kuwert C, *et al.* Dyshidrotic cutaneous T-cell lymphoma. *J Am Acad Dermatol* 1996;34:295–7

171. Duhra P, Ryatt KS. Haemorrhagic pompholyx in bullous pemphigoid. *Clin Exp Dermatol* 1988;13:342–3

172. Beylot-Barry M, Doutre MS, Beylot C. Dyshidrotic pemphigoid. *Ann Dermatol Venereol* 1995;122:81–3

173. Duhra P, Charles-Holmes R. Linear IgA disease with haemorrhagic pompholyx and dapsone-induced neutropenia. *Br J Dermatol* 1991;125:172-4

174. Borradori L, Harms M. Podopompholyx due to pemphigus vulgaris and Trichophyton rubrum infection. Report of an unusual case. *Mycoses* 1994;37:137–9

175. Milgraum SS, Friedman DJ, Ellis CN, *et al.* Pemphigus vulgaris masquerading as dyshidrotic eczema. *Cutis* 1985;35:445–6

176. Davidson CL. Occupational contact dermatitis of the upper extremity. *Occupational Med* 1994;9: 59–74

177. Fischer T. Prevention of irritant dermatitis. *Occupational Med* 1986;1:335-42

178. Schandelmaier F. How do I treat dyshidrosiform eruptions? *Zeitschrift Hautkrankheiten* 1986;61: 735–7

179. Woolner D, Soltani K. Management of hand dermatitis. *Comprehensive Ther* 1994;20:422–6

180. Volden G. Successful treatment of therapy-resistant atopic dermatitis with clobetasol propionate and a hydrocolloid occlusive dressing. *Acta Derm Venereol* 1992;176:126–8

181. Singalavanija S, Frieden IJ. Diaper dermatitis. *Ped Review* 1995;16:142–7

182. Longhi F, Carlucci G, Bellucci R, *et al.* Diaper dermatitis: a study of contributing factors. *Contact Dermatitis* 1992;26:248–52

183. Sires UI, Mallory SB. Diaper dermatitis. How to treat and prevent. *Postgrad Med* 1995;98:79–84, 86

184. Janniger CK, Thomas I. Diaper dermatitis: an approach to prevention employing effective diaper care. *Cutis* 1993;52:153–5

185. Wong DL, Brantly D, Clutter LB, *et al.* Diapering choices: a critical review of the issues. *Ped Nurs* 1992;18:41–54

186. Brook I. Microbiology of secondarily infected diaper dermatitis. *Int J Dermatol* 1992;31:700–2

187. Beacham BE. Common dermatoses in the elderly. *Am Fam Phys* 1993;47:1445–50

188. Fenske NA, Lober CW. Structural and functional changes of normal aging skin. *J Am Acad Dermatol* 1986;15:571–85

189. Ghadially R, Brown BE, Sequeira–Martin SM, *et al.* The aged epidermal permeability barrier. Structural, functional, and lipid biochemical abnormalities in humans and a senescent murine model. *J Clin Invest* 1995;95:2281–90

190. Greist MC, Epinette WW. Cimetidine-induced xerosis and asteatotic dermatitis. *Arch Dermatol* 1982; 118:253–4

191. Sadick NS, McNutt NS, Kaplan MH. Papulosquamous dermatoses of AIDS. *J Am Acad Dermatol* 1990;22:1270–7

192. Healy E, Meenan J, Mulcahy F, *et al.* The spectrum of HIV related skin diseases in an Irish population. *Irish Med J* 1993;86:188–90

193. Duvic M. Papulosquamous disorders associated with human immunodeficiency virus infection. *Dermatol Clin* 1991;9:523–30

194. Lazar AP, Lazar P. Dry skin, water, and lubrication. *Dermatol Clin* 1991;9:45–51

195. Rollins TG. From xerosis to nummular dermatitis. The dehydration dermatosis. *J Am Med Assoc* 1968; 206:637

196. Becker F. Mechanisms, epidemiology and clinical evaluation of venous insufficiency of the lower limbs. *Rev Praticien* 1994;44:726–31

197. Miani S, Boneschi M, La Penna A, *et al* Physiopathology of venous stasis at the microcirculation level. *Minerva Cardioangiol* 1992;40:413–6

198. Scelsi R, Scelsi L, Cortinovis R, *et al.* Morphological changes of dermal blood and lymphatic vessels in chronic venous insufficiency of the leg. *Int Angiol* 1994;13:308–11

199. Bahmer FA. Significance of local factors for the development of contact allergic reactions in patients with chronic venous insufficiency. *Zeitschrift Hautkrankheiten* 1987;62:1662–4

200. Dooms-Goossens A, Degreef H, Parijs M, *et al.* A retrospective study of patch test results from 163 patients with stasis dermatitis or leg ulcers. II. Retesting of 50 patients. *Dermatologica* 1979;159.231–8

201. Frosch PJ, Weickel R. Contact allergy to the preservative bronopol. *Hautarzt* 1987;38:267–70

202. Keilig W. Contact allergy to cetylstearylalcohol (Lanette O) as a therapeutic problem in stasis dermatitis and leg ulcer. *Dermatosen Beruf Umwelt* 1983;31:50–4

203. Lembo G, Balato N, Giordano C, *et al.* Contact sensitization in stasis dermatitis and chronic leg ulcers. Study of 112 patients. *Minerva Med* 1984;75: 1133–5

204. Lindemayr H, Drobil M. Eczema of the lower leg and contact allergy. *Hautarzt* 1985;36:227–31

205. Shupp DL, Winkelmann RK: The role of patch testing in stasis dermatitis. *Cutis* 1988;42:528–30

206. Wilson CL, Cameron J, Powell SM, *et al.* High incidence of contact dermatitis in leg-ulcer patients—implications for management. *Clin Exp Dermatol* 1991;16:250–3

207. Wilkinson SM, English JS. Hydrocortisone sensitivity: clinical features of fifty-nine cases. *J Am Acad Dermatol* 1992;27:683–7

208. Wilkinson SM. Hypersensitivity to topical corticosteroids. *Clin Exp Dermatol* 1994;19:1–11

209. Owens CW, Al-Khader AA, Jackson MJ, *et al.* A severe 'stasis eczema', associated with low plasma zinc, treated successfully with oral zinc. *Br J Dermatol* 1981;105:461–4

210. Torrence BP, Hovanec R, Bartunek C, *et al.* Stasis dermatitis: practical pearls for the dermatologic nurse. *Dermatol Nurs* 1993;5:186–91, 208

211. Zimmet SE. Treatment of stasis dermatitis and ulceration. *Am Fam Phys* 1994;49:1080, 1083

212. Pappert A, Grossman M, DeLeo V. Photosensitivity as the presenting illness in four patients with human immunodeficiency viral infection. *Arch Dermatol* 1994;130:618–23

213. Ophaswongse S, Maibach H. Topical nonsteroidal antiinflammatory drugs: allergic and photoallergic contact dermatitis and phototoxicity. *Contact Dermatitis* 1993;29:57–64

214. Parry EJ, Bilsland D, Morley WN. Photocontact allergy to 4-tert. butyl-4'-methoxy-dibenzoylmethane (Parsol 1789). *Contact Dermatitis* 1995;32:251–2

215. Funk JO, Dromgoole SH, Maibach HI. Sunscreen intolerance. Contact sensitization, photocontact sensitization, and irritancy of sunscreen agents. *Dermatol Clin* 1995;13:473–81

216. Gould JW, Mercurio MG, Elmets CA. Cutaneous photosensitivity diseases induced by exogenous agents. *J Am Acad Dermatol* 1995;33:551–73

217. Gross TP, Ratner L, de Rodriguez O, *et al.* An outbreak of phototoxic dermatitis due to limes. *Am J Epidemiol* 1987;125:509–14

218. Jansen CT, Karvonen J. Polymorphous light eruption. A seven–year follow-up evaluation of 114 patients. *Arch Dermatol* 1984; 120: 862–5

219. Commens C. Polymorphic light eruption sine eruptione and brachioradial pruritus. *Br J Dermatol* 1988; 119:554

220. Dover JS, Hawk JL. Polymorphic light eruption sine eruption. *Br J Dermatol* 1988;118:73–6

221. Rucker BU. Haberle M. Koch HU, *et al.* Ultraviolet light hardening in polymorphous light eruption – a controlled study comparing different emission spectra. *Photodermatol Photoimmunol Photomed* 1991;8: 73–8

222. Leonard F, Morel M, Kalis B, *et al.* Psoralen plus ultraviolet A in the prophylactic treatment of benign summer light eruption. *Photodermatol Photoimmunol Photomed* 1991;8:95–8

223. Murphy GM, Hawk JLM, Magnus IA. Hydroxychloroquine in polymorphic light eruption. a controlled trial with drug and visual sensitivity monitoring. *Br J Dermatol* 1987; 116: 379–86

224. Norris PG, Hawk JLM. Successful treatment of severe polymorphous light eruption with azathioprine. *Arch Dermatol* 1989;125:1377–9

225. Singh G. Atopy in lichen simplex (neurodermatitis circumscripta). *Br J Dermatol* 1973;89:625–7

226. Roberston IM, Jordan JM, Whitlock FA. Emotions and skin (II) – the conditioning of scratch responses in cases of lichen simplex. *Br J Dermatol* 1975;92:407–12

227. Goldblum RW, Piper WN. Artificial lichenification produced by a scratching machine. *J Invest Dermatol* 1954;22:405–15

228. Kinsella LJ, Carney-Godley K, Feldmann E. Lichen simplex chronicus as the initial manifestation of intramedullary neoplasm and syringomyelia. *Neurosurgery* 1992;30(3):418–21

229. Shukla S, Mukherjee S. Lichen simplex chronicus during lithium treatment. *Am J Psychiat* 141:909–10

230. Brunner N, Yawalkar S. A double-blind, multicenter, parallel-group trial with 0.05% halobetasol propionate ointment versus 0.1% diflucortolone valerate ointment in patients with severe, chronic atopic dermatitis or lichen simplex chronicus. *J Am Acad Dermatol* 1991;25:1160–3

231. Datz B, Yawalkar S. A double-blind, multicenter trial of 0.05% halobetasol propionate ointment and 0.05% clobetasol 17-propionate ointment in the treatment of patients with chronic, localized atopic dermatitis or lichen simplex chronicus. *J Am Acad Dermatol* 1991;25:1157–60

232. Bard JW. Flurandrenolone tape in the treatment of lichen simplex chronicus. *J Kent Med Assoc* 1969; 67:668–70

233. Drake LA, Millikan LE. The antipruritic effect of 5% doxepin cream in patients with eczematous dermatitis. Doxepin Study Group. *Arch Dermatol* 1995;131: 1403–8

234. Dean EA, Bernhard JD. Recurrence of lichen simplex chronicus after surgical excision. *Cutis* 1987;40:157–8

235. Kieffer M, Kristensen S, Hallas TE. Prurigo and pets: the benefit from vets. *Br Med J* 1979;1(6177): 1539–40

236. Feuerman EJ, Sandbank M. Prurigo nodularis. Histological and electron microscopical study. *Arch Dermatol* 1975;111:1472–7

237. Harris B, Harris K, Penneys NS. Demonstration by S-100 protein staining of increased numbers of nerves in the papillary dermis of patients with prurigo nodularis. *J Am Acad Dermatol* 1992;26:56–8

238. Vaalasti A, Suomalainen H, Rechardt L. Calcitonin gene-related peptide immunoreactivity in prurigo nodularis: a comparative study with neurodermatitis circumscripta. *Br J Dermatol* 1989;120:619–23

239. Sandbank M. Cutaneous nerve lesions in prurigo nodularis. Electron microscopic study of two patients. *J Cut Pathol* 1976;3:125–32

240. Lindley RP, Payne CM. Neural hyperplasia is not a diagnostic prerequisite in nodular prurigo. A controlled morphometric microscopic study of 26 biopsy specimens. *J Cut Pathol* 1989;16:14–8

241. Rowland Payne CME. Prurigo nodularis. In Bernhard JD, ed. *Itch: Mechanisms and Management of Pruritis*. New York: McGraw Hill, 1994:103–19

242. Miyauchi H, Uehara M. Follicular occurrence of prurigo nodularis. *J Cut Pathol* 1988;15:208–11

243. Nahass GT, Penneys NS. Merkel cells and prurigo nodularis. *J Am Acad Dermatol* 1994;31:86–8

244. Perez GL, Peters MS, Reda AM, *et al.* Mast cells, neutrophils, and eosinophils in prurigo nodularis. *Arch Dermatol* 1993;129:861–5

245. Mattila JO, Vornanen M, Vaara J, *et al.* Mycobacteria in prurigo nodularis: the cause or a consequence? *J Am Acad Dermatol* 1996;34:224–8

246. Miyachi Y, Okamoto H, Furukawa F, *et al.* Prurigo nodularis. A possible relationship to atopy. *J Dermatol* 1980;7:281–3

247. Tanaka M, Aiba S, Matsumura N, *et al.* Prurigo nodularis consists of two distinct forms: early-onset atopic and late-onset non-atopic. *Dermatology* 1995;190:269–76

248. Zelickson BD, McEvoy MT, Fransway AF. Patch testing in prurigo nodularis. *Contact Dermatitis* 1989;20:321–5

249. Rowland Payne CM, Wilkinson JD, McKee PH, *et al.* Nodular prurigo – a clinicopathological study of 46 patients. *Br J Dermatol* 1985;113:431–9

250. Seeburger J, Anderson-Wilms N, Jacobs R. Lennert's lymphoma presenting as prurigo nodularis. *Cutis* 1993;51:355–8

251. Fina L, Grimalt R, Berti E, *et al.* Nodular prurigo associated with Hodgkin's disease. *Dermatologica* 1991;182:243–6

252. Shelnitz LS, Paller AS. Hodgkin's disease manifesting as prurigo nodularis. *Ped Dermatol* 1990;7:136–9

253. McKenzie AW, Stubbing DG, Elvy BL. Prurigo nodularis and gluten enteropathy. *Br J Dermatol* 1976;95:89–92

254. Kundu A, Wade AA, Ilchyshyn A. Prurigo nodularis in an HIV positive man. *Genitourinary Med* 1995;71:129–30

255. Berger TG, Hoffman C, Thieberg MD. Prurigo nodularis and photosensitivity in AIDS: treatment with thalidomide. *J Am Acad Dermatol* 1995;33:837–8

256. Greer KE. Prurigo nodularis and uremia. *South Med J* 1975;68:138–41

257. Heng MC, Allen SG, Kim A, *et al.* Alpha-1 antitrypsin deficiency in a patient with widespread prurigo nodularis. *Australas J Dermatol* 1991;32:151–7

258. Suarez C, Pereda JM, Moreno LM, *et al.* Prurigo nodularis associated with malabsorption. *Dermatologica* 1984;169:211–4

259. Borradori L, Prost C, Wolkenstein P, *et al.* Localized pretibial pemphigoid and pemphigoid nodularis. *J Am Acad Dermatol* 1992;27:863–7

260. Massa MC, Connolly SM. Bullous pemphigoid with features of prurigo nodularis. *Arch Dermatol* 1982;118:937–9

261. Tamada Y, Yokochi K, Oshitani Y, *et al.* Pemphigoid nodularis: a case with 230 kDa hemidesmosomes antigen associated with bullous pemphigoid antigen. *J Dermatol* 1995;22:201–4

262. Amagai N, Stolar E, Williams CM. Unusual widespread type of angiolymphoid hyperplasia with eosinophilia mimicking prurigo nodularis. *J Dermatol* 1993;20:660–1

263. Sarnoff DS, Schiff GM. Widespread cutaneous angiolymphoid hyperplasia with eosinophilia. *J Dermatol Surg Oncol* 1983;9:905–9

264. Noppakun N, Apisarnthanarax P. Multiple cutaneous granular cell tumors simulating prurigo nodularis. *Int J Dermatol* 1981;20:126–9

265. Greither A. Pruritus and prurigo. *Hautarzt* 1980;31:397–405

266. Hudson P, Black MM. Nodular prurigo. *Br J Dermatol* 1976;95 (Suppl 14):79–81

267. Linhardt PW, Walling AD. Prurigo nodularis. *J Fam Pract* 1993;37:495–8

268. Geraldez MC, Carreon-Gavino M, Hoppe G, *et al.* Diflucortolone valerate ointment with and without occlusion in lichen simplex chronicus. *Int J Dermatol* 1989;28:603–4

269. Meyers LN. Use of occlusive membrane in the treatment of prurigo nodularis. *Int J Dermatol* 1989;28:275–6

100

270. Tupker RA, Coenraads PJ, van der Meer JB. Treatment of prurigo nodularis, chronic prurigo and neurodermatitis circumscripta with topical capsaicin. *Acta Derm Venereol* 1992;72:463

271. Waldinger TP, Wong RC, Taylor WB, *et al.* Cryotherapy improves prurigo nodularis. *Arch Dermatol* 1984;120:1598–600

272. Stoll DM, Fields JP, King LE Jr. Treatment of prurigo nodularis: use of cryosurgery and intralesional steroids plus lidocaine. *J Dermatol Surg Oncol* 1983;9:922–4

273. Hann SK, Cho MY, Park YK. UV treatment of generalized prurigo nodularis. *Int J Dermatol* 1990;29:436–7

274. Karvonen J, Hannuksela M. Long term results of topical trioxsalen PUVA in lichen planus and nodular prurigo. *Acta Derm Venereol* 1985;120 (Suppl):53–5

275. Rowland Payne CM. Etretinate and nodular prurigo. *Br J Dermatol* 1988;118:135–6

276. Hirschel-Scholz S, Salomon D, Merot Y, *et al.* Anetodermic prurigo nodularis (with Pautrier's neuroma) responsive to arotinoid acid. *J Am Acad Dermatol* 1991;25:437–42

277. Berth-Jones J, Smith SG, Graham-Brown RA. Nodular prurigo responds to cyclosporin. *Br J Dermatol* 1995;132:795–9

278. van den Broek H. Treatment of prurigo nodularis with thalidomide. *Arch Dermatol* 1980;116:571–2

279. Johnke H, Zachariae H. Thalidomide treatment of prurigo nodularis. *Ugeskrift Laeger* 1993;155:3028–30

280. Winkelmann RK, Connolly SM, Doyle JA, *et al.* Thalidomide treatment of prurigo nodularis. *Acta Derm Venereol* 1984;64:412–7

281. Clemmensen OJ, Olsen PZ, Andersen KE. Thalidomide neurotoxicity. *Arch Dermatol* 1984;120:338–41

282. Wulff CH, Hoyer H, Asboe-Hansen G, *et al.* Development of polyneuropathy during thalidomide therapy. *Br J Dermatol* 1985;112:475–80

# Urticarial diseases

Most patients with urticaria have short-lived, idiopathic disease. Infections, drugs, foods, and contactants may be implicated in some patients. An unfortunate group of patients develop chronic or physical urticaria, which may last months to decades. The mainstay of therapy is continuous histamine-blockade, preferably with minimally sedating agents such as cetirazine, astemazole and loratidine

## Clinical features

Intensely itchy short-lived wheals are found ranging in number from a few to thousands. Wheals consist of erythematous papules, plaques, arcs, and polycyclic forms with peripheral blanching[1] (Figure 45).

- Individual wheals last between one and 24 hours
- Secondary changes including excoriation and purpura may be seen

## Types of urticaria

### Acute urticaria

- Characteristically shows an abrupt onset of one to hundreds of spontaneous wheals which may be associated with dermatographism[2,3]
- This usually clears within 1–6 weeks
- The etiology is occasionally identified

### Chronic urticaria

- Typical short-lived urticarial wheals which last for months to decades
- The natural history suggests that 50% resolve in the first 6 months
- The etiology is not commonly identified, but should be sought in most cases
- It may be due to an autoantibody directed at the mast cell IgE receptor[4–6]

Circulating levels of anti-Fc epsilon RI α auto antibodies are relevant to the pathogenesis of severe chronic urticaria in about 25% of patients

### Adrenergic urticaria

- This is a rare but distinct reported condition in which lesions develop during phases of stress[7]
- Attacks are associated with an increase in the plasma concentrations of noradrenalin, adrenalin, prolactin, and dopamine
- Symptoms can be reproduced by intradermal injection of adrenalin and noradrenalin
- This can be treated successfully with the β-adrenergic blocker, propanolol

### Physical urticaria

- Skin trauma causes mast cells to release histamine and causes a wheal at the site of trauma[8,9]
- A variety of precipitating factors may induce the disease in different patients (see Table 7.1, Figures 46 and 47)
- Patients may present with more than one type of physical urticaria (e.g. heat and cold urticaria)[26]
- Some types, such as aquagenic, cholinergic and cold urticaria, may be associated with angioedema, wheezing, and hypotension
- Treatment consists of minimizing the offending stimulus

**Table 7.1** Summary of urticarial diseases

| Type of urticaria | Precipitating factors | Reaction time | Duration | Diagnostic test | Reported effective treatments |
|---|---|---|---|---|---|
| Symptomatic dermatographism | Stroking or rubbing skin | Minutes | 2–3 hours | Gentle stroking of uninvolved skin | Antihistamines, PUVA[10] |
| Pressure urticaria | Pressure | 3–12 hours | 8–24 hours | Pressure challenge on shoulder – 7kg for 15 min | Topical corticosteroids, sulfasalazine[11] dapsone, and cetirizine |
| Solar urticaria | UV irradiation | 2–5 min | 15 min to 3 hours | Phototesting | Sunscreens, chloroquine, β-carotene, phototherapy, astemizole, terfenidine, cetirizine, doxepin, plasmapheresis[12–16] |
| Cold urticaria | Low temperature | 2–5 min, or up to 3 hours | 1–2 hours, or up to 48 hours | Ice cube to skin for 20 minutes | Cold desensitization, antihistamines such as cyproheptadine and doxepin, ketotifen, terbutaline with aminophylline[17,18] |
| Heat urticaria | High temperature | 2–5 min | 1 hour | Warming of the affected part, e.g. to 43°C for 5 min | Desensitization by repeated exposure to local heat, antihistamines such as astemazole and doxepin[19–21] |
| Cholinergic urticaria | Physical exercise, sweating, hot baths | 2–5 min | 30–60 min | Exercise or hot bath provocation | Antihistamines, ketotifen, or cold water to sweating skin |
| Aquagenic urticaria | Contact with water | Up to 30 min | Hours | Apply water compresses at 35–36°C for 10 min | Antihistamines, phototherapy[22–24] |
| Vibration urticaria | Vibration | 2–5 mins | 60 min | Application of kitchen mixer to forearm | Avoidance of stimuli |

Modified from reference 25

Clinical response to antihistaminic agents is variable

- Patients with symptomatic dermatographism may be difficult to diagnose unless they have recently scratched, or the clinician performs a physical dermatographic challenge

## Angioedema

- Virtually any type of urticaria may be seen in conjunction with angioedema, or angioedema may exist as a singular entity
- Mucous membrane edema may be associated with urticarial wheals on the skin
- Angioedema may be life-threatening due to respiratory compromise and anaphylactic shock
- The same idiopathic, drug, food and physical agents that cause other forms of urticaria may also cause angioedema
- If recurrent and severe, angioedema may rarely be associated with C1-esterase inhibitor deficiency
- Anaphylaxis may be recurrent and life threatening, and patients who experience this reaction pattern should be treated acutely with systemic corticosteroid agents, antihistamines, and epinephrine
- Self-injecting epinephrine kits may be life-saving in the case of severe angioedema and counseling about appropriate use is highly indicated

## Contact urticaria

- Contact with a specific allergen causes histamine release at the contact site with associated itching, redness, and wheals[27]

  Not all patients have visible disease

- Lesions begin within 30 minutes of contact and are limited to areas of direct contact
- Common urticarial contact allergens include rubber[28], cinnamic aldehyde, and sorbic and benzoic acids

- Patients with atopic dermatitis may be more likely to develop this condition
- The most important aspect of treatment in this type of urticaria is avoidance of the allergen

## Urticarial curiosities

- Aquagenic angioedema has been reported in a 21-year-old who experienced persistent swelling of his lips and generalized itching without hives associated with swimming

  Provocative testing with tap water produced transient edema and pruritus

  The reaction spontaneously subsided within a few weeks

- Arthritis or arthralgia (A), hives or urticaria (H) and angioedema (A) consititutes an idiopathic reported triad (the AHA syndrome) which is a diagnosis of exclusion[29]

  It is defined as the absence of associated infection or connective-tissue disease

- Aspartame[30] and caffeine[31,32] have been implicated in inducing urticaria
- Contact urticaria has been reported in different patients due to numerous items; some of the more interesting include: spices, cornstarch[33], globe artichoke[34], litchi fruit[35], kiwi fruit[36], watermelon[37], shitake mushrooms[38], rice[39], buckwheat flour[40], mold on salami casing[41], nickel[42], beef[43], cow milk[44], pork, fish[45], dog saliva[46], tobacco[47], locusts[48], and mouse hair[49]
- A 24-year-old woman developed an acute urticarial reaction secondary to a copper intrauterine contraceptive device[50]

  Allergy to copper was proven by scratch tests and the condition cleared with removal of the intrauterine device

- Dental caries with chronically abscessed teeth was associated with chronic urticaria, and was apparently cleared by extraction of the affected teeth

- Dermatographism may be a poorly recognized cause of vulvar itching[51]
- Earthquake urticaria: acute urticaria was seen in a patient following the 1987 earthquake in Los Angeles, California; psychological stress was hypothesized as the urticaria trigger[52]
- Episodic angioedema with eosinophilia (Gleich syndrome) is a diagnosis of exclusion, as one must make certain the eosinophilia is not a sign of parasitic or allergic reaction[53]
- Ethanol urticaria: a man was reported with onset of urticaria 5–15 minutes after drinking alcoholic beverages of any type[54]

    History was confirmed by a blinded provocatory challenge with 5 ml of ethanol

- Exercise has been reported to cause both urticaria and angioedema[55,56]
- Gallbladder removal helped one patient with chronic urticaria to be free of her disease within 2 days following surgery[57]
- Ganglioneuroblastoma was reported in a 5-year-old boy who had physical urticaria to water, light, and cold for two years[10]

    Left adrenal ganglioneuroblastoma was identified and removed, followed by complete regression of the urticaria

- Latex contact has caused anaphylaxis[58,59]

    Due to a latex vaginal vibrator, oral and vaginal exposure to a condom and rectal exposure to a latex glove

- Menstrual urticaria and anaphylactic angioedema was reported in a patient at each menstruation for a period of 2 years until hysterectomy was performed[60]

    Evaluation showed no hormonal or immunological change

    The only relevant finding was the extraordinarily strong vasodilating action of the menstrual fluid in the patient compared with control fluids

- Philadelphia chromosome positive acute myeloid leukaemia has been associated with painful urticaria[61]
- *Plasmodium vivax* malaria has presented as urticaria[62]
- Postcoital urticaria

    Allergy to penicillin was hypothesized to trigger postcoital urticaria in a woman on three occasions when her sexual partner ingested dicloxacillin[63]

    Human seminal plasma urticaria and anaphylaxis was caused in one patient within 5 minutes of postcoital semen exposure with one partner, but not two former partners; the diagnosis was corroborated by skin prick testing[64]

    Semen may also cause contact urticaria[65]

- Zinc fumes precipitated urticaria and angioedema in a 34-year-old man after he had welded zinc at his job[66]

## Distinguishing features of other conditions with urticarial lesions

Urticaria may be confused with non-urticarial disorders that have different etiologies and treatment. The following is a limited list of conditions to include in the differential diagnosis of urticaria.

- Bullous pemphigoid (see chapter 9: Other itching diseases)

    Typical blisters may not develop for weeks or months

    Lesions last longer than 24 hours

    This condition may respond to topical corticosteroid agents but does not respond to antihistamines

- Dermatitis herpetiformis (see chapter 9: Other itching diseases)

    The delicate, superficial blisters often are scratched away prior to examination

    Lesions last longer than 24 hours

Typical locations include the elbows, knees, and buttocks

This condition does not respond to topical corticosteroid agents or antihistamines

- Erythema multiforme

    Lesions last longer than 24 hours

    Typical locations include mucous membranes, palms and soles; rare sites for urticaria

    Urticarial lesions usually become targetoid within 24 hours

    This condition does not respond to topical corticosteroid agents or antihistamines

- Herpes gestationis (see Chapter 4: Systemic causes of itching)

    Intensely itchy urticarial papules and plaques that usually begins in the second and third trimesters

    Lesions last longer than 24 hours

    Typical bullae develop later

    This condition does not respond to topical corticosteroid agents or antihistamines

- Papular urticaria (insect bites)

    Despite its name, this is not an urticarial condition

    Lesions are small, extremely itchy papules or wheals

    Lesions last longer than 24 hours

    Untouched lesions may have a central punctum whereas well-developed ones may contain small blisters

    It is usually due to arthropod bites

    This condition usually responds to topical corticosteroid agents and systemic antihistaminic agents such as cetirizine

- Polymorphous eruption of pregnancy (see chapter 4: Systemic causes of itching)

    Usually appears in primiparous patients within the striae distensae in the last trimester of pregnancy

Lesions last longer than 24 hours

Small vesicles may often be seen

The etiology is unknown

This condition may respond to topical corticosteroid agents and antihistamines

- Urticaria pigmentosa (see chapter 9: Other itching diseases)

    This condition is not urticarial in the true sense, but may appear urticarial due to mast cell mediators

    Typical lesions have a brown color

    Stroking usually provokes an intense local reaction, and may induce vesiculation

    Lesions last longer than 24 hours

    This is a disease of cutaneous, localized mast cell proliferation

- Urticarial vasculitis

    Purpuric lesions are usually found

    Lesions last longer than 24 hours

    A wide variety of causes of precipitating factors for urticarial vasculitis have been identified, ranging from infections to drugs

    This condition has been reported to be associated with glomerulonephritis

    It does not usually respond as well to topical corticosteroid agents or antihistamines

    Dapsone and other anti-inflammatory agents may be drugs of choice

## Evaluation of the patient with urticaria

### History

Aside from the physical urticarial diseases, the etiology is not commonly discerned. History helps identify the type of urticaria and eliminate non-urticarial diseases, and may help identify cause of eruption[67].

Extensive laboratory evaluation is rarely indicated, instead focus on the history: patients with urticaria are distressed and under duress; they may recall unrelated exposures from earlier decades, and neglect antibiotic therapy instituted a few days ago.

- Duration and prior history – When did this episode start? Has anything like this happened to you before?

  These questions help determine whether this represents an acute or chronic process

  If previous episodes have occurred, this may help identify precipitating factors

- Location – Where are the spots typically located?

  Urticaria limited to the hands and forearms or other localized area may help suggest contact urticaria

  Physical urticarias tend to have limited rather than generalized distributions

- Recent infections – Have you been ill in the past several weeks?

  Note that the onset of urticaria may occur minutes to weeks after the precipitating event

  Infections of the following types may precipitate urticaria:

  Bacterial: focal sepsis including sinusitis and urinary tract infections

  Viral: respiratory infections and hepatitis

  Fungal: vaginal candidiasis

  Parasitic[68]: protozoal and helminth infections

- Drugs – Have you started on new medications in the past month? Have you taken any antibiotics?

  Virtually any medication can cause urticaria, but antibiotics are particularly common

  Look for a good temporal history; often urticarial drug eruptions begin shortly after introduction of a medication

  Discontinuation of the medication may not result in immediate cessation of the eruption; urticaria may persist for weeks

In a patient in whom antibiotics are suspected offenders, remember focal infections can also cause urticaria

Histamine-releasing drugs that can immediately precipitate urticaria (or angioedema) include atropine, codeine, curare, dextran, hydralazine, morphine, pentamidine, and radiocontrast media

Aspirin and non-steroidal anti-inflammatory agents may also precipitate urticaria through other mechanisms, or these agents may exacerbate existing urticaria

- Foods – Do your hives start after eating specific foods?

  Foods are an uncommon cause of urticaria[69]

  Acute or recurrent attacks occur within minutes or hours of ingestion and last for hours to days

  The main foods implicated in urticaria include eggs, nuts, chocolate, fish and shellfish, tomatoes, pork, strawberries, milk, cheese, spices, yeast, and preservatives

- Contactants – Do your hives begin after wearing rubber gloves or other clothing or when you come in contact with anything in particular?

  Contact urticaria usually has a rapid onset following exposure; patients may easily make this association

## Laboratory evaluation

In acute urticaria – a self-limited disease – all laboratory evaluation is optional. In chronic urticaria, laboratory studies are rarely of diagnostic value, but tests such as the following may be indicated:

- Complete blood count with differential: examine for evidence of eosinophilia
- Erythrocyte sedimentation rate: if normal or extremely elevated this may be helpful

- Multichemistry panel: examine for evidence of abnormal protein levels, or hepatic and renal dysfunction
- Urinalysis: examine for evidence of urinary tract infection
- Stool examination for ova and parasites

  Rarely helpful, but virtually any form of intestinal or other parasitosis may induce urticaria

- Radioallergenosorbent tests (RAST): may help identify specific allergies to foods and drugs

  Positive results are frequently irrelevant

  In the vast majority of patients this test bears no fruitful results

- Prick and scratch testing

  Cost-effectiveness and diagnostic value have never been accurately assessed

  Although in select patients these techniques may have value, the vast majority of patients derive no benefit from their use·

  These tests should only be performed by experienced clinicians as interpretation of the results requires clinical skill and severe reactions are possible

## Therapy

The mainstay of urticaria therapy remains long-acting antihistamine therapy[70]. If systemic corticosteroids must be used, the duration of therapy should generally be limited to less than one week. If sedating antihistamines such as hydroxyzine are used, they are best administered at bedtime.

Even if not thought to be directly related to the current eruption, aspirin and nonsteroidal anti-inflammatory agents should be discontinued because they are known exacerbators of urticaria.

### Antihistamines

Because of patient compliance, long-acting antihistamine agents such as astemazole, cetirizine and loratidine are more effective than short-acting agents.

- Antihistamines with intrinsic anti-inflammatory activity such as cetirizine may offer advantages over other antihistaminic agents, but cetirizine is slightly more sedating than loratidine
- Less-sedating antihistamine agents are preferable to older sedating agents
- For a more complete discussion of antihistamines, see chapter 11: Treatment

### Corticosteroids

A controlled trial demonstrated that prednisone 20 mg every 12 hours for 4 days combined with hydroxyzine was more effective than hydroxyzine alone in relieving itching and rash[71].

- When effective, single dose per day schedules of a short-acting corticosteroid agent such as prednisone may not provide 24 hour blockade of symptoms
- Given the significant side-effect profile, long-term systemic corticosteroid agents in chronic urticaria may be an effective treatment, but is rarely a first choice

### Other therapeutic approaches

### Combinations of $H_1$ blockers

- Consider combining minimally sedating antihistamines[72] such as cetirizine[73], loratidine or astemazole with a sedating antihistamine
- Excellent choices may include a bedtime dose of hydroxyzine, chlorpheniramine or doxepin[15,19,74]

## H$_2$ antihistaminic blockers

- Monotherapy with H$_2$ blockers has modest efficacy but is probably less effective than the newer H$_1$ antihistaminic agents[75,76]
- Cimetidine may increase plasma concentrations of H$_1$ antihistamines[77]
- H$_1$ antihistamines such as chlorpheniramine may be combined with agents such as cimetidine or ranitidine to enhance the therapeutic effect[78,79]

  > Addition of H$_2$ blockade decreases itching and whealing

- No published study has compared the addition of H$_2$ agents to the more efficacious newer antihistamines astemazole, cetirizine, and loratidine

## Ketotifen

- Ketotifen, a mast cell stabilizer, is effective in relieving wheals and itching and is more effective than clemastine in chronic urticaria[80,81]
- It is also an effective agent in physical urticaria[82]
- An additional utility of this agent may be in combination with H$_1$ antihistamines in treatment-resistant disease

## Elimination diets

If food is thought to be implicated and the patient is highly motivated, elimination diets may be usefully employed[83].

- Eliminate all foods except chicken and rice with no spices, preservatives, or condiments
- After one week add one simple food, a single spice, or a single food additive per day
- If after several weeks the urticaria continues unabated, food is unlikely to be contributory

## Dapsone

Dapsone is an anti-inflammatory and anti-neutrophilic agent which may benefit some patients with recalcitrant urticaria[84].

- This agent is particularly beneficial in urticarial vasculitis, a related condition
- Doses typically required are 50–100 mg per day in adults

## UVB and PUVA

- Ultraviolet B light (UVB)[85] or Psoralen photochemotherapy (PUVA)[11,86] therapy can be helpful in select patients with recalcitrant disease
- Once therapeutic results have been achieved with 15–20 treatments, maintenance therapy is often required
- Chronic urticaria, solar urticaria, and symptomatic dermatographism are reported to be improved with phototherapy

## Antibiotics

- Working from the hypothesis that chronic antigen stimulation promotes urticaria, treatment with an empiric course of broad spectrum antibiotics and/or antifungal agents has anecdotal support
- Despite no controlled trials demonstrating efficacy, this approach may be employed with limited success

## Topical agents

- Although traditionally thought to play little therapeutic role, oxatomide gel and dechlorpheniramine cream have been shown to decrease itching and erythema, and clobetasol may decrease symptomatic dermatographism[87]
- For extremely limited disease, topical agents may prove beneficial[88,89]

## Miscellaneous therapies reported to be effective

- Sulfasalazine[90]
- Cyclosporin A[91]
- Danazol[92]
- Intravenous immunoglobulin (IVIG)[93]

- Methotrexate[94]
- Nifedipine[95]

- Relaxation therapy[96]
- Stanozolol[97]

---

# References

1. Kobza Black A, Greaves MW, Champion RH, *et al.* The urticarias 1990. *Br J Dermatol* 1991;124:100–8
2. Beltrani VS. Urticaria and angioedema. *Dermatol Clin* 1996;14:171–98
3. Czarnetzki BM. *Urticaria.* Berlin: Springer-Verlag, 1986
4. Grattan CE, Francis DM, Hide M, *et al.* Detection of circulating histamine releasing autoantibodies with functional properties of anti-IgE in chronic urticaria. *Clin Exp Allergy* 1991;21:695–704
5. Hide M, Francis DM, Grattan CE, *et al.* The pathogenesis of chronic idiopathic urticaria: new evidence suggests an auto-immune basis and implications for treatment. *Clin Exp Allergy* 1994;24:624–7
6. Niimi N, Francis DM, Kermani F, *et al.* Dermal mast cell activation by autoantibodies against the high affinity IgE receptor in chronic urticaria. *J Inv Dermatol* 1996;106:1001–6
7. Haustein UF. Adrenergic urticaria and adrenergic pruritus. *Acta Derm Venereol* 1990;70:82–4
8. Duke WW. Urticaria caused specifically by action of physical agents. *J Am Med Assoc* 1924; 83:3–8
9. Greaves MW. The physical urticarias. *Clin Exp Allergy* 1991;21 (Suppl 1):284–9
10. Logan RA, O'Brian TJ, Greaves MW. The effect of psoralen photochemotherapy (PUVA) on symptomatic dermatographism. *Clin Exp Dermatol* 1989; 14:25–8
11. Engler RJ, Squire E, Benson P. Chronic sulfasalazine therapy in the treatment of delayed pressure urticaria and angioedema. *Ann Allergy Asthma Immunol* 1995; 74:155–9
12. Monfrecola G, Nappa P, Pini D. Solar urticaria in the visible spectrum successfully treated with astemizole. *Dermatologica* 1990;180:154–6
13. Diffey BL, Farr PM. Treatment of solar urticaria with terfenadine. *Photo-Dermatol* 1988;5:25–9
14. Neittaanmaki H, Jaaskelainen T, Harvima RJ, *et al.* Solar urticaria: demonstration of histamine release and effective treatment with doxepin. *Photo-Dermatol* 1989;6:52–5
15. Leenutaphong V, Holzle E, Plewig G, *et al.* Plasmapheresis in solar urticaria. *Dermatologica* 1991;182:35–8
16. Torinuki W. Two patients with solar urticaria manifesting pruritic erythema. *J Dermatol* 1992;19:635–7
17. Husz S, Toth-Kasa I, Kiss M, *et al.* Treatment of cold urticaria. *Int J Dermatol* 1994;33:210–3
18. Neittaanmaki H, Myohanen T, Fraki JE. Comparison of cinnarizine, cyproheptadine, doxepin, and hydroxyzine in treatment of idiopathic cold urticaria: usefulness of doxepin. *J Am Acad Dermatol* 1984;11:483–9
19. Higgins EM, Friedmann PS. Clinical report and investigation of a patient with localized heat urticaria. *Acta Dermato-Venereol* 1991;71:434–6
20. Koro O, Dover JS, Francis DM, *et al.* Release of prostaglandin D2 and histamine in a case of localized heat urticaria, and effect of treatments. *Br J Dermatol* 1986;115:721–8
21. Leigh IM, Ramsay CA. Localised heat urticaria treated by inducing tolerance to heat. *Br J Dermatol* 1975; 92:191–4
22. Panconesi E, Lotti T. Aquagenic urticaria. *Clin Dermatol* 1987;5:49–51
23. Parker RK, Crowe MJ, Guin JD. Aquagenic urticaria. *Cutis* 1992;50:283–4
24. Parks A, Camisa C. Aquagenic angioedema. *Cutis* 1986;37:465–6
25. Jorizzo JL, Smith EB. The physical urticarias: an update and review. *Arch Dermatol* 1982;118:194–201
26. Razon S, Vegni M, Schiaffino E, *et al.* Ganglioneuroblastoma and urticaria by physical agents. *Tumori* 1990;76:282–5
27. Kligman AM. The spectrum of contact urticaria. Wheals, erythema, and pruritus. *Dermatol Clin* 1990;8:57–60
28. Heese A, van Hintzenstern J, Peters KP, *et al.* Allergic and irritant reactions to rubber gloves in medical health services. Spectrum, diagnostic approach, and therapy. *J Am Acad Dermatol* 1991;25:831–9
29. McNeil DJ, Kinsella TD, Crawford AM, *et al.* The AHA syndrome: arthritis, hives and angioedema. *Rheumatol Int* 1987;7:277–9
30. Kulczycki A Jr. Aspartame-induced urticaria. *Ann Int Med* 1986;104:207–8

31. Pola J, Subiza J, Armentia A, *et al.* Urticaria caused by caffeine. *Ann Allergy* 1988;60:207–8.

32. Quirce Gancedo S, Freire P, Fernandez Rivas M, *et al.* Urticaria from caffeine. *J Allergy Clin Immunol* 1991; 88:680–1

33. Fisher AA. Contact urticaria due to cornstarch powder. *J Dermatol Surg Oncol* 1987;13:224

34. Quirce S, Tabar AI, Olaguibel JM, *et al.* Occupational contact urticaria syndrome caused by globe artichoke (Cynara scolymus). *J Allergy Clin Immunol* 1996;97:710–1

35. Giannattasio M, Serafini M, Guarrera P, *et al.* Contact urticaria from litchi fruit (Litchi chinensis Sonn.). *Contact Dermatitis* 1995;33:67

36. Veraldi S, Schianchi-Veraldi R. Contact urticaria from kiwi fruit. *Contact Dermatitis* 1990;22:244

37. Temesvari E, Becker K. Contact urticaria from watermelon in a patient with pollen allergy. *Contact Dermatitis* 1993;28:185–6

38. Tarvainen K, Salonen JP, Kanerva L, *et al.* Allergy and toxicodermia from shiitake mushrooms. *J Am Acad Dermatol* 1991;24:64–6

39. Sasai S, Takahashi K, Takahashi K, *et al.* Contact urticaria to rice. *Br J Dermatol* 1995;132:836–7

40. Valdivieso R, Moneo I, Pola J, *et al.* Occupational asthma and contact urticaria caused by buckwheat flour. *Ann Allergy* 1989;63:149–52

41. Maibach HI. Contact urticaria syndrome from mold on salami casing. *Contact Dermatitis* 1995;32:120–1

42. Valsecchi R, Cainelli T. Contact urticaria from nickel. *Contact Dermatitis* 1987;17:187

43. Jovanovic M, Oliwiecki S, Beck MH. Occupational contact urticaria from beef associated with hand eczema. *Contact Dermatitis* 1992;27:188–9

44. Boso EB, Brestel EP. Contact urticaria to cow milk. *Allergy* 1987;42:151–3

45. Melino M, Toni F, Riguzzi G. Immunologic contact urticaria to fish. *Contact Dermatitis* 1987;17:182

46. Mancuso G, Berdondini RM. Contact urticaria from dog saliva. *Contact Dermatitis* 1992;26:133

47. Tosti A, Melino M, Veronesi S. Contact urticaria to tobacco. *Contact Dermatitis* 1987;16:225–6

48. Monk BE. Contact urticaria to locusts. *Br J Dermatol* 1988;118:707–8

49. Karches F, Fuchs T. A strange manifestation of occupational contact urticaria due to mouse hair. *Contact Dermatitis* 1993;28:200

50. Barkoff JR. Urticaria secondary to a copper intrauterine device. *Int J Dermatol* 1976;15:594–5

51. Sherestz EF. Clinical pearl: symptomatic dermatographism as a cause of genital pruritus. *J Am Acad Dermatol* 1995;33:322

52. Sussman G, Stewart JH, Goodman MM. Earthquake urticaria. *Cutis* 1989;43:340

53. Schiavino D, Gentiloni N, Murzilli F, *et al.* Episodic angioedema with eosinophilia (Gleich syndrome). *Allergy Immunopathol* 1990;18:233–6

54. Ting S, Rauls DO, Ashbaugh P, *et al.* Ethanol-induced urticaria: a case report. *Ann Allergy* 1988;60: 527–30

55. Lewis J, Lieberman P, Treadwell G, *et al.* Exercise-induced urticaria, angioedema, and anaphylactoid episodes. *J Allergy Clin Immunol* 1981;68:432–7

56. Duffull SB. Begg EJ. Terfenadine ineffective in the prophylaxis of exercise-induced pruritus. *J Allergy Clin Immunol* 1992;89:916–7

57. Bushkell LL. Chronic urticaria and gallbladder disease: clearing after cholecystectomy. *Arch Dermatol* 1979;115:638

58. Taylor JS, Cassettari J, Wagner W, *et al.*. Contact urticaria and anaphylaxis to latex. *J Am Acad Dermatol* 1989;21:874–7

59. Effendy I, Gieler U, Bischoff R, *et al.* Anaphylaxis due to a latex vaginal vibrator. *Contact Dermatitis* 1992;27:318–9

60. Basomba A, Guerrero M, Campos A, *et al.* Grave anaphylactic-like reaction in the course of menstruation. A case report. *Allergy* 1987;42:477–9

61. Stockley RJ, Daneshmend TK. Painful urticaria heralding the appearance of Philadelphia chromosome positive acute myeloid leukaemia. *Clin Lab Haematol* 1986;8:161–2

62. Maheshwari N, Maheshwari V, Mobashir M. *Plasmodium vivax* malaria presenting with urticaria. *Postgrad Med J* 1989;65:266–7

63. Green RL, Een MA. Postcoital urticaria in a penicillin-sensitive patient: possible seminal transfer of penicillin. *J Am Med Assoc* 1985;254:531

64. Ebo DG, Stevens WJ, Bridts CH, *et al.* Human seminal plasma anaphylaxis (HSPA): case report and literature review. *Allergy* 1995;50:747–50

65. Poskitt BL, Wojnarowska FT, Shaw S. Semen contact urticaria. *J Roy Soc Med* 1995;88:108P–9P

66. Farrell FJ. Angioedema and urticaria as acute and late phase reactions to zinc fume exposure, with associated metal fume fever-like symptoms. *Am J Industr Med* 1987;12:331–7

67. Stafford CT. Urticaria as a sign of systemic disease. *Ann Allergy* 1990;64:264–70

68. Veraldi S, Schianchi-Veraldi R, Gasparini G. Urticaria probably caused by *Endolimax nana*. *Int J Dermatol* 1991;30:376

69. Hannuksela M, Haahtela T. Hypersensitivity reactions to food additives. *Allergy* 1987;42:561–75

70. Kennard CD, Ellis CN. Pharmacologic therapy for urticaria. *J Am Acad Dermatol* 1991;25:176–87

71. Pollack CV Jr, Romano TJ. Outpatient management of acute urticaria: the role of prednisone. *Ann Emerg Med* 1995;26:547–51

72. Jancelewicz Z. Controlled trial of H1 antagonists in the treatment of chronic idiopathic urticaria. *Ann Allergy* 1991;67:433–9

73. Kontou-Fili K, Maniatakou G, Demaka P, *et al*. Therapeutic effects of cetirizine in delayed pressure urticaria: clinicopathologic findings. *J Am Acad Dermatol* 1991;24:1090–3

74. Neittaanmaki H, Fraki JE. Combination of localized heat urticaria and cold urticaria. Release of histamine in suction blisters and successful treatment of heat urticaria with doxepin. *Clin Exp Dermatol* 1988;13:87–91

75. Moscati RM, Moore GP. Comparison of cimetidine and diphenhydramine in the treatment of acute urticaria. *Ann Emerg Med* 1990;19:12–5

76. Farnam J, Grant JA, Guernsey BG, *et al*. Successful treatment of chronic idiopathic urticaria and angioedema with cimetidine alone. *J Allergy Clin Immunol* 1984;73:842–5

77. Salo OP, Kauppinen K, Mannisto PT. Cimetidine increases the plasma concentration of hydroxyzine. *Acta Derm Venereol* 1986;66:349–50

78. Paul E, Bodeker RH. Treatment of chronic urticaria with terfenadine and ranitidine. A randomized double-blind study in 45 patients. *Eur J Clin Pharmacol* 1986;31:277–80

79. Bleehen SS, Thomas SE, Greaves MW, *et al*. Cimetidine and chlorpheniramine in the treatment of chronic idiopathic urticaria: a multi-centre randomized double-blind study. *Br J Dermatol* 1987;117:81–8

80. Kamide R, Niimura M, Ueda H, *et al*. Clinical evaluation of ketotifen for chronic urticaria: multicenter double-blind comparative study with clemastine. *Ann Allergy* 1989;62:322–5

81. McClean SP, Arreaza EE, Lett-Brown MA, *et al*. Refractory cholinergic urticaria successfully treated with ketotifen. *J Allergy Clin Immunol* 1989;83:738–41

82. Huston DP, Bressler RB, Kaliner M, *et al*. Prevention of mast-cell degranulation by ketotifen in patients with physical urticarias. *Ann Int Med* 1986;104:507–10

83. Kemp AS, Schembri G. An elimination diet for chronic urticaria of childhood. *Med J Aust* 985;143:234–5

84. Dayani A, Gould DJ, Campbell S. Delayed pressure urticaria, treatment with dapsone. *J Dermatol Treat* 1992;3:61–2

85. Johnsson M, Falk ES, Volden G. UVB treatment of factitious urticaria. *Photo-Dermatol* 1987;4:302–4

86. Olafsson JH, Larko O, Roupe G, *et al*. Treatment of chronic urticaria with PUVA or UVA plus placebo: a double-blind study. *Arch Dermatol Res* 1986;278:228–31

87. Locci F, Del Giacco GS. Treatment of chronic idiopathic urticaria with topical preparations: controlled study of oxatomide gel versus dechlorpheniramine cream. *Drugs Under Exp Clin Res* 1991;17:399–403

88. Barlow RJ, Macdonald DM, Black AK, *et al*. The effects of topical corticosteroids on delayed pressure urticaria. *Arch Dermatol Res* 1995;287:285–8

89. Lawlor F, Black AK, Murdoch RD, *et al*. Symptomatic dermographism: wealing, mast cells and histamine are decreased in the skin following long-term application of a potent topical corticosteroid. *Br J Dermatol* 1989;121:629–34

90. Jaffer AM. Sulfasalazine in the treatment of corticosteroid-dependent chronic idiopathic urticaria. *J Allergy Clin Immunol* 1991;88:964–5

91. Fradin MS, Ellis CN, Goldfarb MT, *et al*. Oral cyclosporin for severe chronic idiopathic urticaria and angioedema. *J Am Acad Dermatol* 1991;25:1065–7

92. Wong E, Eftekhari N, Greaves MW, *et al*. Beneficial effects of danazol on symptoms and laboratory changes in cholinergic urticaria. *Br J Dermatol* 1987;116:553–6

93. O'Donnel BF, Barlow RJ, Kobza Black A, *et al*. Response of severe chronic urticaria to intravenous immunoglobulin (IVIG). *Br J Dermatol* 1994;131 (Suppl 44):23–4

94. Weiner MJ. Methotrexate in corticosteroid-resistant urticaria. *Ann Int Med* 1989;110:848

95. Bressler RB, Sowell K, Huston DP. Therapy of chronic idiopathic urticaria with nifedipine: demonstration of beneficial effect in a double-blinded, placebo-controlled, crossover trial. *J Allergy Clin Immunol* 1989;83:756–63

96. Shertzer CL, Lookingbill DP. Effects of relaxation therapy and hypnotizability in chronic urticaria. *Arch Dermatol* 1987;123:913–6

97. Brestel EP, Thrush LB. The treatment of glucocortimcosteroid-dependent chronic urticaria with stanozolol. *J Allergy Clin Immunol* 1988;82:265–9

# Localized itching 8

Certain skin sites have a predilection for specific diseases which may present as localized pruritus. Discussing the site of itching rather than separating the many diseases helps the clinician to understand the differential diagnosis and, sometimes, the multifactorial nature of these processes

## Anal itching (pruritus ani)

### Predisposing factors

Predisposing factors include poor or excessive hygiene, fecal residue, excessive moisture, scratching behavior and topical medications.

- Half of patients in one series[1] had poorly formed stools or incomplete stool evacuation with resultant frequent soiling; diarrhea can exacerbate the problem.

  > Dietary control of aberrant bowel habits may help

- Anal sphincter function may be abnormal in some patients[2,3]
- Excessive sweating and obesity may predispose towards intertriginous dermatitis due to bacterial and/or candidal overgrowth
- Feelings of shame and guilt may exacerbate the condition
- Patients tended to worsen the problem by application of topical agents and overzealous cleaning; contact sensitivity to local anesthetic agents is well-recognized
- Rare causes

  > Although neoplastic conditions such as extra-mammary Paget's and cutaneous T-cell lymphoma may result in itching, these malignancies are rare and should generally only be considered in treatment-refractory disease[4]

  > Intravenous doses of hydrocortisone sodium phosphate can cause burning or itching in the anorectal area[5]

Some medications may irritate the enteric or rectal mucosa and may contribute to itching including colchicine, mineral oil and quinidine

Diets rich in certain foods such as popcorn may mechanically irritate the area

Coffee has been hypothesized to exacerbate the condition, as has beer, chocolate, citrus fruit, pork, soda, spices, tea and tomatoes[6]

Symptomatic dermatographism may be an occasional cause and would prompt effective treatment with non-sedating antihistamines

### Physical examination

Search for:
- Parasites[7] (especially *Enterobius vermicularis* (pinworms) and *Entamoeba histolytica*)
- Trauma
- Hemorrhoids
- Infections including candidiasis, tinea, erythrasma, herpes, and others
- Anal fissure[8]
- Mucosal prolapse
- Fistulas
- Neoplasia (including warts)
- Active dermatitis or psoriasis
- Underlying skin disease (e.g. lichen sclerosis, psoriasis, etc.)

### Treatment

The essentials of the treatment consist of keeping the perianal skin scrupulously clean and dry[9–11].

- Stop vigorous cleaning and all over-the-counter preparations including cleaning pads, detergents, soaps and cleaning solutions[6]
- Allow only water
- If patients are not allergic to the fragrances, recommend use of pre-moistened wipes

Stool softeners or bran supplements may help patients with irregular bowel habits. If there are no objective findings to the contrary, reassure patients that there is no evidence of serious internal disease, infection or cancer.

- If it seems appropriate, advise dietary discretion with avoidance of potentially offending foods[6]

Use of mild to moderate potency topical corticosteroid ointments for several weeks benefits patients; however, long-term use of topical corticosteroids, especially medium to high potency corticosteroids, may produce permanent atrophy[12].

- If lichenification is present, using a stronger potency agent for limited periods is acceptable to penetrate the thickened epidermis
- Unless there are no alternatives, avoid long-term (>1–2 months) use of topical corticosteroid agents due to real risk of skin atrophy
    This rule is particularly important for patients using potent or superpotent topical corticosteroids
- If candidiasis is present or suspected, topical therapy with nystatin powder or ointment or alternatively an azole antifungal agent should be used

For patients with intractable pruritus ani[13]:

- Reconsider the initial diagnosis and review all of the contactants[14]
    Epicutaneous patch testing to identify allergens if appropriate

Even exotic contactants can cause anal itching: Ginkgo tree proctitis has been reported[15], as has sensitivity to fragrance in toilet tissue[16]

- Consider neoplastic and structural etiologies[17]
- Although not a first-line treatment, reported effective treatments include[18]:

    Ablation with helium–neon laser or cryosurgery[19,20]

    Intracutaneous injection of methylene blue (methylthionine chloride) 0.5%

    Intralesional triamcinolone injection may be beneficial[21]

- Consider the psychological factors which may chronify the condition[22,23]
- Listen to the patient, provide support, and accept how uncomfortable and even disabling this condition can be[6]
- Consider adding a systemic antipruritic agent such as doxepin or amitriptyline to decrease aberrant sensations and provide a calming effect

    If neuropsychiatric disease is perceived to be an important part of this condition, appropriate pharmacologic and psychologic intervention may be necessary

## Eyelid itching

Eyelid itching may be due to a number of inflammatory dermatoses, the differentiation of which depends upon the presenting signs and symptoms.

### Airborne allergen blepharitis

Eyelid dermatitis may be due to pollen and other allergens, and is seen associated with conjunctival inflammation. The key to diagnosis is to examine the conjuctivae for injection and other signs of inflammation and to perform an appropriate history[24,25].

Systemic antihistamines, especially the minimally sedating or non-sedating antihistamines, can help, i.e., astemazole, cetirizine and lorati-dine. Topical agents are clearly helpful and one or more agents can be used.

- Ketorelac tromethamine ophthalmic solu-tion, a non-steroidal anti-inflammatory agent, inhibits prostaglandin synthesis and is effective in decreasing itching of seasonal allergic conjunctivitis
- Cromolyn sodium ophthalmic solution stabilizes mast cells and also aids the itching of seasonal allergic conjunctivitis
- Topical corticosteroid agents are available for cutaneous or ophthalmic use

  Cutaneous agents are reviewed in chapter 11: Treatment. They are appropriate for eyelids but not conjuctivae

  Ophthalmic agents may be used on both eye-lids and conjunctivae

  Note that long-term use of ocular cortico-steroid agents may predispose the patient towards the development of eyelid atrophy, cataracts and glaucoma

### Behavior modification

Advise patients to avoid scrubbing, scratching and rubbing and the use of harsh cleansing agents and exfoliants.

### Contact dermatitis

Unilateral or bilateral itching, redness, and lichenification suggest this disorder, but identi-fying a contactant responsible is a formidable challenge.

### Eye cosmetics

Eye cosmetics may be the cause of either irritant or allergic contact dermatitis[26,27].

- Eye cosmetics include eye shadows, eye shadow setting creams, under-eye conceal-ers, eye-liners, mascaras, artificial eyelashes, eyebrow pencils[28], and eye makeup removers[29]

- Vehicles, preservatives and stabilizers are potential causes
- Nickel in an eye pencil, in an eyelash curler[30], and in contact lens cleaner[31,32] were identified as causative in different patients

  Patients using contact lenses are exposed to an entire array of solutions with active ingre-dients and preservatives

- Nail polish and other potential contact allergens may cause contact dermatitis of the eyelid but not elsewhere
- Allergy to cosmetics, toiletries and frag-rances may occur after prolonged use
- Topical medicaments including lanolin and neomycin are particularly likely to cause allergic contact dermatitis (Figure 48)

As with all other conditions, patients may inad-vertently make the condition worse by overly enthusiastic scrubbing technique, the use of harsh cleansers or gritty scrubs, and the applica-tion of exfoliants. Patch testing may help iden-tify the mysterious allergen, and should be performed in most patients with treatment-resistant, chronic blepharitis[33].

- Patch test reactions are particularly likely to nickel sulphate, methylchloroisothiazoli-none/methylisothiazolinone, fragrance-mix, cinnamic alcohol, diazolidinyl urea, and neomycin sulfate[34,35]

### Seborrheic dermatitis

Seborrheic dermatitis is not confined to the scalp, but may involve the ears, eyebrows, eye-lids, lateral nose, central chest, and other loca-tions (see Figure 8.1).

- Disease of the eyelids may be associated with conjunctivitis

Clues to this diagnosis include evident sebor-rheic dermatitis elsewhere: thick, adherent

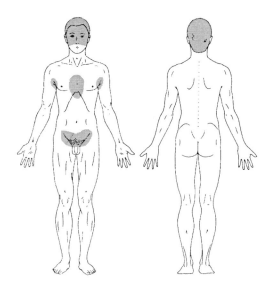

**Figure 8.1** Areas typically affected by seborrheic dermatitis

scale. The pathogenesis of seborrheic dermatitis is unknown, but it may be related to colonization with *Malessezia furfur*.

### Treatment
- Gentle scrubbing of the lids with baby shampoo and water may help remove crusts
- Topical antifungal creams or shampoos (e.g. ketoconazole) may also diminish seborrheic dermatitis severity, but should not be instilled into the eyes

### Atopic dermatitis

Atopic dermatitis may occur anywhere on the cutaneous surface, and the eyelids are particularly likely to become irritated given their sensitivity and the numerous cosmetics and other agents applied.

- Atopic patients have lowered itch thresholds, and often rub to the point of lichenification
- Low-potency topical corticosteroid ointments applied for limited periods can decrease itching, scaling and lichenification

### Miscellaneous causes of eyelid itching
- Sjogren's syndrome[36]
- Pediculosis
- Lichen planus of the eyelids is a rare event[37]
- Lupus erythematosus
- Psoriasis vulgaris

## Scalp itching

The differential diagnosis of scalp itching is extensive[38] and the following conditions may play a role.

### Atopic dermatitis

The scalp is a common site for atopic dermatitis, especially in children[39].

- It is not uncommon for atopic patients to have active dermatitis confined to the occipital scalp

Therapy is similar to other dermatitic conditions in the use of mild to medium potency corticosteroid solutions or ointments as the mainstay of therapy.

### Contact dermatitis

Patients often recall an inciting event and subsequent chronic scratching or rubbing. Irritant or allergic contact dermatitis may be precipitated by permanent wave solutions, relaxing solutions, hair coloring agents, home hair-care products, and other contactants[39].

- Epicutaneous patch testing may be useful in allergic contact dermatitis if the suspected potential allergen is not otherwise identified
- Therapy may consist of:

  Coal tar shampoo or shampoo admixed with corticosteroid agents

  Topical corticosteroid agents ranging from mild-potency agents such as fluocinolone oil under occlusion overnight to clobetasol solution daily

## Folliculitis

May be seen in association with seborrheic dermatitis or as an independent itchy condition Folliculitis can respond to systemic or topical antistaphylococcal therapy.

## Lichen simplex chronicus

Any disease entity that itches can be chronified through scratching or rubbing behavior, and the scalp is no exception. A common site is the posterior scalp, and this condition may be associated with traumatic, usually reversible, hair loss.

■ Therapy may consist of:

Potent or superpotent topical corticosteroid agents which may also be used under occlusion with a shower cap

Intralesional corticosteroid injections are also occasionally helpful

## Neurotic excoriations

Patients typically present with persistent scratching signs such as excoriations without primary lesions.

■ Some patients with seborrheic dermatitis and other pruritic primary dermatoses have no evident erythema or scale, yet have visible excoriations
■ Neurotic excoriation is a diagnosis of exclusion, and assumes one has treated subclinical dermatitis with appropriate interventions

The use of neuropsychiatric systemic agents, especially those with antihistaminic effect, may prove useful. If obsessive–compulsive behavior constitutes a major part of the patient's problem, imipramine can be a useful agent.

■ Some patients who have no primary skin disease and have no excoriations nevertheless complain of intense itching

Some of these patients may have psychogenic itching, whereas others may have primary neurologic disease such as mononeuritis multiplex

Differentiation of these disorders is challenging to the clinician

## Pediculosis

Although pediculosis is most common in school children, it may be seen in all ages[40].

■ The author was infested while serving in his dermatology residency!

See further discussion in chapter 5: Infections, infestations, bites and stings.

## Psoriasis

At times, psoriasis can be difficult to differentiate from seborrheic dermatitis. It appears with characteristic bright erythematous scaling patches and plaques[41].

■ Therapy may consist of:

Coal tar shampoo with or without salicylic acid

Topical corticosteroid agents ranging from mild-potency agents such as fluocinolone oil under occlusion overnight to clobetasol solution daily

Topical vitamin D analogs such as calcipotriene[42]

Ultraviolet phototherapy – facilitated with the use of scalp UVB wands

## Seborrheic dermatitis

This may present without visible erythema, scale, hair casts, or other objective findings, or may have the characteristic mild erythema, greasy scale and excoriations[43,44] (Figures 49–51).

119

- Therapy may consist of:

    Therapeutic shampoos containing selenium sulfide, zinc pyrithione, coal tar, salicylic acid, cetrimide, chloroxine, or ketoconazole may help, as may shampoos mixed with mild corticosteroid agents such as fluocinolone

    Topical corticosteroid agents ranging from mild-potency agents such as fluocinolone oil under occlusion overnight to clobetasol solution daily

    Ointments and solutions of topical azole antifungal agents[45] or lithium succinate[46] may help

## Other rare or uncommonly itchy dermatoses[38]

- Acne keloidalis
- Angiosarcoma
- Book lice (*Liposcelis mendax*) infestations[47]
- Dermatomyositis[48]
- Dissecting cellulitis (perifolliculitis abscedens et suffodiens)
- Eosinophilic pustulosis[49]
- Ectodermal dysplasia, ectrodactyly, cleft lip/palate syndrome[50]
- Fiberglass dermatitis
- Hailey-Hailey disease[51]
- Histiocytosis X[52]
- Lichen planus and planopilaris
- Lupus erythematosus
- Neuropsychiatric diseases
- Pityriasis rubra pilaris
- Scabies, particularly crusted in the immunocompromised host[53-55]
- Tinea capitis (common but itching is uncommon)

## Scrotal itching

Predisposing factors include poor or excessive hygiene, excessive moisture, scratching behavior, and topical medications (Figure 52). To treat, keep the scrotal skin scrupulously clean and dry and stop the use of all over-the-counter preparations, cleaning pads, detergents, soaps and cleaning solutions except water. A mild to moderate corticosteroid cream or ointment should be prescribed on a temporary basis[56].

## Predisposing factors

- Excessive sweating and obesity may predispose towards intertriginous dermatitis due to bacterial and/or candidal overgrowth[57]
- The barrier function of the scrotum is poor, and thus percutaneous penetration of irritants and allergens is enhanced

    Topical agents that do not produce irritant reaction elsewhere on the skin readily produce scrotal irritant dermatitis[58]

- Feelings of shame and guilt may exacerbate the condition
- Patients tended to worsen the problem by application of topical agents and overzealous cleaning; contact sensitivity to local anesthetic agents is well-recognized
- Although neoplastic conditions such as extramammary Paget's may result in itching[59], these malignancies are rare and should generally only be considered in treatment-refractory disease
- Riboflavin deficiency was said to be a cause of scrotal dermatitis in a study in southern China[60]

## Physical examination

Search for:

- Neoplasia (e.g. Bowenoid papulosis, Paget's disease[59], idiopathic calcinosis of the scrotum[61])
- Active atopic, contact or seborrheic dermatitis
- Psoriasis
- Condyloma acuminata
- Fungal infections

- Candidiasis is most commonly found
- Tinea infections may occasionally be seen
- White piedra has been reported to cause scrotal itching[62]
- Other underlying skin disease (e.g. balanitis xerotica obliterans, etc.)
- Parasites including *Enterobius,* pediculosis or scabies

## Treatment

The essentials of the treatment consist of keeping the scrotal skin scrupulously clean and dry.

- Stop vigorous cleaning and all over-the-counter preparations including cleaning pads, detergents, soaps and cleaning solutions
- Allow only warm water as a cleansing agent and suggest patting dry with a soft towel
- If there are no objective findings to the contrary, reassure patients that there is no evidence of serious internal disease, infection or cancer

Mild to moderate potency topical corticosteroid ointment for several weeks benefits patients, however, long-term use of topical corticosteroids, especially medium to high potency corticosteroids, may produce permanent atrophy.

- If lichenification is present, using a stronger potency agent for limited periods is acceptable to penetrate the thickened epidermis
- If candidiasis is present or suspected, topical therapy with nystatin powder or ointment or an azole antifungal agent should be used

For patients with intractable scrotal itching:

- Reconsider the initial diagnosis and review all of the contactants, including clothing that contacts the area
- Avoid use of fragrances in cleansing products, detergents, and fabric softeners

- Epicutaneous patch testing can help to identify relevant allergens
- Consider adding a systemic antipruritic agent such as doxepin or amitriptyline to decrease aberrant sensations and provide a calming effect
- Use of extremely constricting underwear should be discouraged

## Notalgia paresthetica

Other names for this condition include subscapular pruritus, posterior pigmented pruritic patch, hereditary localized pruritus[63,64]. It typically involves a unilateral isolated sensory neuropathy involving the posterior primary rami of thoracic nerves T2 through T6. There is an increase in the sensory epidermal innervation in the affected skin areas in notalgia paresthetica, which could contribute to the symptoms[65].

- Clinically, it presents as unilateral localized itching of the back overlying the scapulae

  Chronic scratching behavior may create lichenification, hyperpigmentation, and macular amyloidosis in the distribution of the itching[63,66–68]

- Anecdotal experience suggests potent corticosteroid agents or topical local anesthetics (2.5% lidocaine and 2.5% prilocaine) may help, and experimental evidence suggests that it may respond to topical capsaicin[69–71]
- Recurrence following cessation of therapy is typical

## Solar pruritus (brachioradial pruritus)

This is an uncommon condition affecting the lateral aspects of one or both arms. It is primarily seen in Caucasian people living in the tropics or subtropics with outdoor occupations or avocations[72–74].

■ It may be the same condition as forearm neuropathy and pruritus as described by Massey and Massey[75]

This seems to be a benign neuropathy. Roentgenographic evidence of cervical vertebral osteoarthritis may be found in some patients. Biopsy specimens are non-specific, so it does not seem to be a primary skin condition. Clinically, the itching is usually bilateral and affects the lateral aspects of the arm with no primary lesions.

■ Since there are no primary lesions, this excludes polymorphous light eruption, solar urticaria, chronic actinic dermatitis etc., which all have active lesions

> Polymorphous light eruption sine eruption has been reported, but may represent solar pruritus[76]

■ In one study[77], the most commonly affected area was the elbow area superficial to the brachioradialis and extensor carpi longus muscles, but extension of the pruritus to include the forearm and/or upper arm was common

■ Solar pruritis is more common in areas of intense solar exposure, but sunshine may not be pathogenic

When considering treatment, capsaicin has been found to be beneficial[77,78] and systemic doxepin or amitriptyline may also be beneficial.

## Vulvar itching

Itching of the female genitalia maybe due to a wide variety of conditions including vaginitis, irritant or allergic contact dermatitis (mucositis), lichen sclerosus et atrophicus, other primary skin diseases, and neoplasia. Although chronic genital itching may have a psychiatric overlay and has some similarities with chronic pain syndromes, the majority of patients have organic diseases[79].

■ Patients with this distressing, embarrassing problem may compound the problem by avoiding professional help for months or years

■ Alternatively, despite real symptoms they may be told they have no active disease and there is nothing that can be done

■ Spending a moment to listen to patients may one of your most valuable interventions

Contact sensitivity is a common cause of vulvar itching (Figure 53). If suspected, reconsider the initial diagnosis and review all of the contactants. Epicutaneous patch testing may help identify the allergens and may be appropriate in all patients with chronic vulvar itching[80]. Consider allergy to:

■ Fragrances in laundry products, vaginal perfumes, douches, soaps and other cleansing products; even sensitivity to fragrance in sanitary pads[81,82] has been reported to cause itching

■ Preservatives, fragrances or active ingredients in creams, ointments and other topical agents

> Note that patients can be allergic to individual topical corticosteroid, antibacterial, and antifungal agents

■ Active ingredients, preservatives, or devices used for contraception

■ A drug hypersensitivity reaction to enalapril has been reported as localized vulvovaginal itching[83]

■ Allergy to consort allergens ranging from colognes and other cosmetics, toiletries and fragrances used by sexual partner(s)

■ Allergy to semen[84,85] and partner's sweat contents have been reported

> A patient reported severe vulvar itching following three episodes of intercourse due to sensitivity to the drug thioridazine in her sexual partner's semen[86]

Examine for evidence of:

- Diabetes – pruritus vulvae is three times more likely in diabetic women, and it may be a sign of poor diabetes control[87]
- Parasites (*Trichomonas, Enterobius*, scabies and lice, in particular (Figure 54))
- *Enterobius vermicularis* live adult worms have been found in the high vagina[88]
- Trauma (may be a sign of repetitive excoriation, sexual abuse, etc.)
- Neoplasia
- Active dermatitis
- Candidiasis or tinea infections
- Underlying skin disease (e.g. lichen sclerosis et atrophicus, psoriasis, etc.)

Diagnostic tests may help establish the diagnosis and guide appropriate therapy:

- Potassium hydroxide and wet mount
- Cultures
- Skin biopsy – perform a full thickness skin biopsy (punch or excision) of anogenital lesions that do not respond to conventional therapy
- Epicutaneous patch testing

## Treatment

### Candidal and fungal infections

Three-quarters of all women will experience at least one yeast infection in their life; this may occur during pregnancy. Common yeast organisms include *Candida albicans, C. tropicalis* and *C. glabrata*; non-albicans species are more resistant to imidazole agents.

- Infection responds to appropriate antifungal therapy which can be administered intravaginally (e.g. terconazole suppository at bedtime for 3 nights) or with systemic fluconazole or itraconazole (100 mg/day for 7 days)
- Chronic candidiasis should alert the physician to search for diabetes or human immunodeficiency virus infection
- Some susceptible patients may benefit from a single 100 mg fluconazole dose during each menstrual period to decrease the risk of recurrence; alternatively one week each month of daily fluconazole therapy may be indicated

### Condyloma

Investigation of partners may be useful, but frequently partners are infected with different human papilloma virus types than are causing the active disease. Weakly destructive techniques including ablation with laser, cryosurgery, trichloroacetic acid, podofilox or excision may be effective[89]. The techniques are reviewed in major texts of gynecology and dermatology.

### Bacterial infections

Gonorrhea, chlamydia, T-mycoplasma infection, and other infections may cause vaginal itching and should be considered in the differential diagnosis[90,91]. Therapies are reviewed in major texts of gynecology and dermatology.

*Bacterial vaginosis*

- Previously called *Haemophilus vaginalis, Gardnerella vaginalis*, and nonspecific vaginitis; now it is recognized as a condition with greater than normal quantities of anaerobic bacteria
- Bacterial vaginosis is most commonly seen in reproductive-aged women
- Metronidazole vaginal gel one applicator full twice daily for 5 days or clindamycin vaginal cream one applicator full at bedtime for 7 days
- Metronidazole 500mg orally twice daily for 7 days or 2000mg as a single oral dose

### Trichomonas

Infection results in signs and symptoms of vaginitis and this can be diagnosed in the office setting by performing a microscopic evaluation.

Note this pathogen has been declining in prevalence over the past two decades[90].

- Metronidazole vaginal gel one applicator full twice daily for 5 days or metronidazole 2000 mg as a single oral dose; treat the sexual partner with the same oral dose

### Irritant or allergic dermatitis

If possible, work to remove any potential irritants or allergens, and advise discontinuation of excessive bathing and douching behavior.

- Irritant or allergic dermatitis should respond to the use of mild-potency topical corticosteroid ointments for several weeks
- Long-term use of topical corticosteroids, especially medium to high potency corticosteroids, may produce permanent atrophy
- When recalcitrant, brief courses of systemic corticosteroids may provide needed relief

### Lichen sclerosus (et atrophicus)

- See Figures 8.2, 55, 56
- Clobetasol ointment applied twice daily for two weeks to two months often produces rapid response
- Topical testosterone proprionate has been reported effective[92], but may be less effective than clobetasol[93]; it also has risk of androgenizing effects
- In one study[94], nine out of 12 patients had severe itching relieved by cryosurgery

### Psoriasis and other dermatoses

Typical signs and symptoms of psoriasis, lichen planus, and other chronic itchy dermatoses are usually found elsewhere in patients with vulvar psoriasis; and treatment is typical for the same condition elsewhere.

- Realization that the anogenital skin may be affected by the same conditions that occur elsewhere should make the clinician examine beyond the site of chief complaint

- Other rare skin conditions may cause vulvar itching or burning including pemphigus, benign familial pemphigus, pemphigoid, linear IgA disease, angiolymphoid hyperplasia with eosinophilia[95], and dermatitis herpetiformis

### Vulvar vestibulitis

This is the sensation of severe burning, pain, or rawness on vestibular touch or vaginal entry; itching may be a component of this discomfort.

- Irritants may play a major role
- Orifices of Skene's and Bartholin's glands are erythematous, itchy, and painful
- Topical benzocaine or lidocaine ointment, topical corticosteroid agents and intralesional interferon may be effective
- Occasionally destructive techniques such as cryosurgery and vestibulectomy with vaginal advancement may be required

### Intractable vulvar itching

Educate patients that all skin diseases are treatable but cure cannot always be expected.

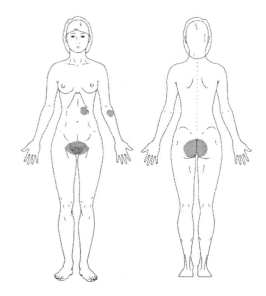

**Figure 8.2** Lichen sclerosus et atrophicus

■ Effective management is defined by whether a topical or systemic agent reliably controls outbreaks or symptoms when it is used

At some point, consider cessation of all topical therapies and use of systemic prednisone (1 mg/kg/day for 2 weeks combined with fluconazole 100 mg/day for two weeks); this may offer dramatic relief.

■ Contact sensitivity is possible to topical products, intravaginal products, and anything that contacts the genital area
■ Consider replacing all topical agents with systemic equivalents

Readdress the issue of neoplastic processes; biopsy or rebiopsy if necessary[96,97]. Rare causes of anogenital pruritus include cloacogenic carcinoma[98], extramammary Paget's disease, basal cell carcinoma[99], squamous cell carcinoma, vulvar intraepithelial neoplasia, pseudolymphoma[100] and syringoma[101,102].

■ If there are no objective findings to the contrary, reassure patients that there is no evidence of serious internal disease, infection or cancer
■ Other rare reports of vulvar itching include:

Itching as a manifestation of seasonal allergic disease[103]

Itching due to food allergy[104]

Itching due to symptomatic dermatographism[105]

Itching due to enalapril ingestion[83]

Although not first-line treatments, reported effective treatments include:

■ Systemic antipruritic agents including amitriptyline or doxepin in doses ranging from 10 to 100 mg per day

Note that four weeks of therapy may be required to achieve the desired therapeutic effect, and patient education about this expectation may help decrease anxiety

■ Absolute alcohol injection in the vulva[106,107]
■ Treatment of pruritus vulvae by means of $CO_2$ laser[108] or the flashlamp-excited dye laser[109]
■ 78% of patients in one study[110] achieved more than one month's relief with subcutaneous injection of triamcinolone acetonide

### Essential (dysesthetic) vulvodynia

This is a diagnosis of exclusion and should only be considered after long-term evaluation and empiric therapeutic intervention[79]. Also known as pudendal neuralgia, it is defined as essentially constant pain or itch in the area supplied by the pudendal nerve[111].

■ Physical findings are rarely seen, and many of the findings are secondary to scratching or rubbing behavior and application of irritants or allergens
■ Treatment involves systemic antipruritic agents including amitriptyline or doxepin in doses ranging from 10–100 mg daily

Note that 4 weeks of therapy may be required to achieve the desired therapeutic effect and patient education about this expectation may help decrease anxiety

Anticonvulsant therapy with carbamazepine or diphenylhydantoin may also be effective

### Psychogenic vulvar itching

Like essential vulvodynia, this is a diagnosis of exclusion and should only be considered after long-term evaluation and empiric therapeutic intervention.

■ Symptoms may include itching or burning sensations, and signs may include redness, burning and discomfort[112]
■ Depression may be the most common psychiatric disease responsible, but occasionally this may be due to schizophrenia, dementia, or personality disorders

# References

1. Smith LE, Henrichs D, McCullah RD. Prospective studies on the etiology and treatment of pruritus ani. *Dis Colon Rectum* 1982;25:358–63

2. Allan A, Ambrose NS, Silverman S, *et al.* Physiological study of pruritus ani. *Br J Surg* 1987; 74:576–9

3. Farouk R, Duthie GS, Pryde A, *et al.* Abnormal transient internal sphincter relaxation in idiopathic pruritus ani: physiological evidence from ambulatory monitoring. *Br J Surg* 1994;81:603–6

4. Stevens HP, Ostlere LS, Rustin MH. Perianal bowenoid papulosis presenting with pruritus ani. *Br J Dermatol* 1993;129:648–9

5. Novak E, Gilbertson TJ, Seckman CE, *et al.* Anorectal pruritus after intravenous hydrocortisone sodium succinate and sodium phosphate. *Clin Pharmacol Therapeutics* 1976;20:109–12

6. Aucoin EJ. Pruritus ani. *Postgrad Med* 1987;82:76–80

7. Gilman RH, Marquis GS, Miranda E. Prevalence and symptoms of *Enterobius vermicularis* infections in a Peruvian shanty town. *Trans Roy Soc Trop Med Hyg* 1991;85:761–4

8. Petros JG, Rimm EB, Robillard RJ. Clinical presentation of chronic anal fissures. *Am Surgeon* 1993;59:666–8

9. Alexander-Williams J. Pruritus ani. What to do, what not to do to control this infernal itch. *Postgrad Med* 1985;77:56–9,62,65

10. Bassford T. Treatment of common anorectal disorders. *Am Fam Phys* 1992;45:1787–94

11. Daniel GL, Longo WE, Vernava AM III. Pruritus ani. Causes and concerns. *Dis Colon Rectum* 1994; 37:670–4

12. Goldman L, Kitzmiller KW. Perianal atrophoderma from topical corticosteroids. *Arch Dermatol* 1973; 107:611–2

13. Eusebio EB, Graham J, Mody N. Treatment of intractable pruritus ani. *Dis Colon Rectum* 1990;33: 770–2

14. Handfield-Jones SE, Cronin E. Contact sensitivity to lignocaine. *Clin Exp Dermatol* 1993;18:342–3

15. Becker LE, Skipworth GB. Ginkgo-tree dermatitis, stomatitis, and proctitis. *J Am Med Assoc* 1975;231: 1162–3

16. Brody RS. Irritation from scented toilet tissue. *J Am Med Assoc* 1983;249:473

17. Hill VA, Hall-Smith P, Smith NP. Cutaneous T-cell lymphoma presenting with atypical perianal lesions. *Dermatology* 1995;190:313–6

18. Pirone E, Infantino A, Masin A, *et al.* Can proctological procedures resolve perianal pruritus and mycosis? A prospective study of 23 cases. *Int J Colorectal Dis* 1992;7:18–20

19. Detrano SJ. Cryotherapy for chronic nonspecific pruritus ani. *J Dermatol Surg Oncol* 1984;10:483–4

20. Matsiak IuO, Varyvoda IM, Slobodian IeR, *et al.* The use of low-intensity laser therapy under sanatorium-health resort conditions in proctology patients. *Vrachebnoe Delo* 1993;5–6:150–2

21. Minvielle L, Hernandez VL. The use of intralesional triamcinolone hexacetonide in treatment of idiopathic pruritus ani. *Dis Colon Rect* 1969;12:340–3

22. Koblenzer CS. Pruritus ani. In *Psychocutaneous Disease*, Orlando: Grune & Stratton, 1987:220–221

23. Magni G, Pirone E, Dodi G. Two cases of psychogenic pruritus ani in the same family. *Ann Gastroenterol Hepatol* 1987;23:233–4

24. Friedlaender MH. A review of the causes and treatment of bacterial and allergic conjunctivitis. *Clin Therap* 1995;17:800–10

25. Granstein RD. Skin and mucous membrane disorders. In Albert D, Jakobiec F, Robinson N, eds. *Principles and Practice of Ophthalmology*, Vol 5. Philadelphia: WB Saunders, 1994;3154–9

26. Bartunek CK, Brodell LP, Brodell RT. The skin and the eye: a multidisciplinary approach. *Dermatol Nursing* 1996;8.263–279,284

27. Dooms-Goossens A. Cosmetics as causes of allergic contact dermatitis. *Cutis* 1993;52:316–20

28. Zemba C, Romaguera C, Vilaplana J. Allergic contact dermatitis from nickel in an eye pencil. *Contact Dermatitis* 1992;27:116

29. Ross JS, White IR. Eyelid dermatitis due to cocamidopropyl betaine in an eye make-up remover. *Contact Dermatitis* 1991;25:64

30. Brandrup F. Nickel eyelid dermatitis from an eyelash curler. *Contact Dermatitis* 1991;25:77

31. Vilaplana J, Romaguera C, Grimalt F. Contact dermatitis from nickel and cobalt in a contact lens cleaning solution. *Contact Dermatitis* 1991;24:232–3

32. Yorav S, Ronnen M, Suster S. Eyelid contact dermatitis due to Liquifilm wetting solution of hard contact lenses. *Contact Dermatitis* 1987 17:314–5

33. Fisher AA. Part II: The management of eyelid dermatitis in patients with 'status cosmeticus', the cosmetic intolerance syndrome. *Cutis* 1990;46: 199–201

34. Nethercott JR, Nield G, Holness DL. A review of 79 cases of eyelid dermatitis. *J Am Acad Dermatol* 1989; 21:223–30

35. Valsecchi R, Imberti G, Martino D, *et al.* Eyelid dermatitis: an evaluation of 150 patients. *Contact Dermatitis* 1992;27:143–7

36. Katayama I, Koyano T, Nishioka K. Prevalence of eyelid dermatitis in primary Sjogren's syndrome. *Int J Dermatol* 1994;33:421–4

37. Itin PH, Buechner SA, Rufli T: Lichen planus of the eyelids. *Dermatology* 1995;191:350–1

38. Bernhardt JD. The itchy scalp. *J Ger Dermatol* 1996;3:8–12

39. Goh CL. Eczema of the face, scalp and neck: an epidemiological comparison by site. *J Dermatol* 1989; 16:223–6

40. Elgart ML. Pediculosis. *Dermatol Clin* 1990;8: 219–28

41. Farber EM, Nall L. Natural history and treatment of scalp psoriasis. *Cutis* 1992;49:396–400

42. Green C, Ganpule M, Harris D, *et al.* Comparative effects of calcipotriol (MC903) solution and placebo (vehicle of MC903) in the treatment of psoriasis of the scalp. *Br J Dermatol* 1994;130:483–7

43. Janniger CK, Schwartz RA. Seborrheic dermatitis. *Am Fam Phys* 1995;52.149–55,159–60

44. Osment LS. Dermatoses of the scalp. *J Fam Pract* 1979;8:1217–33

45. Sei Y, Hamaguchi T, Ninomiya J, *et al.* .Seborrhoeic dermatitis: treatment with anti-mycotic agents. *J Dermatol* 1994;21:334–40

46. Anonymous. A double-blind, placebo-controlled, multicenter trial of lithium succinate ointment in the treatment of seborrheic dermatitis. Efalith Multi-center Trial Group. *J Am Acad Dermatol* 1992;26: 452–7

47. Burgess I, Coulthard M, Heaney J. Scalp infestation by *Liposcelis mendax. Br J Dermatol* 1991;125:400–1

48. Kasteler JS, Callen JP. Scalp involvement in dermatomyositis. Often overlooked or misdiagnosed. *J Am Med Assoc* 1994;272:1939–41

49. Taieb A, Bassan-Andrieu LB, Maleville J. Eosinophilic pustulosis of the scalp in childhood. *J Am Acad Dermatol* 1992;27:55–60

50. Trueb RM, Bruckner-Tuderman L, Wyss M, *et al.* Scalp dermatitis, distinctive hair abnormalities and atopic disease in the ectrodactyly-ectodermal dysplasia-clefting syndrome. *Br J Dermatol* 1995;132: 621–5

51. Marren P, Burge S. Seborrhoeic dermatitis of the scalp – a manifestation of Hailey-Hailey disease in a predisposed individual? *Br J Dermatol* 1992;126: 294–6

52. Lookingbill DP. Histiocytosis X confined to the skin of the scalp. *J Am Acad Dermatol* 1984;10:968–9

53. Alinovi A, Pretto ME. Scabietic infestation of the scalp: a clue for puzzling relapses. *J Am Acad Dermatol* 1994;31:492–3

54. Duran C, Tamayo L, de la Luz Orozco M, *et al.* Scabies of the scalp mimicking seborrheic dermatitis in immunocompromised patients. *Ped Dermatol* 1993;10:136–8

55. Hubler WR Jr. Epidemic Norwegian scabies. *Arch Dermatol* 1976;112:179–81

56. Kantor GR. What to do about pruritus scroti. *Postgrad Med* 1990;88:95–102

57. Woskoff A, Carabelli S, Hoffman M. Dermatitis of the scrotum. *Medicina Cutanea Ibero-Latino-Americana* 1982;10:37–40

58. Fisher AA. Unique reactions of scrotal skin to topical agents. *Cutis* 1989;44:445–7

59. Satoh Y, Kanbayashi H, Azuma A, *et al.* An autopsy case of Paget's disease of the scrotum with general metastasis. *Gan No Rinsho – Jap J Cancer Clin* 1987; 33:1294–301

60. Lo CS. Riboflavin status of adolescents in southern China: average intake of riboflavin and clinical findings. *Med J Aust* 1984;141:635–7

61. Moskovitz B, Bolkier M, Ginesin Y, *et al.* Idiopathic calcinosis of scrotum. *European Urol* 1987;13:130–1

62. Benson PM, Lapins NA, Odom RB. White piedra. *Arch Dermatol* 1983;119:602–4

63. Bernhard JD. Macular amyloidosis, notalgia paresthetica and pruritus: three sides of the same coin? *Dermatologica* 1991;183:53–4

64. Massey EW, Pleet AB. Localized pruritus-notalgia paresthetica. *Arch Dermatol* 1979;115:982–3

65. Springall DR, Karanth SS, Kirkham N, *et al.* Symptoms of notalgia paresthetica may be explained by increased dermal innervation. *J Invest Dermatol* 1991;97:555–61

66. Goulden V, Highet AS, Shamy HK. Notalgia paraesthetica—report of an association with macular amyloidosis. *Clin Exp Dermatol* 1994;19:346–9

67. Pena-Penabad MC, Garcia-Silva J, Armijo M. Notalgia paraesthetica and macular amyloidosis: cause-effect relationship? *Clin Exp Dermatol* 1995; 20:279

68. Weber PJ, Poulos EG. Notalgia paresthetica. Case reports and histologic appraisal. *J Am Acad Dermatol* 1988;18:25–30

69. Wallengren J. Treatment of notalgia paresthetica with topical capsaicin. *J Am Acad Dermatol* 1991;24: 286–8

70. Leibsohn E. Treatment of notalgia paresthetica with capsaicin. *Cutis* 1992;49:335–6

71. Wallengren J, Klinker M. Successful treatment of notalgia paresthetica with topical capsaicin: vehicle-controlled, double-blind, crossover study. *J Am Acad Dermatol* 1995;32:287–9

72. Waisman M. Solar pruritus of the elbows (brachioradial summer pruritus). *Arch Dermatol* 1968;98: 481–5

73. Walcyk PJ, Elpern DJ. Brachioradial pruritus: a tropical dermopathy. *Br J Dermatol* 1986;115:177–80

74. Heyl T. Brachioradial pruritus. *Arch Dermatol* 1983;119:115–6

75. Massey EW, Massey JM. Forearm neuropathy and pruritus. *South Med J* 1986;79:1259–60

76. Commens C. Polymorphic light eruption sine eruptione and brachioradial pruritus. *Br J Dermatol* 1988;119:554

77. Knight TE, Hayashi T. Solar (brachioradial) pruritus: response to capsaicin cream. *Int J Dermatol* 1994; 33:206–9

78. Goodless DR, Eaglstein WH. Brachioradial pruritus: treatment with topical capsaicin. *J Am Acad Dermatol* 1993;29:783–4

79. Lynch PJ, Edwards L. *Genital Dermatology*. New York: Churchill Livingstone, 1994

80. Lewis FM, Harrington CI, Gawkrodger DJ. Contact sensitivity in pruritus vulvae: a common and manageable problem. *Contact Dermatitis* 1994;31:264–5

81. Borgatta L. Sensitivity to deodorant sanitary pads. *J Am Med Assoc* 1978;240:1239–40

82. Eason EL, Feldman P. Contact dermatitis associated with the use of Always sanitary napkins. *Can Med Assoc J* 1996;154:1173–6

83. Heckerling PS. Enalapril and vulvovaginal pruritis. *Ann Int Med* 1990;112:217–22

84. Freeman S. Woman allergic to husband's sweat and semen. *Contact Dermatitis* 1986;14:110–2

85. Mikkelsen EJ, Henderson LL, Leiferman KM, *et al.* Allergy to human seminal fluid. *Ann Allergy* 1975; 34:239–43

86. Sell MB. Sensitization to thioridazine through sexual intercourse. *Am J Psychat* 1985;142;271–9

87. Neilly JB, Martin A, Simpson N, *et al.* Pruritus in diabetes mellitus: investigation of prevalence and correlation with diabetes control. *Diabetes Care* 1986;9:273–5

88. Deshpande AD. *Enterobius vermicularis* live adult worms in the high vagina. *Postgrad Med J* 1992;68:690–1

89. Kehoe S, Luesley D. Pathology and management of vulval pain and pruritus. *Curr Opin Obstet Gynecol* 1995;7:16–9

90. Levine GI. Sexually transmitted parasitic diseases. Primary Care. *Clin Office Pract* 1991;18:101–28

91. Chan L. Investigation and treatment of vaginal discharge and pruritus vulvae. *Singapore Med J* 1989;30:471–2

92. Ayhan A, Urman B, Yuce K, *et al.* Topical testosterone for lichen sclerosus. *Int J Gynaecol Obstet* 1989;30:253–5

93. Cattaneo A, De Marco A, Sonni L, *et al.* Clobetasol vs. testosterone in the treatment of lichen sclerosus of the vulvar region. *Minerva Ginecol* 1992;44:567–71

94. August PJ, Milward TM. Cryosurgery in the treatment of lichen sclerosus et atrophicus of the vulva. *Br J Dermatol* 1980;103:667–70

95. Scurry J, Dennerstein G, Brenan J. Angiolymphoid hyperplasia with eosinophilia of the vulva. *Aust NZ J Obstet Gynaecol* 1995;35:347–8

96. Lavery HA. Vulval dystrophies: new approaches. *Clin Obstet Gynaecol* 1984;11:155–69

97. McKay M. Vulvitis and vulvovaginitis: cutaneous considerations. *Am J Obstet Gynecol* 1991;165: 1176–82

98. Lee KC, Su WP, Muller SA. Multicentric cloacogenic carcinoma: report of a case with anogenital pruritus at presentation. *J Am Acad Dermatol* 1990;23: 1005–8

99. Goldstein AI, Kent DR. All vulvar lesions should be biopsied. Basal cell carcinoma – an example of the futility of diagnosis by gross appearance. *Am J Obstet Gynecol* 1975;121:173–4

100. Minderhoud-Bassie W, Chadha-Ajwani S, Huikeshoven FJ. Vulvar pseudolymphoma. *Eur J Obstet Gynecol Reprod Biol* 1992;47:167–8

101. Carter J, Elliott P. Syringoma – an unusual cause of pruritus vulvae. *Aust NZ J Obstet Gynaecol* 1990;30: 382–3

102. Greaves MW, Young AW Jr, Herman EW, *et al.* Syringoma of the vulva: incidence, diagnosis, and cause of pruritus. *Obstet Gynecol* 1980;55:515–8

103. Dhaliwal AK, Fink JN. Vaginal itching as a manifestation of seasonal allergic disease. *J Allergy Clin Immunol* 1995;95:780–2

104. Hardy JS. Pubic itching due to food allergy. *Ann Allergy* 1994;72:546

105. Sherertz EF. Clinical pearl: symptomatic dermatographism as a cause of genital pruritus. *J Am Acad Dermatol* 1994;31:1040–1

106. Sutherst JR. Treatment of pruritus vulvae by multiple intradermal injections of alcohol. A double-blind study. *Br J Obstet Gynaecol* 1979;86:371–3

107. Clouser JK, Friedrich EG Jr. A new technique for alcohol injection in the vulva. *J Reprod Med* 1986; 31:971–2

108. Ovadia J, Levavi H, Edelstein T. Treatment of pruritus vulvae by means of CO2 laser. *Acta Obstet Gynecol Scand* 1984;63:265–7

109. Reid R, Omoto KH, Precop SL, *et al.* Flashlamp-excited dye laser therapy of idiopathic vulvodynia is safe and efficacious. *Am J Obstet Gynecol* 1995;172: 1684–96

110. Kelly RA, Foster DC, Woodruff JD. Subcutaneous injection of triamcinolone acetonide in the treatment of chronic vulvar pruritus. *Am J Obstet Gynecol* 1993;169:568–70

111. Anonymous. Vulvovaginitis – Causes and therapies. *National Institute of Child Health and Human Development and the International Society for the Study of Vulvar Disease*, 1995

112. Cotterill JA. Dermatological non–disease: a common and potentially fatal disturbance of cutaneous body image. *Br J Dermatol* 1981;104:611–9

# Other itching diseases 9

This chapter discusses the diseases commonly associated with itching, including psoriasis, lichen planus, the mastocytoses, and the autoimmune blistering diseases. Some autoimmune blistering diseases, such as dermatitis herpetiformis, have itching as a characteristic feature, whereas other pathogenically related diseases such as pemphigus typically have no itching. Special mention of cutaneous T-cell lymphoma and parapsoriasis will be made as these are notoriously itchy conditions. Virtually any disease with cutaneous inflammation may itch, and scratching may perpetuate the diseases through lichenification

## Bullous pemphigoid

### Pathophysiology

Patients with bullous pemphigoid demonstrate circulating autoantibodies which react with an antigen located in the lamina lucida region of the basement membrane zone. Complement activation by these autoantibodies initiates influx and activation of mast cells along with other inflammatory cells[1,2].

Tissue injury with damage and eventual destruction of the basement membrane occurs as a result of the release of inflammatory mediators.

### Clinical features

Most commonly this is a disease of the elderly. The usual appearance is that of generalized or localized, large, tense bullae on either an erythematous base or normal skin(Figure 57).

- Itching may be absent or intense, and itching may precede the development of skin lesions[3]
- Bullous pemphigoid may be an itchy dermatosis without large blisters[4]

    Generalized itching may be a presenting sign of pemphigoid[5]

Urticarial, dyshidrosiform, or eczematous lesions may be seen[6,7]

Pemphigoid nodularis consists of prurigo-like lesions with scattered hyperpigmented nodules and plaques, and may precede the onset of blistering by some months

- Diagnosis is made by means of biopsy with direct immunofluorescence studies

### Treatment

Conservative treatment may be accomplished with systemic and topical corticosteroids. Severe disease may require immunosuppressive agents such as methotrexate, azathioprine and cyclophosphamide[8,9].

- Following successful treatment of bullous pemphigoid, the itching may persist for prolonged periods[3]

## Cutaneous T-cell lymphoma (mycosis fungoides)

Cutaneous T-cell lymphoma encompasses a constellation of diseases of malignant clonal lymphocytes that initially are epidermotropic, but lose this skin-affinity over time. This uncommon neoplastic disease may be intensely itchy and may masquerade for years or decades as chronic dermatitis[10,11].

- Virtually any longstanding, recalcitrant inflammatory dermatosis may seem to evolve into a cutaneous T-cell lymphoma[12]
- Analogously, a number of conditions may be mistaken for cutaneous T-cell lymphoma including pseudolymphoma, drug eruptions, and allergic contact dermatitis[13]

### Clinical appearance

Erythematous to plum-colored, scaling patches and plaques are seen in early disease (Figures 58–60).

- Atypical clinical presentations have included eruptions that are pigmented purpura-like[14], granulomatous, hypopigmented, verrucous, psoriasisform, and pustular[15]

Within months to decades, progression to tumor is seen. Lymphadenopathy and infiltration of internal organs may occur at any time, but is usually a late manifestation. An erythrodermic variant, the Sézary syndrome, has a worse prognosis and may be associated with a leukemic infiltrate[16].

- The number of Sézary cells in the blood is neither sensitive nor specific for the diagnosis of the syndrome

The diagnosis is made histopathologically. However, early diagnosis may not be possible clinically or histopathologically, as the early features of cutaneous T-cell lymphoma overlap with numerous other conditions[17,18].

### Treatment

No modality or combination of modalities has clearly shown to be therapeutically superior, and no systemic therapy cures patients with cutaneous T-cell lymphoma. Although not currently curable, the following treatment modalities improve this condition, relieve itching and may induce remission, but none has been shown in comparative trials to be superior to others:

- Topical corticosteroids
- Topical chemotherapy with mechlorethamine or carmustine[19,20]
- Psoralen photochemotherapy (PUVA)[21]
- Radiation including Grenz rays or electron beam radiation[22,23]
- Systemic chemotherapy with retinoids, interferon alpha, interleukin-2 fusion toxin, temozolomide, and others[24,25]
- Photopheresis

## Dermatitis herpetiformis

### Epidemiology

This is a disease that most commonly affects those between 15 and 50 years, but may commence at any age. It is more common in those of European origin. Patients are at increased likelihood of having human lymphocyte antigens (HLA)-B8 and -DR3.

### Pathophysiology

Gluten-sensitive enteropathy indistinguishable from that of celiac disease occurs frequently in this group of patients, and this gluten sensitivity is thought to be related to disease development and progression[26].

- Circulating anti-gliadin antibodies are present in half of patients, but their significance is unknown
- IgA deposits in the skin bind to reticulin fibers and disappearance of this autoantibody correlates with improvement of dermatitis herpetiformis

  One hypothesis is that gliadin binds to reticulin fibers as gluten–antigluten immune complexes, damaging the fibers and making them immunogenic

## Clinical appearance

Itching is found on symmetrical extensor elbow surfaces, buttocks, extensor knees, back and face (Figures 61, 62). Although this is a blistering disease characterized by small vesicles on an erythematous base, because of active scratching blisters are uncommonly observed[26,27].

- The itching can be particularly intense with little visible clinically, and patients have been misdiagnosed as having neurotic excoriations
- Diagnosis is made by means of biopsy with direct immunofluorescence studies

    Granular deposits of IgA at the dermoepidermal junction are pathognomonic

## Treatment

Gluten-free diets may provide complete or partial response, but must be strictly followed for two or more years to achieve successful results.

- Gluten restriction may allow dapsone (or other agent) dosage reduction and is highly advisable for all those willing to modify their diets [28]

    Dietary intervention may reverse the immunopathologic findings and result in loss of IgA[29]

- The risk of lymphoma, another itchy disorder, is greater in patients with dermatitis herpetiformis, and there is some evidence that gluten-free diets may lessen the long-term risk of lymphoma[30]

Dapsone is particularly effective at 100 mg or more per day.

- This agent requires careful monitoring for hematologic side-effects and should be used judiciously in those with glucose-6-phosphate dehydrogenase deficiency

Sulfapyridine may also be effective and this agent can also cause hematologic and other side-effects.

# Eosinophilic pustular folliculitis (Ofuji's disease)

Eosinophilic pustular folliculitis is a rare skin disease of unknown etiology originally reported in normal Japanese patients, but now is commonly seen in many geographic areas in immunocompromised patients[31,32].

- Most commonly it is observed in adult patients with acquired immunodeficiency syndrome[33]
- It can also be seen in non-Hodgkin's lymphoma, B-cell chronic lymphatic leukemia, and other myeloproliferative disorders[34–36]
- An infantile or childhood form of this condition is also occasionally seen[37,38]

## Pathology

To date demonstration of pathogenic organisms has been unsuccessful, and thus this condition may represent a multifactorial disorder.

- *Pseudomonas* infection of the hair follicle has been shown to be the cause of the disease in a few patients by repeated cultures and response to antibacterial therapy
- Fungal eosinophilic pustular folliculitis has been hypothesized on the basis of demonstration of histopathologic hyphae in select patients and response to ketoconazole or itraconazole[39,40]

## Clinical features

Eosinophilic pustular folliculitis is characterized by the spontaneous development of recurrent, sterile papules, pustules, and plaques on the face, trunk, arms, and occasionally the palms and soles[41].

- Tinea-like annular lesions may be seen
- Itching may be so severe that primary pustules are not identified

Reported effective treatments have included:

- Acemetacin[42]
- Cetirizine[43]
- Cyclosporin[44]
- Dapsone[45]
- Ketoconazole[40]
- Indomethacin[46]
- Interferon-alpha 2b[47]
- Isotretinoin[48]
- Itraconazole[40]
- Metronidazole[49]
- Topical corticosteroids (only modestly effective)[31]
- Phototherapy with psoralen photochemotherapy or ultraviolet B[50,51]

## Infantile acropustulosis

This is an uncommon, idiopathic, pustular dermatosis primarily seen in among black male infants of 2 to 12 months of age, which may persist for as long as 2 years[52–58].

- Distal extremities bear recurrent crops of 1–3mm itchy papules and pustules
- This disease is typically not as itchy as scabies with which it may be easily confused
- Infantile acropustulosis is diagnosed histopathologically

### Treatment

Treatment is not always required if minimally symptomatic. A variable response to topical corticosteroids is typical.

- Dapsone may be effective in doses up to 2mg/kg/day
- High dose sedating antihistamines may also help

## Lichen planus

This is best remembered by a mnemonic: lichen planus is the disease of Ps[59–62].

- Pruritic: itching is extraordinarily severe, yet excoriations are rarely seen (Figure 63)
- Peripheral: the distribution tends to be acral (wrists and ankles) rather than central (Figure 9.1)
- Planar: lesions tend to be shiny, flat-topped papules
- Polygonal: lesions tend to be polygonal rather than round or ovoid
- Phenomenon of Koebner: trauma to the skin induces the skin disease in the distribution of the trauma, thus linear clusterings are occasionally seen (Figure 64)
- Private parts: the penis and vulva are commonly involved
- Purple: the lesions have a characteristic violaceous-red hue, with fine white, lacy lines, Wickham's striae are found on individual lesions in both the skin and mucosae[63] (Figure 65)
- Pigmentation: particularly in darkly pigmented patients, hyperpigmentation follows the papules and may be persistent
- Persistence: skin lesions typically last about a year, and 85% clear within 18 months

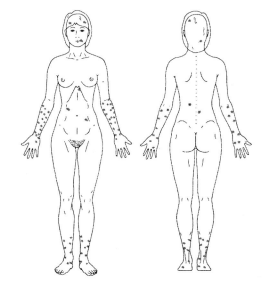

**Figure 9.1** Typical distribution of lichen planus

## Other features

Ulceration may occasionally be seen acrally. Mucous membrane involvement is common, but often asymptomatic.

- Oral ulcers may cause stinging and pain
- Vaginal lesions may cause itching, burning, pain, and dispareunia[64]

Lichen planus occasionally presents asymptomatically. The pathogenesis is idiopathic, but evidence is mounting that it is immunologically mediated. A number of medications have either been associated with lichen planus or have produced lichenoid drug eruptions that present similarly.

- These agents include chloroquine, gold, chlorothiazine, demeclocycline, hydrochlorthiazide, penicillamine, phenothiazine, quinacrine, streptomycin and tetracycline

### Treatment

- Potent or superpotent topical corticosteroid agents are usually effective for minimizing itching and flattening lesions
    - On mucous membranes, super-potent topical corticosteroid gels work well as does triamcinolone in a base designed for the oral mucosa (Orabase)
- Sedating antihistaminic agents at bedtime provide temporary relief
- Systemic corticosteroids are occasionally useful for limited times when the eruption is severe and the planned therapeutic duration is short
- Oral retinoids including etretinate and isotretinoin have some efficacy with recalcitrant disease
- The author has anecdotal successful experience with low-dose weekly methotrexate
- Other reported successful therapies have included

Cyclophosphamide
Cyclosporin, topical
Dapsone
Griseofulvin (although reported effective, this agent is of dubious value)
Interferon alfa-2b[65]
Metronidazole
Psoralen photochemotherapy[66]

## Linear IgA bullous dermatosis

This is a rare acquired blistering disease of childhood characterized by large individual or grouped bullae, also known as chronic bullous disease of childhood[67].

- Although itching is noted to occur, itch severity is not as severe as in dermatitis herpetiformis, thus further discussion will be avoided in this text

## Mastocytosis

Mastocytosis is the collective name for a group of clinical syndromes whose signs and symptoms are due to the infiltration of various tissues by mast cells and to the release of chemical mediators by these cells. The skin is the most frequently affected organ and itching is the most common symptom[68,69].

- About half of children with urticaria pigmentosa may experience resolution of lesions and symptoms by adolescence

Systemic mastocytosis most commonly results from mast cells in the gut, bone, liver, and spleen.

- Uncommonly, myelodysplasia may eventuate in mast cell leukemia[69]

The Darier's sign, pathognomonic for mastocytosis, is the name for the whealing or blistering that occurs when lesions are rubbed (Figure 66)

- This is more likely to be demonstrated in discrete mastocytotic lesions rather than on broad surface infiltration as is seen in telangiectasia macularis eruptiva perstans

Skin manifestations include[70–73]:

- Urticaria pigmentosa (Figures 9.2 and 67)
- Solitary mastocytoma

    A pink to erythematous or yellow papule or nodule

- Diffuse cutaneous mastocytosis

    Involved skin has a yellow, thickened appearance, or it can be diffusely involved with tiny papules

- Telangiectasia macularis eruptiva perstans (Figure 68)

    Telangiectasia, erythema and brown pigmentation may cover large portions of the body surface area

### Treatment

- For localized skin disease, superpotent topical corticosteroid agents may result in rapid improvement
- $H_1$ and $H_2$ antihistamines help to control itching and the hypersecretion of gastric acid that may occur
- Ketotifen, a mast cell stabilizer, treatment may be very effective
- Azelastine, a novel antiallergic medication, is superior to chlorpheniramine in suppressing skin responses to histamine and morphine sulfate and in suppressing pruritus in patients with mastocytosis[74]
- Psoralen photochemotherapy may help diffusely involved patients

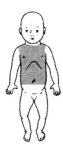

**Figure 9.2** Urticaria pigmentea (Mastocytosis) in a new born

## Parapsoriasis

The term parapsoriasis refers to a group of chronic asymptomatic or mildly symptomatic scaly dermatoses of unknown etiology[75,76]. There are numerous parapsoriasis diseases, some of which are actually cutaneous T-cell lymphoma.

- Cutaneous T-cell lymphoma is notoriously difficult to diagnose early (see below)

### Small plaque parapsoriasis

- Clinically characterized by round to ovoid, scaly plaques on the trunk and proximal aspect of extremities
- Typically, small plaque disease is not itchy and is described to distinguish this from other conditions

### Large plaque parapsoriasis

- Characterized by large (>10 cm), ill-defined, irregularly shaped erythematous to brown macules or plaques, usually associated with some epidermal atrophy (Figure 69)

    Pigmentary changes, telangiectasia, and fine scaling are commonly seen

    Atrophy is almost always seen

- Large-plaque parapsoriasis and its variant, retiform parapsoriasis, have a strong tendency to develop into cutaneous T-cell lymphoma[77]

### Pityriasis lichenoides chronica and pityriasis lichenoides et varioliformis acuta

These are benign, generally non-pruritic disorders without recognized association with cutaneous T-cell lymphoma, although anecdotal reports suggest progression to this condition may occur[78].

- Pityriasis lichenoides et varioliformis acuta

presents as erythematous to brown, hemorrhagic scaly papules that predominate on the trunk and flexural extremities

- Pityriasis lichenoides chronica presents as fine scaly macules and papules on the trunk and extremities

## Pityriasis rosea

This is not a rare nor unusual disease, but its etiology remains obscure. The first manifestation often is a larger and more distinct lesion (herald patch) than the rest of the lesions which will follow in one or more weeks[79–81].

- The herald patch is absent in 20–25% of cases

One or more weeks later there is a rapid onset of truncal, ovoid, erythematous macules and papules that follow the relaxed skin tension lines, often with fine scaling at the periphery.

- Characteristically, the eruption is confined to the trunk, the base of the neck and the upper limbs (Figure 70)
- New lesions continue to develop for several weeks
- Macules and papules fade after 3–6 weeks, but some clear in 1 or 2 weeks and a few persist for as long as 2 months
- Pityriasis rosea may be atypical in appearance or distribution

    Unilateral pityriasis has been reported

    Papulovesicular, vesicular, pustular, and erythema multi-forme-like lesions may be seen

- Secondary syphilis should be considered in the differential diagnosis but can usually be distinguished by the absence of palm, sole and mucous membrane lesions
- Treatment is supportive with reassurance, topical corticosteroids and emollients[82]

    For particularly symptomatic disease, use of phototherapy may be highly effective

Controversy exists about its utility given a recent, small, controlled trial demonstrating poor response to UVB[83]

## Pityriasis rubra pilaris

This is an idiopathic disease that often begins seemingly innocuously as scalp itching, and progresses to a devastating erythroderma within 2 months[84].

- The disease may resolve spontaneously within a few months to a year or more, although persistent cases do occur
- The acute self-resolving form seems to be the most frequent in children, compared to adults

    Since juvenile pityriasis rubra pilaris has a relatively rapid course and often has a spontaneous resolution, unless the disease is persistent it seems unnecessary to use potentially harmful drugs[85,86]

Clinically, patients generally have salmon-colored or erythematous thick, disabling plaques on the palms and soles, which extend beyond the dorsopalmar and plantar junctions.

- Circumscribed psoriasiform scaly patches on the elbows and knees may also be seen
- An exfoliative erythroderma associated with diffuse follicular plugging
- A biopsy is used to help confirm this diagnosis

### Treatment

- Etretinate is more effective than isotretinoin, although isotretinoin results in occasional clearing[87,88]
- Methotrexate is also known to improve the disease[89]

    The author has anecdotally used combined methotrexate and etretinate with a high response rate

- Topical corticosteroid agents, phototherapy, and other antipsoriatic approaches are generally unhelpful[90]

## Psoriasis

Although not typically regarded as an itching disease, research shows that about two-thirds of sufferers report moderate to severe itching. Itching may chronify psoriasis through mechanisms of lichenification and the phenomenon of Koebner[91].

- Psoriatic patients with symptoms of depression may be more likely to itch severely than psoriatics without itching

### Clinical features

The appearance of a typical psoriatic lesion is characteristic with a vibrant red color, silvery white scale, and variable thickness (Figures 71–73). Although any surface may be involved, typically affected skin areas include elbows, knees, scalp, natal cleft, and umbilicus. Diagnostic nail features may include pits, the oil drop sign, and nail plate hypertrophy.

### Treatment

#### Corticosteroid agents

These may be particularly helpful in decreasing the itching of psoriatic lesions.

- Medium to ultra-high potency agents are required to decrease the inflammation and thereby relieve the itching[92]
- If used on the scalp, corticosteroid solutions and oils are preferred over other vehicles
- Caution should be exercised in long-term treatment with these agents as tachyphylaxis and cutaneous atrophy are known sequelae[93]
- Although systemic corticosteroids have been employed their role is limited[94]

#### Phototherapy

These modalities may be the most effective treatment in many patients, but are time consuming and costly (note that all phototherapeutic modalities predispose to cutaneous carcinogenesis)[95].

- Ultraviolet B (UVB): this therapy is effective in most patients
- Psoralen photochemotherapy (PUVA): this remains the most effective phototherapy technique in clearing psoriatic lesions and relieving itching, but must be administered in physicians' offices
- Heliotherapy: solar irradiation in the summer months may be particularly beneficial if used judiciously around the noon hour

#### Non-corticosteroid topical psoriatic agents

- Calcipotriene: this is a synthetic vitamin $D_3$ analog with anti-inflammatory and antipsoriatic activity

  Should be used for 8 to 12 weeks to achieve results

  Synergy with topical corticosteroids and phototherapy has been demonstrated

- Tazerotene: this is a synthetic retinoid with anti-inflammatory and antipsoriatic activity

  Should be used for 8 to 12 weeks to achieve results

- Anthralin (dithranol): this is a synthetic compound with marked antipsoriatic activity within 4 to 8 weeks[96]

  This product should be used cautiously because it stains skin and clothing and is irritating

- Coal tar: this is a distillate of tar with thousands of active and inactive components; has significant anti-inflammatory and antipsoriatic properties

  Tars are problematic as they stain clothing, are potentially irritating and have a striking odor

- Capsaicin: this is a natural compound from hot peppers that may decrease cutaneous inflammation and improve psoriasis

  One-third of patients may not tolerate this agent because of its transient burning properties

### Systemic agents

- Methotrexate: this agent taken once weekly acts as a folate antagonist and decreases the cutaneous inflammatory response[97,98]

  Although highly effective in doses ranging from 5–25 mg weekly, it is potentially hepatotoxic and may suppress hematopoiesis

- Cyclosporin: this potent anti-inflammatory agent has demonstrated antipsoriatic activity and may result in rapid clearing

  Note it is potentially nephrotoxic, precipitates hypertension and may increase opportunistic infections

- Retinoids: this class of antiproliferative agents includes isotretinoin, acitretin, and etretinate; acitretin and etretinate have demonstrated antipsoriatic activity[99–101]

  Etretinate: an antiproliferative agent that can be used alone or in combination with PUVA with main side-effects including reversible alopecia, cheilitis, elevated serum lipids and liver transaminases

  Acitretin: a metabolite of etretinate with similar side-effects but markedly shorter half-life

- Sulfasalazine: this anti-inflammatory agent is not extremely potent in the majority of patients, but may serve as an adjunct to other treatments

- Miscellaneous agents: severely affected psoriatic patients refractory to other systemic approaches may respond to second- or third-line agents including hydroxyurea[102], oral antibiotics, or systemic corticosteroids

## Transient and persistent acantholytic dermatosis (Grover's disease)

This idiopathic self-limited dermatosis occurs in middle-aged to elderly people. The diagnosis is made clinically and histopathologically. The evolution may be acute or chronic, and primary lesions consist of intensely itchy discrete papules and papulovesicles distributed mainly on the chest, back, and thighs[103,104] (Figure 74).

- The disease duration is typically less than 3 months, but it can persist for several years[105]
- Four different histopathologic types are recognized (Darier-like, pemphigus vulgaris-like, Hailey–Hailey-like, and spongiotic)

### Treatment

- Mild disease can be treated with generous quantities of topical corticosteroid agents
- Severe disease may require systemic retinoid agents including etretinate, acitretin, or isotretinoin or psoralen photochemotherapy (PUVA)
- An anecdotal report exists which claims therapeutic response with topical selenium sulfide[106]

# References

1. Anhalt GJ, Morrison LH. Bullous and cicatricial pemphigoid. *J Autoimmunity* 1991;4:17–35
2. Anhalt GJ. Pemphigoid. Bullous and cicatricial. *Dermatol Clin* 1990;8:701–16
3. Bingham EA, Burrow D, Sanford JC. Prolonged pruritis and bullous pemphigoid. *Clin Exp Dermatol* 1984;9:564–70
4. Morrison LH, Diaz LA, Anhalt GJ. Bullous pemphigoid. In Wojnarowska F, Briggaman RA, eds. *Management of Blistering Diseases.* London: Chapman and Hall Medical, 1990;63–82
5. Barker DJ. Generalized pruritis as the presenting feature of bullous pemphigoid. *Br J Dermatol* 1983;109:237–9
6. Ross JS, McKee PH, Smith NP, *et al.* Unusual variants of pemphigoid: from pruritis to pemphigoid nodularis. *J Cut Pathol* 1992;19:212–6
7. Torrelo A, Espana A, Moreno R, *et al.* Dyshidrosiform pemphigoid. *Med Cut Ibero-Latino-Am* 1990; 18:189–90
8. Huilgol SC, Black MM. Management of the immunobullous disorders. I. Pemphigoid. *Clin Exp Dermatol* 1995;20:189–201
9. Korman N. Bullous pemphigoid. *J Am Acad Dermatol* 1987;16:907–24
10. Abel EA, Wood GS, Hoppe RT. Mycosis fungoides: clinical and histologic features, staging, evaluation, and approach to treatment. *Ca Cancer J Clin* 1993;43:93–115
11. Koh HK, Charif M, Weinstock MA. Epidemiology and clinical manifestations of cutaneous T-cell lymphoma. *Hematol Oncol Clin North Am* 1995;9: 943–60
12. Fransway AF, Winkelmann RK. Chronic dermatitis evolving to mycosis fungoides: report of four cases and review of the literature. *Cutis* 1988;41:330–5
13. Fisher AA. Allergic contact dermatitis mimicking mycosis fungoides. *Cutis* 1987;40:19–21
14. Barnhill RL, Braverman IM. Progression of pigmented purpura-like eruptions to mycosis fungoides: report of three cases. *J Am Acad Dermatol* 1988;19: 25–31
15. Camisa C, Aulisio A. Pustular mycosis fungoides. *Cutis* 1994;54:202–4
16. Duangurai K, Piamphongsant T, Himmungnan T. Sézary cell count in exfoliative dermatitis. *Int J Dermatol* 1988;27:248–52
17. Kuzel TM, Roenigk HH Jr, Rosen ST. Mycosis fungoides and the Sézary syndrome: a review of pathogenesis, diagnosis, and therapy. *J Clin Oncol* 1991;9: 1298–313
18. Payne CM, Grogan TM, Spier CM, *et al.* A multidisciplinary approach to the diagnosis of cutaneous T-cell lymphomas. *Ultrastruct Pathol* 1992;16:99–125
19. Lorincz AL. Cutaneous T-cell lymphoma (mycosis fungoides). *Lancet* 1996;47:871–6
20. Vonderheid EC. Topical mechlorethamine chemotherapy. Considerations on its use in mycosis fungoides. *Int J Dermatol* 1984;23:180–6
21. Honig B, Morison WL, Karp D. Photochemotherapy beyond psoriasis. *J Am Acad Dermatol* 1994;31:775–90
22. Jones GW, Hoppe RT, Glatstein E. Electron beam treatment for cutaneous T-cell lymphoma *Hematol Oncol Clin North Am* 1995;9:1057–76
23. MacDonald RH, Russell AR. Mycosis fungoides: its management with superficial X-rays and strontium 90 therapy compared. *Br J Dermatol* 1971;85: 388–93
24. Bunn PA Jr, Hoffman SJ, Norris D, *et al.* Systemic therapy of cutaneous T-cell lymphomas (mycosis fungoides and the Sézary syndrome). *Ann Int Med* 1994;121:592–602
25. Mielke V, Staib G, Sterry W. Systemic treatment for cutaneous lymphomas. *Rec Results Cancer Res* 1995; 139:403–8
26. Fry L. Dermatitis herpetiformis. In Wojnarowska F, Briggaman RA, eds. *Management of Blistering Diseases.* London: Chapman and Hall Medical, 1990;139–60
27. Smith EP, Zone JJ. Dermatitis herpetiformis and linear IgA bullous dermatosis. *Dermatol Clin* 1993;11: 511–26
28. Garioch JJ, Lewis HM, Sargent SA, *et al.* 25 years' experience of a gluten-free diet in the treatment of dermatitis herpetiformis. *Br J Dermatol* 1994;131: 541–5
29. Hall RP. Dietary management of dermatitis herpetiformis. *Arch Dermatol* 1987;123:1378–80
30. Sigurgeirsson B, Agnarsson BA, Lindelof B. Risk of lymphoma in patients with dermatitis herpetiformis. *Br Med J* 1994;308:13–5
31. Moritz DL, Elmets CA. Eosinophilic pustular folliculitis. *J Am Acad Dermatol* 1991;24:903–7
32. Ofuji S, Ogino A, Horio T, *et al.* Eosinophilic pustular folliculitis. *Acta Derm Venereol* 1970;50:195–203

33. Ferrandiz C, Ribera M, Barranco JC, *et al.* Eosinophilic pustular folliculitis in patients with acquired immunodeficiency syndrome. *Int J Dermatol* 1992;31:193–5

34. Evans TR, Mansi JL, Bull R, *et al.* Eosinophilic folliculitis occurring after bone marrow autograft in a patient with non-Hodgkin's lymphoma. *Cancer* 1994; 73:2512–4

35. Lambert J, Berneman Z, Dockx P, *et al.* Eosinophilic pustular folliculitis and B-cell chronic lymphatic leukaemia. *Dermatology* 1994;189 (Suppl 2):58–9

36. Patrizi A, Di Lernia V, Neri I, *et al.* Eosinophilic pustular folliculitis (Ofuji's disease) and non–Hodgkin lymphoma. *Acta Derm Venereol* 1992;72:146–7

37. Darmstadt GL, Tunnessen WW Jr, Swerer RJ. Eosinophilic pustular folliculitis. *Pediatrics* 1992;89: 1095–8

38. Garcia-Patos V, Pujol RM, de Moragas JM. Infantile eosinophilic pustular folliculitis. *Dermatology* 1994; 189:133–8

39. Dyall-Smith D, Mason G. Fungal eosinophilic pustular folliculitis. *Aust J Dermatol* 1995;36:37–8

40. Haupt HM, Stern JB, Weber CB. Eosinophilic pustular folliculitis: fungal folliculitis? *J Am Acad Dermatol* 1990;23:1012–4

41. Brenner S, Wolf R, Ophir J. Eosinophilic pustular folliculitis: a sterile folliculitis of unknown cause? *J Am Acad Dermatol* 1994;31:210–2

42. Nishijima S, Sugiyama T, Nakagawa M, *et al.* Two cases of eosinophilic pustular folliculitis treated by acemetacin. *J Dermatol* 1994;21:779–82

43. Harris DW, Ostlere L, Buckley C, *et al.* Eosinophilic pustular folliculitis in an HIV-positive man: response to cetirizine. *Br J Dermatol* 1992;126:392–4

44. Taniguchi S, Tsuruta D, Hamada T. Eosinophilic pustular folliculitis responding to cyclosporin. *Br J Dermatol* 1994;131:736–8

45. Steffen C. Eosinophilic pustular folliculitis (Ofuji's disease) with response to dapsone therapy. *Arch Dermatol* 1985;121:921–3

46. Lee ML, Tham SN, Ng SK. Eosinophilic pustular folliculitis (Ofuji's disease) with response to indomethacin. *Dermatology* 1993;186:210–2

47. Mohr C, Schutte B, Hildebrand A, *et al.* Eosinophilic pustular folliculitis: successful treatment with interferon-alpha. *Dermatology* 1995;191:257–9

49. Smith KJ, Skelton HG, Yeager J, *et al.* Metronidazole for eosinophilic pustular folliculitis in human immunodeficiency virus type 1-positive patients. *Arch Dermatol* 1995;131:1089–91

50. Breit R, Rocken M. A classical form of eosinophilic pustular folliculitis – successful therapy with PUVA. *Hautarzt* 1991;42:247–50

51. Porneuf M, Guillot B, Barneon G, *et al.* Eosinophilic pustular folliculitis responding to UVB therapy. *J Am Acad Dermatol* 1993;29:259–60

52. Findlay RF, Odom RB. Infantile acropustulosis. *Am J Dis Child* 1983;137:455–7

53. Jarratt M, Ramsdell W. Infantile acropustulosis. *Arch Dermatol* 1979;115:834–6

54. Jennings JL, Burrows WM. Infantile acropustulosis. *J Am Acad Dermatol* 1983;9:733–8

55. Kahana M, SchewachMillet, Feinstein A. Infantile acropustulosis. *Clin Exp Dermatol* 1987;12:291–2

56. McFadden N, Falk ES. Infantile acropustulosis. *Cutis* 1985;36:49–51

57. Palungwachira P. Infantile acropustulosis. *Australasian J Dermatol* 1989;30:97–100

58. Pizzi de Parra N, Larralde de Luna M, Cicioni V, *et al.* Infantile acropustulosis. Considerations on 11 cases. *Med Cutanea Ibero-Latino-Am* 1987;15:135–9

59. Black MM. Lichen planus and lichenoid disorders. In Champion RH, Burton JL, Ebling FJG, eds. *Textbook of Dermatology*, 5th edn. Oxford: Blackwell Scientific Publications, 1992:1675–98

60. Fellner MJ. Lichen planus. *Int J Dermatol* 1980;19:71–75

61. Samman PD. Lichen planus: an analysis of 200 cases. *Trans Rep St John's Hosp Dermatol Soc* 1961;46:36–8

62. Singh OP, Kanwar AJ. Lichen planus in India: an appraisal of 441 cases. *Int J Dermatol* 1976;15:752–6

63. Rivers JK, Jackson R, Orizaga M. Who was Wickham and what are his striae? *Int J Dermatol* 1986;25:611–13

64. Edwards L. Vulvar lichen planus. *Arch Dermatol* 1989;125:1677–80

65. Hildebrand A, Kolde G, Luger TA, *et al.* Successful treatment of generalized lichen planus with recombinant interferon alfa-2b. *J Am Acad Dermatol* 1995; 33:880–3

66. Ortonne JP, Thivolet J, Sannwald C. Oral photochemotherapy in the treatment of lichen planus (LP): clinical results, histological and ultrastructural observations. *Br J Dermatol* 1978;99:77–88

67. Marsden RA. Linear IgA disease of childhood (chronic bullous disease of childhood). In Wojnarowska F, Briggaman RA, eds. *Management of*

*Blistering Diseases*. London: Chapman and Hall Medical, 1990;119–25

68. Fine J. Mastocytosis. *Int J Dermatol* 1980;19:117–23

69. Marney SR Jr. Mast cell disease. *Allergy Proceed* 1992;13:303–10

70. Greaves MW. Mastocytosis. In Champion RH, Burton JL, Ebling FJG, eds. *Textbook of Dermatology*, 5th edn. Oxford: Blackwell Scientific Publications, 1992;2065–72

71. Kettelhut BV, Metcalfe DD: Pediatric mastocytosis. *J Invest Dermatol* 1991;96:15S–18S

72. Parks A, Camisa C. Reddish-brown macules with telangiectasia and pruritus. Urticaria pigmentosa-telangiectasia macularis eruptiva perstans (TMEP) variant, with systemic mastocytosis. *Arch Dermatol* 1988;124:429–30, 432–3

73. Tay YK, Giam YC. Cutaneous mastocytosis in Singapore. *Singapore Med J* 1993;34:425–9

74. Friedman BS, Santiago ML, Berkebile C, *et al.* Comparison of azelastine and chlorpheniramine in the treatment of mastocytosis. *J Allergy Clin Immunol* 1993;92:520–6

75. Benmaman O, Sanchez JL. Comparative clinico-pathological study on pityriasis lichenoides chronica and small plaque parapsoriasis. *Am J Dermatopathol* 1988;10:189–96

76. Piamphongsant T. Parapsoriasis and related conditions. *Ann Acad Med Singapore* 1988;17:486–91

77. Lambert WC. Premycotic eruptions. *Dermatol Clin* 1985;3:629–45

78. Fortson JS, Schroeter AL, Esterly NB. Cutaneous T-cell lymphoma (parapsoriasis en plaque). An association with pityriasis lichenoides et varioliformis acuta in young children. *Arch Dermatol* 1990;126:1449–53

79. Cavanaugh RM Jr. Pityriasis rosea in children. A review. *Clin Ped* 1983;22:200–3

80. Parsons JM. Pityriasis rosea update: 1986. *J Am Acad Dermatol* 1986;15:159–67

81. Truhan AP. Pityriasis rosea. *Am Fam Phys* 1984;29:193–6

82. Weigand DA. How I treat pityriasis rosea. *Postgrad Med* 1968;44:269–70

83. Leenutaphong V, Jiamton S. UVB phototherapy for pityriasis rosea: a bilateral comparison study. *J Am Acad Dermatol* 1995;33:996–9

84. Cohen PR, Prystowsky JH. Pityriasis rubra pilaris: a review of diagnosis and treatment. *J Am Acad Dermatol* 1989;20:801–7

85. Piamphongsant T, Akaraphant R. Pityriasis rubra pilaris: a new proposed classification. *Clin Exp Dermatol* 1994;19:134–8

86. Gelmetti C, Schiuma AA, Cerri D, *et al.* Pityriasis rubra pilaris in childhood: a long-term study of 29 cases. *Ped Dermatol* 1986;3:446–51

87. Borok M, Lowe NJ. Pityriasis rubra pilaris. Further observations of systemic retinoid therapy. *J Am Acad Dermatol* 1990;22:792–5

88. Dicken CH. Isotretinoin treatment of pityriasis rubra pilaris. *J Am Acad Dermatol* 1987;16:297–301

89. Anderson FE. Pityriasis rubra pilaris treated with methotrexate. *Aust J Dermatol* 1966;8:183–5

90. Dicken CH. Treatment of classic pityriasis rubra pilaris. *J Am Acad Dermatol* 1994;31:997–9

91. Farber EM, Nall LM. The natural history of psoriasis in 5,600 patients. *Dermatologica* 1974;148:1–18

92. Nilsson JE, Gip LJ. Systemic effects of local treatment with high doses of potent corticosteroids in psoriatics. *Acta Derm Venereol* 1979;59:245–8

93. Du Vivier A, Stoughton RB. Tachyphylaxis to the action of topically applied corticosteroid. *Arch Dermatol* 1975;111:581–3

94. Cohen HJ, Baer RL. Triamcinolone and methyl prednisolone in psoriasis. Comparison of their intralesional and systemic effects. *J Invest Dermatol* 1960;34:271–5

95. LeVine MJ, Parrish JA. Outpatient phototherapy of psoriasis. *Arch Dermatol* 1980;116:552–4

96. Runne U, Kunze J. Short-duration ('minutes') therapy with dithranol for psoriasis. *Br J Dermatol* 1982;106:135–9

97. Roenigk HH, Auerbach R, Maibach HI, *et al.* Methotrexate in psoriasis: revised guidelines. *J Am Acad Dermatol* 1988;19:145–6

98. Zachariae H. Psoriasis and the liver. In Roenigk HH, Maibach HI, eds. *Psoriasis*. New York: Marcel Dekker, 1985; 47–64

99. Parker S, Coburn P, Lawrence C *et al.* A randomised double–blind comparison of PUVA-etretinate and PUVA-placebo in the treatment of chronic plaque psoriasis. *Br J Dermatol* 1984;110:215–20

100. Lowe NJ, Roenigk H, Voorhees JJ. Etretinate. Appropriate use in severe psoriasis. *Arch Dermatol* 1988;124:527–8

101. Morison WL. Etretinate and psoriasis. *Arch Dermatol* 1987;123:879–81

102. Touraine R, Revuz J, Tulliez M. Psoriasis and hydroxyurea. *Br J Dermatol* 1972;86:102

103. Grover RW. Transient acantholytic dermatosis. *Arch Dermatol* 1971;104:26–37
104. Chalet M, Grover R, Ackerman AB. Transient acantholytic dermatosis: a reevaluation. *Arch Dermatol* 1977;113:431–5
105. Simon RS, Bloom D, Ackerman AB. Persistent acantholytic dermatosis: a variant of transient acantholytic dermatosis (Grover disease). *Arch Dermatol* 1976; 112:1429–31
106. Segal R, Alteras I, Sandbank M. Rapid response of transient acantholytic dermatosis to selenium sulfide treatment for pityriasis versicolor. *Dermatologica* 1987;175:205–7

# Curious itching conditions

10

In organizing a book on itching, these disorders do not seem to fit anywhere else except a chapter on curious conditions. Many of the conditions listed in the chapter are uncommon or rare; others are reasonably common, yet are infrequently recognized. For other itch curiosities, see chapter 4: Systemic conditions, and chapter 7: Urticaria

## Acne itch

- Itching at the site of active acne has been described[1]

    Itching may also begin as topical and systemic acne therapy begin to work, and this itching may last as long as 4 weeks

- Patients with acne vulgaris and subclinical dermographism relate that their acne produces the symptoms of itching, burning, soreness, and/or tenderness[2,3]

    Antihistamines may help the signs and symptoms of the condition

- Another form of itching acne, acne solaria, is said to appear and relapse after sun exposure, is almost always itchy and is preferably localized on the upper anterior chest, the deltoid regions and the shoulders[4]

    The use of greasy or oily sun protectors promotes the development of this condition

## Aquagenic pruritus

Aquagenic itching may be a common and trivial condition or a severe and disabling symptomatic disorder. Transient and trivial itching occurs in a substantial proportion of the population.

- One survey study[5] shows a population prevalence of 45%, and of those affected 33% report a family history of water-related itching

    This condition is not the same as the severe, intense itching of true aquagenic itching

- Aquagenic itching of the elderly generally occurs while the skin is being dried following bathing in women with dry skin[6,7]

    Winter exacerbations are known to occur

    This condition in the elderly generally responds to short-duration bathing and emollient application

True aquagenic itching is a disease in which severe, generalized, itchy, prickling skin discomfort is evoked by contact with water at any temperature without observable skin change[6,8].

- Skin discomfort usually develops within minutes of water contact, but may begin 2 to 15 minutes after water exposure has ceased, and last from 10 to 120 minutes
- Fresh water, sea water, and sweating may all provoke the itching reaction
- Sparing of the palms, soles, and scalp is characteristic
- In most aquagenic pruritus sufferers the disease starts before the age of 30, and in about half will persist for over 10 years

Little is known about its etiology and pathogenesis.

- Increased levels of blood histamine and cutaneous mast cell degranulation are present prior to water exposure and they increase still further with water challenge[8]

    Arguing against histamine pathogenesis is the usual lack of response to antihistaminic agents, and the absence of wheal and flare

- Abnormalities in fibrinolytic activity have been noted and are of unknown significance[9]

Aquagenic pruritus has been reported in association with a number of systemic conditions:

- Acute lymphoblastic leukemia[10]
- Hemachromatosis[11]
- Hypereosinophilic syndrome[12]
- Juvenile xanthogranuloma[13]
- Metastatic cervical squamous cell carcinoma[14]
- Myelodysplastic syndrome[14]
- Polycythemia rubra vera[15]

### Treatment

- The least expensive treatment is sodium bicarbonate added to the bath water – this has been known to fail[6]

    500 mg of sodium bicarbonate may be required with each bath to raise the pH to 8

- Sponge baths or rapid, warm showers may minimize itching
- Hydrophobic emollients may be helpful in aquagenic itching of the elderly, but are not typically helpful in true aquagenic itching
- Topical capsaicin treatment may be effective, but generalized use of this preparation is not typically practical[16,17]
- Partial relief may be obtained in about half of patients with oral antihistamine therapy
- UVB and PUVA have been reported effective in refractory disease[18,19]

    Tolerance may occur to treatments, and continued phototherapy may be required to maintain response

- Systemic corticosteroid agents have also been reported effective but this is unlikely to be a rational long-term strategy[20]
- In polycythemia rubra vera, aspirin, α-interferon and other approaches may be indicated
- Propranolol has anecdotal reported success[21]

### Atmoknesis

This is a frequent problem rarely mentioned by patients and is defined as itching which is provoked by open exposure of the skin to air[22].

- Atmoknesis occurs in many patients with underlying itchy skin diseases including psoriasis and atopic dermatitis, but may rarely be seen in some patients with underlying systemic causes of generalized pruritus, such as hepatobiliary disease

### Cervical rib itching

- Itching from compression of a cervical nerve by a cervical rib has been reported[23]
- This must be exceedingly rare

### Ciguatera fish poisoning

Ciguatera is the commonest form of poisoning resulting from eating fish in the tropics. It is due to the formation of ciguatoxin by a dinoflagellate, *Gambierdiscus toxicus*, loosely attached to algae growing on coral reefs. The toxin, which is harmless to fish, is ingested by small herbivorous fish and passes up the food chain as these are eaten by carnivores.

- In addition to intense itching, the toxic effects include gastroenteritis, peripheral neuropathy and central nervous system dysfunction[24]
- Most cases are mild, but occasionally the disease is severe or fatal[25]

### Dogger bank itch (weed rash)

This is allergic dermatitis due to contact with microscopic marine organisms, *Alcyonidium gelatinosum*, *Alcyonidium hirsutum*, and *Electra pilosa*, which form coralliform, encrusting and filamentous colonies attached to the sea-floor. A sea-weed, *Sargassum muticum*, may also be responsible.

- Occurs mostly in fishermen who work in the North Sea[26,27]
- Contact with the organism occurs when the bryzoan is hauled aboard fishing vessels with other contents of the net[28]
- Contact may cause a disabling allergic contact dermatitis
- One hapten has been identified as the (2-hydroxyethyl) dimethylsulfoxonium ion[29,30]
- Use of protective clothing diminishes contact

## Elderly itching (senile pruritus)

Itching in the elderly is a symptom that is as diverse as all of the subjects reviewed in this text, as the elderly are subject to all skin diseases to which other adults are subject, as well as distinct conditions of aging skin. Nevertheless, there are conditions more common in the elderly that can give rise to severe itching, and there is a true idiopathic itching in the elderly[31].

### Predisposing factors for itching in the elderly

The epidermis of elderly patients appears more asteatotic (dry) than normal, is thinner than normal, and has poor barrier function. Asteatosis results from a series of factors:

- The amount of lipid produced in the skin does not seem to change in aging, but the composition of the lipid changes

    Sebum secretion is highest in young adults and then declines steadily throughout life in both men and women[32]

    The increased occurrence of dry skin in the elderly has been shown to be unrelated to the sebum secretion rate

- In some itching patients, particularly those with asteatosis, one can demonstrate increased intracorneal cohesion and altered skin surface contour parameters[33]

The epidermis has approximately 50% fewer cell layers in older than younger individuals, accompanied by an increased size of corneocytes[34].

- With age the sebum-derived triglycerides decrease markedly, and the fatty acid concentrations in the skin decline

The dermal–epidermal interface becomes flattened with advancing age, leading to less area for fluid exchange from below[35].

- There are fewer superficial dermal capillaries, resulting in less vascular transudation

    Slowed dermal clearance of irritants and allergens undoubtedly contributes to clinical disease

- Behavioral factors can exacerbate the asteatosis[36,37]

    Excessive use of soaps, detergents and other solvents, hot water, and vigorous scrubbing of the skin can remove any vestige of a protective lipid barrier

Cutaneous cellular turnover and repair are much slower, and the time required to recover from insults is prolonged. Paradoxically, there is an age-dependent decrease in the incidence of allergic contact dermatitis, with decreased sensitization to new allergens and waning responses in previously sensitized subjects[38].

- Elicitation of allergic contact dermatitis is still possible, but the typical clinical appearance may be blunted[39]
- Thus older individuals are not only more vulnerable to environmental insults but through lack of distinct symptoms they fail to recognize that they are being adversely affected

The elderly are more likely than their younger counterparts to have systemic diseases which can potentially cause itching[40], and take more medications that can also potentially cause itching.

Some problems which are more likely to occur in the elderly include asteatotic dermatitis, stasis dermatitis[41–43] (see chapter 6: Common dermatitis diseases), and idiopathic elderly itching.

### Idiopathic elderly itching

This is a diagnosis of exclusion, and in the author's opinion a diagnosis that should only be invoked when empiric treatment has failed for the common dermatitides and when systemic causes of itching have been excluded by careful evaluation. The pathophysiology is unknown.

- Bernhard[44] has hypothesized that this may represent a form of phantom itch. The logic behind this hypothesis is as follows:

  The central nervous system (CNS) can intrinsically generate the sensation of itch

  The CNS expects a certain amount of input from peripheral nerve fibers

  With aging, peripheral nerve fibers can degenerate, sending less signal to the CNS

  The CNS compensates by making its own signals

- Clinically, one sees normal skin, often with secondary changes of rub and scratch
- Treatment is difficult

  Ultraviolet light phototherapy, doxepin, topical emollients with anesthetic agents may help

- The author would be grateful for any information on a universally effective treatment for this disorder

### Epidermolysis bullosa itching

- A family with dominant dystrophic epidermolysis bullosa has been reported[45] in whom linear lichenified lesions and troublesome pruritus were prominent features
- A 46-year-old woman with the Dowling-Meara variant of epidermolysis bullosa simplex presented with worsening, recurrent, itchy, circinate crops of clear and hemorrhagic herpetiform blisters affecting her trunk and limbs[46]
- Other types of epidermolysis bullosa may also itch, perhaps by the same mysterious mechanisms by which surgical and other scars itch

### External magnetic fields

- Paroxysmal attacks of itching constitute a rare sensory symptom of multiple sclerosis, and two women with this disease were reported[47] to have itching which occurred at the onset of treatment with external picoTesla range magnetic fields and coincident with the process of neurologic recovery

  An explanation for this phenomenon escapes the author

### Gum (gingiva) itching

- Two patients were reported[48] in the dental literature with gingival recession and itching that were related to intrinsic psychiatric disease
- Psychologically, the oral cavity is related directly or symbolically to the major human instincts and passions

### Judo-jogger's itch

- In a single patient report[49], itchy ankles and wrists occurred when jogging, but only if the jogging episode followed a judo session by one day

  This condition most likely represents another clinical condition

### Keloids

- Patients have related on occasion that their keloids or hypertrophic scars itch, particularly when they are actively growing[50] (Figure 75)

## Localized itching from central nervous system disease

- See section on focal central nervous system diseases within chapter 4: Systemic causes of itching

## Macular and lichen amyloidosis

- Lichen amyloidosis is said to be a papular, intensely pruritic cutaneous idiopathic amyloidosis, whereas macular amyloidosis has similar symptoms, but has no papular component[51,52]

  Reports exist of lichen amyloidosis of the vulva[53] and nipple[54], and other reports of the effectiveness of phototherapy[55] and dermabrasion[56]

- The amyloid in lichen amyloidosis is not derived from immunoglobulins or serum proteins but is derived from keratin peptides of necrotic keratinocytes, likely deposited in the dermis as the result of chronic scratching or rubbing[57–62]

  Lichen amyloidosis shows typical histologic signs of chronic scratching

- Treatment of lichen amyloidosis should not be directed at removing amyloid nor should patients undergo extensive evaluation for systemic amyloidosis
- Non-pruritic lichen amyloidosis has been reported[63], but patient histories of itching are notoriously unreliable
- These disease entities likely represent other well or poorly recognized clinical conditions[64–66]

## Mercury exposure itching

- Mercury intoxication can cause widespread itching dermatitis, with anorexia, weight loss, and photosensitivity[67]

  Sweating, scaling, erythematous palms in children may be a clue for mercury toxicity, especially if associated with other symptoms as noted above

- Mercury hypersensitivity is a very rare allergic response to mercury and other constituents of dental amalgam or to vaccines containing merthiolate as a preservative[68,69]

  Stomatitis on mucosa adjacent to amalgam dental restorations, often clinically resembling lichen planus is the most common sign[70,71]

  Dental workers may also be subject to being exposed to mercury-containing compounds on their exposed hands[72]

  Other reported symptoms include dermatitis, urticaria, erythema, edema and itching, occurring primarily on the face, neck, limbs and upper torso

  Hypersensitivity can be confirmed through patch testing to mercury metal, ammoniated mercury, and mercuric chloride[73,74]

  Clinical response to amalgam removal is exceptionally difficult to gauge given the tremendous placebo effect of this intervention

## *Mucuna pruriens*–associated itching

- Contact with the legume *Mucuna pruriens* (cowhage) may induce intense itching and dermatitis upon contact[75,76]
- The 10–13 cm fruiting pod bears about 5000 spicules, each of which is capable of inducing several hours of itching upon penetration of the epidermis
- Mucunain, a protein isolated from the spicules, has peptidase activity and is the presumed pruritogen[77]
- Dried spicules remain potent itch-inducers, and these have been a component of itching powder

## Nasal itching as atypical angina

- Nasal pruritus has been reported to be a manifestation of angina in coronary artery disease[78]

## Nevus and tumor itching

### Epidermal nevi

- Epidermal nevi, especially inflammatory linear verrucous epidermal nevi (ILVEN), may itch intensely[79] (Figure 76)
- In about 75% of cases, dermatitic epidermal naevi have their onset during the first 5 years of life
- They are characterized by itching which may be intense
- The lesions are linear and comprise eczematous or psoriasiform papules most commonly located on the leg, and may be from a few cm to the length of the limb
- Optimal treatment is destruction or excision, anti-inflammatory agents may provide temporary relief

### Melanocytic nevi

- Itching in melanocytic nevi may be a sign of recent trauma, but may also rarely indicate malignant transformation

### Melanoma

- In one study of presenting complaints for melanoma, itching was noted in 24%, whereas bleeding and crusting were noted in 18% of cases[80]
- Patients with itching melanomas are less likely to promptly seek medical attention than those with bleeding or ulceration[81]

### Seborrheic keratoses

- Seborrheic keratoses frequently itch, especially when subjected to repetitive trauma

### Other miscellaneous neoplasms with itch potential

- Angiokeratomas may itch[82]
- Eccrine poromas may itch and this itching can signal malignant transformation[83]
- Eruptive xanthomas
- Dermatofibromas[84]
- Follicular basal cell nevus with comedo-like lesions (a rare hamartoma)[85]

## Notalgia paresthetica

See chapter 8: Localized itching

## Paroxysmal itching

- In a single case report, a 72-year-old woman had daily, sudden, intense itching with no skin lesions, which prompted secondary excoriation[86]

  Although no etiology was identified, there was a temporal association with the onset of her itching and the death of her husband

- Paroxysmal itching may also be seen in multiple sclerosis[87]

## Peculiar persistent pruritic affection of the skin

- In a single report[88], this is the phenomenon of an itch that attacks a small area and is relieved by a single scratch or pinch
- This condition most likely represents puncta pruritica

## Phantom itching

- Physicians are often familiar with phantom pain following amputation, but itching may not be unusual[89]

  Phantoms occupy definite position in space, may be capable of movement, and are most commonly described as tingling

- Phantom breast itching sensations following mastectomy are quite common[90,91]
- A single amputation patient completed a brief sensation and pain log, consisting of quantitative and qualitative scales, for 28 days after amputation[92]

  She experienced phantom limb sensations, which spread from her toes to encompass her entire leg by day 10 after surgery

  The quality of sensations remained relatively constant and was described as itching and tingling

The duration and frequency of these episodes decreased throughout the 28 days

- In one bizarre recorded case of a bilateral below-the-knee amputee, severe bilateral phantom itching could only be relieved by 'scratching' phantom feet[93]

  The patient mimicked the act of scratching over the anatomic areas where his feet had been

  He 'scratched' behind closed doors so 'nobody would believe he was crazy'

## Post-cellulitis itching

- A friend related his mysterious intermittent itching which episodically occurs in the area confined to where he previously had cellulitis
- This may occur by similar mechanisms as are involved in itching surgical wounds

## Post-herpetic itching

- Post-herpetic neuralgia most commonly presents with pain or burning sensations, but may present with itching
- Although this condition is rarely reported, it is not uncommonly encountered among the elderly[94,95]

## Postmenopausal itch

- Widespread itching is known associated with the postmenopausal syndrome
- Hormone replacement therapy may ameliorate the itching

## Premenstrual itching

- Recurrent menstrual-associated cholestasis may induce itching[96]

## Prurigo pigmentosa

- Apparently rare elsewhere, this predominantly Japanese disorder has itchy erythematous papules or reticulate plaques of the trunk and neck which result in postinflammatory hyperpigmentation[97–99]
- This idiopathic condition generally responds to dapsone or minocycline

## Pruritic cheilitis

- Cheilitis of benign lymphoplasia has been reported as pruritic cheilitis in which there are varying degrees of itching of the vermilion border[100]
- Histologically, the condition was characterized by a dense lymphocytic infiltrate with numerous lymphoid follicles containing well-differentiated germinal centers

## Pruritus prohibitus

- This is reported as the self-resolving itch that you cannot scratch due to social limitations[101]
- At least a few people may not limit their scratching behavior, and in a single extreme case this has resulted in incarceration[102]

## Puncta pruritica

- This is defined as a chronic, idiopathic condition characterized by the occurrence of one or more intensely itchy pinpoint spots in clinically normal skin that are characteristically improved by fingernail pressure or pinching the skin[103–107]
- Most patients need only reassurance
- Many patients may have other clinically recognizable conditions
- Prurigo nodularis differs in having visible, palpable lesions

## Purpura itching

- The sudden onset of markedly pruritic, purpuric lesions with a clinical appearance similar to the progressive pigmented purpuric dermatoses has been reported[108]

- The itching is severe and unremitting and may lead to depression and loss of sleep
- This condition most likely represents another clinical condition with the artifact of secondary excoriation

## Radiation-induced itching

- Scaling, erythema, and itching often occur with external beam radiation at doses of 2000–2800 centiGray[109]

  At this dose there is destruction of the sebaceous glands and altered skin regeneration within the field

## Referred itch (Mitempfindungen)

- Scratching an irritation may produce a well localized itch, prick or tingle elsewhere[110,111]
- Scratch (stimulus points) and referred itch (referral points) are ipsilateral and scratching the site of the referred itch does not cause the original spot to itch
- The mechanism is unknown but it may be thalamic

## Sauna itch

- Atopic dermatitis and cholinergic urticaria may be exacerbated by the heat of the sauna[112,113]
- When used correctly, sauna exposure uncommonly causes itching

## Seawater-induced itching

- This was described as itching shortly after immersion of any part of the body into seawater, and the 'immersed part becomes blotchy and itchy'[114]
- This appears to be a physical urticaria specific to seawater from the description, but insufficient information is given to make this diagnosis with certainty

## Sea algae toxin dermatitis

- A seaweed dermatitis is caused by the organism *Lyngbya majuscula Gomont* that occurs in persons who have swum off the coast of Oahu in Hawaii
- Experimentally, cutaneous inflammation was induced by debromoaplysiatoxin, a purified toxin extracted from the organism[115]

  By topical application, the toxin was found to produce an irritant pustular folliculitis in humans and to cause a severe cutaneous inflammatory reaction in rabbits and in hairless mice

## Subacute prurigo (itchy red bump disease)

There are clearly a few patients with itchy, recurrent or persistent, symmetric, erythematous papular dermatitis present on the extensor aspects of the limbs, buttocks and trunk that cannot be explained by atopic dermatitis, dermatitis herpetiformis, folliculitis, insect bites, prurigo nodularis, and other nosologic designations[116–119] (Figure 77).

- Some of these patients have an atopic history, whereas others do not seem to have this predisposition
- Most commonly the condition occurs in young to middle-aged patients and women are more frequently affected
- This is a diagnosis of exclusion and careful evaluation for all other diagnostic possibilities is critical

Non-specific anti-inflammatory and antipruritic treatment has been suggested, including:

- Topical and systemic corticosteroid agents
- Sedating antihistaminic agents at bedtime
- Dapsone
- Phototherapy

## Tattoo itching

Itching may be localized to tattoos on the basis of an allergic dermatitis or photoallergic reaction (Figure 78). Multiple colors in tattoos have been reported to cause these reactions including black (carbon and other pigments[120]), red (mercury or cadmium[121–123]), purple (manganese[124,125]), yellow (cadmium[126]), green (chromium[127–129]), and blue (cobalt[130]).

- Cadmium sulfide, a yellow pigment that is also used to intensify red color, is a photosensitizer[131]
- Mercury in the form of cinnabar has been suspected to form itching, swelling, and eczematous changes within the red parts of the tattoos within seconds to hours of

vaccinations containing thimerosol, a complex organic mercurial compound, as a preservative[132]

Treatment with potent topical corticosteroids is generally effective, but does not prevent the next episode.

## Wound itching

- The skin commonly itches following surgical intervention, often months to years following the surgical procedure
- Itching also occurs in burns
- Although in the author's experience this is a common complaint, it is seldom discussed in the medical literature, and rarely requires intervention[133–138]

## References

1. Yee KC, Cunliffe WJ. Itching in acne – an unusual complication of therapy. *Dermatology* 1994;189:117–9
2. Fisher DA. A syndrome of acne vulgaris and subclinical dermographic urticaria. *Cutis* 1991;47:429–32
3. Levine MI. A syndrome of acne vulgaris and subclinical dermographism. *Cutis* 1992;49:25
4. Padilha-Goncalves A, Alvimar Ferreira J. Solar acne. *Med Cut Ibero Lat Am* 1977;5:271-4
5. Potasman I, Heinrich I, Bassan HM: Aquagenic pruritus. prevalence and clinical characteristics. *Isr J Med Sci* 1990;26:499–503
6. Menagé H du P, Greaves MW. Aquagenic pruritus. *Semin Dermatol* 1995;14:313–6
7. Bircher AJ. Water-induced itching. *Dermatologica* 1990;181:83–7
8. Steinman HK, Greaves MW. Aquagenic pruritus. *J Am Acad Dermatol* 1985;13:91–6
9. Lotti T, Steinman HK, Greaves MW, *et al.* Increased cutaneous fibrinolytic activity in aquagenic pruritus. *Int J Dermatol* 1986;25:508–10
10. Ratnaval RC, Burrows NP, Marcus RE, *et al.* Aquagenic pruritus and acute lymphoblastic leukemia. *Br J Dermatol* 1993;129:346–9
11. Nester JE. Hemachromatosis and pruritus. *Ann Int Med* 1983;98:1026
12. Newton JA, Singh AK, Greaves MW, *et al.* Aquagenic pruritus associated with the hypereosinophilic syndrome. *Br J Dermatol* 1990;122:103–6
13. Handfield-Jones SE, Hills RJ, Ive FA, *et al.* Aquagenic pruritus associated with juvenile xanthogranuloma. *Clin Exp Dermatol* 1993;18:253–5
14. Ferguson JE, August PJ, Guy AJ. Aquagenic pruritus associated with metastatic squamous cell carcinoma of the cervix. *Clin Exp Dermatol* 1994;19:257–8
15. Abdel-Naser MB, Gollnick H, Orfanos CE. Aquagenic pruritus as a presenting symptom of polycythemia vera. *Dermatology* 1993;187:130–3
16. Lotti T, Teofoli P, Tsampau D. Treatment of aquagenic pruritus with topical capsaicin cream. *J Am Acad Dermatol* 1994;30:232–5
17. Hautmann G, Teofoli P, Lotti T. Aquagenic pruritus, PUVA and capsaicin treatments. *Br J Dermatol* 1994;131:920–1
18. Menagé H du P, Norris PG, Hawk JLM, *et al.* The efficacy of psoralen photochemotherapy in the treatment of aquagenic pruritus. *Br J Dermatol* 1993;129:163–5
19. Smith RA, Ross JS, Staughton RC. Bath PUVA as a treatment for aquagenic pruritus. *Br J Dermatol* 1994;131:584
20. Carson TE. Aquagenic pruritus: effective treatment with intramuscular triamcinolone acetonide. *Cutis* 1991;48:382

21. Thomsen K. Aquagenic pruritus responds to propranolol. *J Am Acad Dermatol* 1990;22:697

22. Bernhard JD. Nonrashes. 5. Atmoknesis: pruritus provoked by contact with air. *Cutis* 1989;44:143–4

23. Rongioletti F. Pruritus as presenting sign of cervical rib. *Lancet* 1992;339:55

24. Allsop JL, Martini L, Lebris H, *et al.* Neurologic manifestations of ciguatera. Three cases with a neurophysiologic study and examination of one nerve biopsy. *Revue Neurol* 1986;142:590–7

25. Hampton MT, Hampton AA. Ciguatera fish poisoning. *J Am Acad Dermatol* 1989;20:510–1

26. Newhouse ML: Dogger bank itch: survey of trawlermen. *Br Med J* 1966;5496:1142–5

27. Newhouse ML. Dogger bank itch among Lowestoft trawlermen. *Proc Roy Soc Med* 1966;59:1119–20

28. Jeanmougin M, Lemarchand-Venencie F, Hoang XD, *et al.* Occupational eczema with photosensitivity caused by contact with Bryozoa. *Ann Dermatol Venereol* 1987;114:353–7

29. Carle JS, Christophersen C. Dogger bank itch. 4. An eczema-causing sulfoxonium ion from the marine animal, *Alcyonidium gelatinosum* [Bryozoa]. *Toxicon* 1982;20:307–10

30. Carle JS, Thybo H, Christophersen C. Dogger bank itch (3). Isolation, structure determination and synthesis of a hapten. *Contact Dermatitis* 1982;8:43–7

31. Fleischer AB Jr. Pruritus in the elderly. *Advances Dermatol* 1995;10:41–59

32. Downing DT, Stewart ME, Strauss JS. Changes in sebum secretion and the sebaceous gland. *Clin Ger Med* 1989;5:109–14

33. Long CC, Marks R. Stratum corneum changes in patients with senile pruritus. *J Am Acad Dermatol* 1992; 27:560–4

34. Gilchrest BA. Pruritus in the elderly. *Semin Dermatol* 1995;14:317–319

35. Grove GL. Physiologic changes in older skin. *Clin Ger Med* 1989;5:115–25

36. Fleischer AB Jr. Pruritus in the elderly: management by senior dermatologists. *J Am Acad Dermatol* 1993;28:603–9

37. Beauregard S. Gilchrest BA. A survey of skin problems and skin care regimens in the elderly. *Arch Dermatol* 1987;123:1638–43

38. Kwangsukstith C, Maibach HI. Effect of age and sex on the induction and elicitation of allergic contact dermatitis. *Contact Dermatitis* 1995;33:289–98

39. Sauder DN. Effect of age on epidermal immune function. *Clin Ger Med* 1989;5:149–60

40. Duncan WC, Fenske NA. Cutaneous signs of internal disease in the elderly. *Geriatrics* 1990;45:24–30

41. Kurban RS, Kurban AK. Common skin disorders of aging: diagnosis and treatment. *Geriatrics* 1993;48: 30–1, 35–6, 39–42

42. Yap KB, Siew MG, Goh CL. Pattern of skin diseases in the elderly seen at the National Skin Centre (Singapore) 1990. *Sing Med J* 1994;35:147–50

43. Levine N. 'Winter itch': what's causing this rash? *Geriatrics* 1996;51:20

44. Bernhard JD. Phantom itch, pseudophantom itch, and senile pruritus. *Int J Dermatol* 1992;31:856–7

45. Goulden V, Handfield–Jones S, Neild V, *et al.* Linear prurigo simulating dermatitis artefacta in dominant dystrophic epidermolysis bullosa. *Br J Dermatol* 1993;129:443–6

46. McGrath JA, Burrows NP, Russell Jones R, *et al.* Epidermolysis bullosa simplex Dowling-Meara troublesome blistering and pruritus in an adult patient. *Dermatology* 1993;186:68–71

47. Sandyk R. Paroxysmal itching in multiple sclerosis during treatment with external magnetic fields. *Int J Neuroscience* 1994;75:65–71

48. Aksoy N. Psychosomatic diseases and dentistry (report of two psychoneurotic cases). *Ankara Universitesi Dis Hekimligi Fakultesi Dergisi* 1990;17:141–3

49. Sullivan SN. Judo-jogger's itch. *New Engl J Med* 1979;300:866

50. Rudolph R. Wide spread scars, hypertrophic scars, and keloids. *Clin Plastic Surg* 1987;14:253–60

51. Kibbi AG, Rubeiz NG, Zaynoun ST, *et al.* Primary localized cutaneous amyloidosis. *Int J Dermatol* 1992;31:95–8

52. Brownstein MH, Hashimoto K. Macular amyloidosis. *Arch Dermatol* 1972;106:50–7

53. Gorodeski IG, Cordoba M, Shapira A, *et al.* Primary localized cutaneous lichen amyloidosus of the vulva. *Int J Dermatol* 1988;27:259–60

54. Ganor S, Dollberg L. Amyloidosis of the nipple presenting as pruritus. *Cutis* 1983;31:318

55. Hudson LD. Macular amyloidosis: treatment with ultraviolet B. *Cutis* 1986;38:61–2

56. Wong CK, Li WM. Dermabrasion for lichen amyloidosus. Report of a long-term study. *Arch Dermatol* 1982;118:302–4

57. Black MM, Jones EW. Macular amyloidosis. A study of 21 cases with special reference to the role of the epidermis in its histogenesis. *Br J Dermatol* 1971;84: 199–209

58. Iwasaki K, Mihara M, Nishiura S, *et al.* Biphasic amyloidosis arising from friction melanosis. *J Dermatol* 1991;18:86–91

59. Leonforte JF. Origin of macular amyloidosis. Apropos of 160 cases. *Annales Dermatologie Venereol* 1987;114:801–6

60. Sumitra S, Yesudian P. Friction amyloidosis: a variant or an etiologic factor in amyloidosis cutis? *Int J Dermatol* 1993;32:422–3

61. Weyers W. Lichen amyloidosus – disease entity or the effect of scratching. *Hautarzt* 1995;46:165–72

62. Wong CK, Lin CS. Friction amyloidosis. *Int J Dermatol* 1988;27:302–7

63. Kuligowski ME, Chang A. Non-itchy lichen amyloidosus. *Int J Dermatol* 1992;31:747

64. Bernhard JD. Macular amyloidosis, notalgia paresthetica and pruritus: three sides of the same coin? *Dermatologica* 1991;183:53–4

65. Cerroni L, Kopera D, Soyer HP, *et al.* Notalgia paresthetica, "posterior pigmented pruritic patch" and macular amyloidosis. Three stages of a disease. *Hautarzt* 1993;44:777–80

66. Goulden V, Highet AS, Shamy HK. Notalgia paraesthetica – report of an association with macular amyloidosis. *Clin Exp Dermatol* 1994;19:346–9

67. von Muhlendahl KE. Intoxication from mercury spilled on carpets. *Lancet* 1990;336:1578–79

68. Handley J, Todd D, Burrows D. Mercury allergy in a contact dermatitis clinic in Northern Ireland. *Contact Dermatitis* 1993;29:258–61

69. Kawai K, Zhang XM, Nakagawa M, *et al.* Allergic contact dermatitis due to mercury in a wedding ring and a cosmetic. *Contact Dermatitis* 1994;31:330–1

70. Ulukapi I. Mercury hypersensitivity from amalgam: report of case. *ASDC J Dent Children* 1995;62:363–4

71. Veien NK. Stomatitis and systemic dermatitis from mercury in amalgam dental restorations. *Dermatol Clinics* 1990;8:157–60

72. Kanerva L, Komulainen M, Estlander T, *et al.* Occupational allergic contact dermatitis from mercury. *Contact Dermatitis* 1993;28:26–8

73. Namikoshi T, Yoshimatsu T, Suga K, *et al.* The prevalence of sensitivity to constituents of dental alloys. *J Oral Rehab* 1990;17:377–81

74. Pambor M, Timmel A. Mercury dermatitis. *Contact Dermatitis* 1989;20:157

75. Anonymous. Mucuna pruriens-associated pruritus-New Jersey. *J Am Med Assoc* 1986;255:313

76. Denman ST. Wuepper KD. Histologic and biochemical characteristics of Mucuna pruriens. *Clin Res* 1982;30:581

77. Shelley WB, Arthur RP. Studies on cowhage (*Mucuna pruriens*) and its pruritogenic protease, mucunain. *Arch Dermatol* 1955;73:399

78. Reichstein RP, Stein WG. Nasal pruritus as atypical angina? *New Engl J Med* 1983;309:667

79. Dellon AL, Luethke R, Wong L, *et al.* Epidermal nevus: surgical treatment by partial-thickness skin excision. *Ann Plastic Surg* 1992;28:292–6

80. du Vivier AW, Williams HC, Brett JV, *et al.* How do malignant melanomas present and does this correlate with the seven–point check-list? *Clin Exp Dermatol* 1991;16:344-7

81. Cassileth BR, Lusk EJ, Guerry D IV, *et al.* 'Catalyst' symptoms in malignant melanoma. *J Gen Int Med* 1987;2:1–4

82. Miwa N, Kobayashi T, Kanzaki T, *et al.* Angiokeratoma corporis circumscriptum naeviforme with transepidermal elimination. *J Dermatol* 1993;20: 247–51

83. Pylyser K, De Wolf-Peeters C, Marien K. The histology of eccrine poromas: a study of 14 cases. *Dermatologica* 1983;167:243–9

84. Veraldi S, Bocor M, Gianotti R, *et al.* Multiple eruptive dermatofibromas localized exclusively to the buttock. *Int J Dermatol* 1991;30:507–8

85. Crivellato E, Trevisan G, Grandi G, *et al.* Bilateral follicular basal cell nevus with comedo-like lesions. *Acta Derm Venereol* 1983;63:77–9

86. Hazelrigg DE. Paroxysmal pruritus. *J Am Acad Dermatol* 1985;13:839–40

87. Yamamoto M, Yabuki S, Hayabara T, *et al.* Paroxysmal itching in multiple sclerosis: a report of three cases. *J Neurol Neurosurg Psychiatry* 1981;44: 19–22

88. Waisman M. Peculiar pruritus. *Arch Dermatol* 1978;114:968

89. Bernhard JD. Phantom itch, pseudophantom itch, and senile pruritus. *Int J Dermatol* 1992;31:856–7

90. Lierman LM. Phantom breast experiences after mastectomy. *Oncol Nurs Forum* 1988;15:41–4

91. Staps T, Hoogenhout J, Wobbes T. Phantom breast

sensations following mastectomy. *Cancer* 1985; 56:2898–901

92. McGrath PA, Hillier LM. Phantom limb sensations in adolescents: a case study to illustrate the utility of sensation and pain logs in pediatric clinical practice. *J Pain Symptom Manag* 1992;7:46–53

93. Jacome D. Phantom itching relieved by scratching phantom feet. *J Am Med Assoc* 1978;240:2432

94. Darsow U, Lorenz J, Bromm B, *et al*. Pruritus circumscriptus sine materia: a sequel of postherpetic neuralgia. Evaluation by quantitative psychophysical examination and laser-evoked potentials. *Acta Derm Venereol* 1996;76:45–7

95. Liddell K. Letter: Post-herpetic pruritus. *Br Med J* 1974;4:165

96. Dahl MG. Premenstrual pruritus due to recurrent cholestasis. *Trans St Johns Hosp Dermatol Soc* 1970; 56:11–3

97. Aso M, Miyamato T, Morimura T, *et al*. Prurigo pigmentosa successfully treated with minocycline. *Br J Dermatol* 1989;120: 705–8

98. Joyce AP, Horn TD, Anhalt GJ. Prurigo pigmentosa. Report of case and review of literature. *Arch Dermatol* 1989;125:1551–4

99. Liu MT, Wong CK. Prurigo pigmentosa. *Dermatology* 1994;188:219–21

100. Guoqi X, Yiming H, Huibao S, *et al*. Pruritic cheilitis. Six cases of a rarely seen benign lymphoplasia. *Oral Surg, Oral Med, Oral Pathol* 1983;55:359–62

101. Bernhard JD. Nonrashes. 3. Pruritus prohibitus. *Cutis* 1982;29:358–9

102. Weinstein BR, Bernhard JD. Incarceration for excoriation. *Cutis* 1990;46:240

103. Boyd AS, Zemstov A, Nelder KH. Puncta pruritica. *Int J Dermatol* 1992;31:370

104. Crissey JT. Puncta pruritica. *Int J Dermatol* 1991;30: 722–4

105. Crissey JT. Puncta pruritica. *Int J Dermatol* 1992;31: 166

106. Schamberg IL. Peculiar persistent pruritic affection of the skin. *Arch Dermatol* 1977;113:986

107. Toomey N. Itch points (puncta pruritica). *Arch Dermatol* 1922;5:744–7

108. Pravda DJ. Moynihan GD. Itching purpura. *Cutis* 1980;25:147–51

109. Hassey KM, Rose CM. Altered skin integrity in patients receiving radiation therapy. *Oncol Nurs Forum* 1982;9:44–50

110. Evans PR. Referred itch (Mitempfindungen). *Br Med J* 1976;2:839–41

111. Richter CP. Mysterious form of referred sensation in man. *Proc Nat Acad Sci USA* 1977;74:4702–5

112. Hannuksela M, Vaananen A. The sauna, skin and skin diseases. *Ann Clin Res* 1988;20:276–8

113. Markkola L, Mattila KJ, Koivikko MJ. Sauna habits and related symptoms in Finnish children. *Eur J Ped* 1989;149:221–2

114. Buckholtz GA, Lockey RF. Seawater-induced itching. *J Am Med Assoc* 1991;266:3040

115. Solomon AE, Stoughton RB. Dermatitis from purified sea algae toxin (debromoaplysiatoxin). *Arch Dermatol* 1978;114:1333–5

116. Jorizzo JL, Gath S, Smith EB. Prurigo: a clinical review. *J Am Acad Dermatol* 1981;4:723–9

117. Mali JWH. Prurigo simplex subacuta: a group of cases with atopic background. *Acta Derm Venereol* 1967;47:304–8

118. Sherertz EF, Jorizzo JL, White WL, *et al*. Papular dermatitis in adults: subacute prurigo, American style? *J Am Acad Dermatol* 1991;24:697–702

119. Uehara M, Ofuji S. Primary eruption of prurigo simplex subacuta. *Dermatologica* 1976;153:49–56

120. Tope WD, Arbiser JL, Duncan LM. Black tattoo reaction: the peacock's tale. *J Am Acad Dermatol* 1996;35:477–8

121. Anonymous. The case of the itching tattoo. *Ann Int Med* 1967;67:1116–7

122. Davis RG. Hazards of tattooing. Report of two cases of dermatitis caused by sensitization to mercury (cinnabar). *US Armed Forces Med J* 1960;11:261–80

123. Goldstein N. Mercury-cadmium sensitivity in tattoos. A photoallergic reaction in red pigment. *Ann Int Med* 1967;67:984–9

124. Schwartz RA, Mathias CG, Miller CH, *et al*. Granulomatous reaction to purple tattoo pigment. *Contact Dermatitis* 1987;16:198–202

125. Nguyen LW, Allen HB,. Reactions to manganese and cadmium in tattoos. *Cutis* 1979;23:71–2

126. Tindall JP, Smith JG. Unusual reactions in yellow tattoos: microscopic studies on histologic dections. *South Med J* 1962;55:792–5

127. Bjornberg A. Allergic reaction to chrome in green tattoo markings. *Acta Derm Venereol* 1959;39:23–9

128. Heileson B. Chromium allergy as the possible cause of eczema tattooing. *Acta Derm Venereol* 1953;33: 255

129. Lowenthal LJA. Reactions in green tattoos. *Arch Dermatol* 1960;82:237–43

130. Bjornberg A. Allergic reaction to cobalt in light blue tattoo markings. *Acta Derm Venereol* 1941;41:260–3

131. Bjornberg A. Reactions to light in yellow tattoos from cadmium sulfide. *Arch Dermatol* 1963;88:83–7

132. Kravitz P. Influenza vaccine and itchy tattoos. *Ann Int Med* 1978;88:428

133. Bell L, McAdams T, Morgan R, *et al.* Pruritus in burns: a descriptive study. *J Burn Care Rehab* 1988;9: 305–8

134. Herman LEU. Itching in scars. In Bernhard JD, ed. *Itch. Mechanisms and Management of Pruritus.* New York: McGraw Hill, 1994;153–60

135. Phillips LG, Robson MC. Pruritus in burns. *J Burn Care Rehab* 1988;9:308–9

136. Ramirez OM. The anchor subperiosteal forehead lift. *Plastic Reconstructive Surg* 1995;95:993–1003

137. Ship AG, Weiss PR, Mincer FR, *et al.* Sternal keloids: successful treatment employing surgery and adjunctive radiation. *Ann Plastic Surg* 1993;31:481–7

138. Smith S. Pruritus in burns. *J Burn Care Rehab* 1988; 9:309–10

# Treatment

## 11

Each patient and disease should be considered as unique; accordingly there are no therapies that work for all patients in all conditions. The treatments outlined below are guidelines to help clinicians understand agents and their efficacy in a broad fashion

## Topical treatment

Topical agents are extremely important in therapeutic intervention[1,2]. Note that essentially all topical agents have risks of sensitization and side-effects (see also chapter 6: Common dermatitis diseases).

### Vehicles

Unlike systemic agents, topical drugs for dermatologic use are generally incorporated into a vehicle, a simple or highly complex drug-delivery system. Ideal vehicles promote release of the active drug and facilitate penetration through the epidermal barrier. Types of vehicles include:

- Solutions (aqueous, alcoholic, and oil-based)
- Lotions (oil in water and water in oil)
- Semisolid preparations (ointments, creams and gels)
- Shake lotions (solid suspended in water)

Choice of therapeutic vehicle for treating any given patient and condition should take into account a number of factors including:

- Patient preference (some prefer creams, others ointments)
- Body site treated (solutions may be best for hairy scalps)
- Disease pathophysiology (drying creams may be superior in vesicular contact dermatitis)
- Method of application (ointments may be easier to use under plastic occlusion)

- Hypersensitivity to specific vehicle ingredients (e.g. allergy to ethylenediamine or Kathon CG)

### Anesthetics

Anesthetic agents decrease sensations in both pain and itch receptors, accordingly they may provide not only itch relief, but relief of tingling and other dysesthesias. A number of anesthetic agents exist including benzocaine, camphor, lidocaine, menthol, pramoxine, and a mixture of prilocaine and lidocaine.

- No comparative studies clearly demonstrate one agent as better than another, but all appear relatively safe
- Benzocaine, lidocaine, and similar '-caine' anesthetics are likely to be more potent antipruritic agents than pramoxine, menthol and camphor

  Anesthetics such as benzocaine are extraordinarily rapid antipruritic agents

  Although previously thought to be common sensitizers, only rarely do anesthetics sensitize; their sensitization potential may approximate that of topical corticosteroid agents

  Recent evidence[3] suggests that menthol acts by decreasing cutaneous nerve activity, but not by decreasing skin temperature

  A eutectic mixture of the local anesthetics lidocaine and prilocaine (EMLA) has well-documented antipruritic activity[4]

- These agents may be found alone or combined together in various products

## Antihistamines

Antihistamines including diphenhydramine, dimetindene, doxepin and promethazine are available as itch relievers. Their mode of action probably involves histamine blockade and possibly anesthesia, but this has not been well-studied.

- Dimetindene[5] and especially doxepin[6] have been well established as reasonably safe and effective antipruritic agents
- By contrast, there are essentially no published data suggesting any efficacy for diphenhydramine

Side-effects such as drowsiness and xerostomia occur when large portions of the body surface area are covered or young children are treated.

- Rarely, visual and auditory hallucinations following topical applications have been reported due to exceedingly high blood levels of diphenhydramine[7]
- Intoxication may occur with promethazine[8]

Allergic contact sensitization may be more common with this class of agents than other antipruritic agent types.

## Capsaicin

Capsaicin has been demonstrated to relieve itching[9–12], but large numbers of patients experience stinging and burning from its use. Its putative mode of action is via depletion of substance P and other neuropeptides. Capsaicin must be used several times daily in order to achieve the desired effects, and it is apparently free of systemic toxicity.

## Corticosteroids

These are highly effective anti-inflammatory agents that are elegant and rarely cause irritation or sensitization. The mode of action is multifactorial[13,14].

- Topical glucocorticoid treatment can suppress histamine release from dermal mast cells and can decrease the numbers of mast cells present
- Analogous to systemic corticosteroids, these agents exert a broad range of anti-inflammatory activities that are discussed below with systemic corticosteroid agents

These are usually the agents of choice in treating atopic, contact and irritant dermatitis[6]. With the possible exception of newer 'soft molecule' corticosteroids, the higher the potency, the greater the efficacy and the greater the risk of side-effects (Box 11.1).

- Characteristics of 'soft molecules'[15]:

  High lipophilicity (enhances penetration)

  High corticosteroid binding affinity (decreases amount of drug required)

  Rapid single-step degradation to inactive metabolites (reduces systemic toxicity of active metabolites; application to large body surface areas does not affect plasma cortisol levels)

- Examples of 'soft molecules' include:

  Fluticasone proprionate

  Methylprednisolone aceponate[16,17]

Corticosteroids may be used under plastic film or hydrocolloid dressing occlusion to enhance penetration. Prolonged use of any topical corticosteroid agent may induce tachyphylaxis[18,19].

### Side-effects from topical corticosteroids

In a large meta-analysis[20] adverse reactions were found to be mild and transient. 'Common' side-effects (1% or less) include irritation, itching, burning, dryness, scaling and vesicle formation.

*Cutaneous atrophy[21]*

- Reversible or permanent; may be more common in older agents than 'soft molecules' (Figures 79, 80)

```
┌─────────────────────────────────────────────────────────────────────────────┐
│                                                                               │
│  Box 11.1  Corticosteroid potency (US trade names)*                           │
│                                                                               │
│  Group I            Betamethasone diproprionate (Diprolene ointment, gel, solution)
│  Superhigh potency  Clobetasol (Temovate cream, ointment, emollient cream, gel, solution)
│                     Diflorasone diacetate (Psorcon ointment)**               │
│                     Halobetasol (Ultravate cream, ointment)                  │
│                                                                               │
│  Group II           Amcinonide (Cyclocort ointment)                          │
│  Potent             Betamethasone diproprionate (Diprolene A cream)          │
│                     Desoximetasone (Topicort cream, ointment gel)            │
│                     Diflorasone diacetate (Florone ointment or Psorcon cream)│
│                     Fluocinonide (Lidex cream, ointment, gel, solution)      │
│                     Halcinonide (Halog cream, ointment, solution)            │
│                     Mometasone furoate (Elocon ointment)                     │
│                                                                               │
│  Group III          Amcinonide (Cyclocort cream, lotion)                     │
│  Mid-potency        Betamethasone diproprionate (Diprosone cream)            │
│                     Betamethasone valerate (Valisone ointment)               │
│                     Diflorasone diacetate (Florone or Maxiflor cream)        │
│                     Fluocinonide (Lidex E cream)                             │
│                     Fluticasone proprionate (Cutivate ointment)             │
│                     Triamcinolone acetonide (Aristocort A ointment)         │
│                                                                               │
│  Group IV           Fluocinolone acetonide (Synalar ointment)               │
│  Mid-potency        Flurandrenolide (Cordran ointment)                      │
│                     Hydrocortisone valerate (Westcort ointment)             │
│                     Mometasone furoate (Elocon cream)                        │
│                     Triamcinolone acetonide (Aristocort and Kenalog cream)  │
│                                                                               │
│  Group V            Betamethasone diproprionate (Diprosone lotion)          │
│  Mid-potency        Betamethasone valerate (Valisone cream)                 │
│                     Fluocinolone acetonide (Synalar cream)                   │
│                     Flurandrenolide (Cordran SP cream)                       │
│                     Fluticasone proprionate (Cutivate cream)                │
│                     Hydrocortisone butyrate (Locoid cream)                   │
│                     Hydrocortisone valerate (Westcort cream)                 │
│                     Triamcinolone acetonide (Kenalog lotion)                │
│                                                                               │
│  Group VI           Aclometasone diproprionate (Aclovate cream, ointment)  │
│  Mild potency       Betasmethasone valerate (Valisone Lotion)               │
│                     Desonide (Desowen or Tridesilon cream, ointment, lotion)│
│                     Fluocinolone acetonide (Synalar solution, Dermasmoothe FS oil)
│                                                                               │
│  Group VII          Hydrocortisone, Dexamethasone, Flumethasone, Prednisolone, or
│  Low potency        Methylprednisolone                                       │
│                                                                               │
│  *Partial list of generic names listed in alphabetical order within groups with select trade names
│  **Less potent than Group I                                                  │
│                                                                               │
└─────────────────────────────────────────────────────────────────────────────┘
```

- Skin fragility
- Ecchymoses
- Telangiectasia
- Stellate pseudoscars
- Ecchymoses
- Striae

*Acneiform eruptions*
- Acne
- Folliculitis
- Perioral dermatitis
- Rosacea

*Miscellaneous reported side-effects*
- Hirsutism
- Reduced wound healing
- Glaucoma
- Intrauterine growth retardation[22]

*Allergic contact dermatitis*
- Vehicle: most products contain occasionally sensitizing preservatives
- Drug allergy to topical corticosteroid agents is well-documented[23], and one may become cross-sensitized to multiple corticosteroid agents

*Hypothalamic–pituitary–adrenal suppression*
- Much more common with superpotent agents than with any other class[24]

  > 7 g daily of clobetasol propionate or betamethasone dipropionate was sufficient to suppress morning plasma cortisol levels in 20% of patients; 2 g daily may suppress morning plasma cortisol levels

- Even hydrocortisone may suppress morning plasma cortisol levels
- Newer corticosteroid agents, i.e. fluticasone proprionate and methylprednisolone aceponate[17], are rapidly inactivated in a single hydrolytic metabolic step and are hepatically cleared in the first-pass; accordingly 'soft molecules' may be systemically safer than older, slowly-degraded species

*Miscellaneous systemic effects (theoretically possible, rarely, if ever, observed)*
- Cushing's syndrome
- Growth retardation
- Hypertension
- Muscle wasting

## Cooling agents

Shake lotions, for example calamine and alcohol, can provide temporary relief of itching and are reasonable safe[25].

- Menthol acts more as an anesthetic than a cooling agent, but provides a sensation of cooling
- Applications of large quantities of most shake lotions is cosmetically inelegant
- Application of large quantities of alcohol is potentially irritating to skin and transcutaneous absorption in children is problematic

## Coal tar

Coal tar is not a single ingredient, but a variable mixture of thousands of active and inactive chemicals. Although some of the molecular forms in tar are undoubtedly carcinogenic and systemically absorbed in minute quantities, tars are considered generally safe and have minimal toxicity.

- Folliculitis and itching are occasional side-effects
- Purified coal tars have a less unpleasant odor and are less likely to stain clothing
- Tars may be incorporated into gels, solutions, creams, ointments, and shampoos

## Crotamiton

Although this agent is an effective scabicide[26,27], in a double-blind, paired-comparison trial, there was no significant difference in itch relief between crotamiton lotion and its vehicle.

- Some patients anecdotally report that this agent is highly effective

## Emollients

Although emollients are not generally considered antipruritic agents, they can provide significant relief from itching[28]. Additionally they can help restore an impaired cutaneous barrier, a common finding in inflammatory dermatoses. Addition of other agents, including lactic acid and urea, enhances the activity of the emollient.

- Ammonium lactate 12% lotion of cream is particularly efficacious in asteatotic dermatitis and in restoring the normal barrier function of the skin
- Emollients can be easily combined with virtually any other topical or systemic regimen

## Tacrolimus (FK 506)

This agent was first employed systemically for prevention of transplant rejection. The molecules of the drug are small enough to allow transcutaneous absorption[29].

- As an immunosuppressant, it is about 100 times more potent than cyclosporin A
- The agent inhibits development of experimental allergic contact dermatitis[30]
- Initial studies suggest that topical tacrolimus 0.1% ointment is a rapid, effective antipruritic and anti-inflammatory agent in atopic dermatitis with negligible toxicity[31]

   In an open study of 50 atopic patients with facial dermatitis, itching was reduced within 3 days, but one-third of patients developed detectable blood levels of tacrolimus, ranging to 0.9ng/ml

- Tacrolimus works well compared with placebo

   A randomized, double-blind, multi-center study which compared 0.03%, 0.1% and 0.3% tacrolimus ointment with vehicle alone was performed in patients suffering from moderate to severe atopic dermatitis. The ointment was applied twice daily.

   After 3 weeks of treatment, the median percentage decrease in the dermatitis severity score was 66.7% for the 54 patients receiving 0.03% tacrolimus, 83.3% for the 54 patients receiving 0.1% tacrolimus, 75.0% for the 51 patients receiving 0.3% tacrolimus, and 22.5% for the 54 patients receiving vehicle only

   A sensation of burning at the site of application was the only adverse event that was significantly more frequent with tacrolimus than with vehicle alone. Throughout the study, most patients in the three tacrolimus groups had blood concentrations of tacrolimus below 0.25ng/ml, a clinically insignificant value

   In this placebo-controlled trial the short-term application of tacrolimus ointment is effective in the treatment of atopic dermatitis, with the sensation of burning being the main side-effect[32]

- In several open and randomized studies performed in the dermatology center of the Wake Forest University School of Medicine, many patients were induced into remission who had not responded to other topical and systemic agents

## Sodium cromoglycate

10% sodium cromoglycate was more effective than placebo in atopic dermatitis[33] and may improve itching, sleep disturbance, inflammation and lichenification[34].

- This agent has not been extensively tested for itching, but is quite safe

## Bathing agents

Virtually any agent or group of agents can be incorporated into bathing regimens, and bathing itself may improve itching

- Rice bran broth bathing improves itching in most patients with atopic dermatitis[35]
- Biweekly water bath hyperthermia has been tried in psoriasis with demonstrated improvement in psoriatic lesions, and hot water alone may help itching[36]

  Hot water may also disrupt the epidermal barrier, leaving the skin more susceptible to irritant contact dermatitis

- Miscible bath oils or vegetable oils may provide hydration to the skin and are as effective as topical emollient lotions
- Colloidal oatmeal baths are an age-old remedy that many find soothing for generalized itching
- Tar baths can be given with miscible coal tar with satisfying results
- Sodium bicarbonate baths may help some patients[37,38]

## Systemic therapy

There are no specific systemic antipruritic systemic agents that help all patients. Most antipruritic agents act centrally by a property or mechanism related to sedation.

Anti-inflammatory drugs including corticosteroids and cyclosporin decrease inflammation and their attendant inflammatory mediators. Antihistamines ($H_1$ receptor antagonists) have a peripheral antipruritic action only in the uncommon case where itch is due to histamine release, as in urticaria.

### Placebo

Placebo response in itching conditions is quite marked.

- Epstein and Pinski[39] demonstrated that with four successive, different placebo agents, itch relief from one or more agents was achieved by 66%

  The first placebo agent used was the most effective

To a large extent, many systemic antipruritic agents may work primarily by placebo mechanism. Rather than assuming this is a limitation, the author believes that the placebo response is a clear demonstration of the powerful central nervous system modulation of itch.

### Charcoal

Oral charcoal helps relieve the itching of renal disease[40,41] and cholestatic liver disease. It may have utility in a broad range of itchy disorders.

### Corticosteroid agents

Corticosteroid agents profoundly affect lymphocyte and monocyte function and can suppress inflammation resulting from mechanical, infectious, and immunologic stimuli.

- Corticosteroids decrease elaboration and release[42] of vasoactive and chemoattractive factors, decrease secretion of destructive enzymes, and decrease recruitment of other inflammatory cells
- Corticosteroids indirectly inhibit phospholipase A2 through induction of the protein lipocortin[43]
- Inflammatory mediators affected by corticosteroids include prostaglandins, interleukins (IL-1, IL-2, IL-3, IL-6), interferon, granulocyte/monocyte colony stimulating factor, leucotrienes, and tumor necrosis factor alpha

  The above mediators orchestrate key aspects of the inflammatory response, and suppression of these mediators profoundly affects the inflammatory process at multiple levels

Systemic corticosteroids are excellent anti-inflammatory agents but do not provide itch relief in non-inflammatory itching conditions such as in renal or hepatic disease. Whenever possible, these agents are best given for a limited time rather than as chronic therapy.

**Table 11.1** Comparison of various systemic corticosteroid agents

| Agent | Anti-inflammatory potency | Mineralocorticoid potency | Biologic half-life (hours; oral or i.v.) | Equivalent dose (mg) |
|---|---|---|---|---|
| Betamethasone | 25 | 0 | 36–72 | 0.75 |
| Cortisol | 1 | 1 | 8–12 | 20 |
| Dexamethasone | 25 | 0 | 36–72 | 0.75 |
| Methylprednisolone | 5 | 0.5 | 12–36 | 4 |
| Prednisolone | 4 | 0.8 | 12–36 | 5 |
| Prednisone | 4 | 0.8 | 12–36 | 5 |
| Triamcinolone | 5 | 0 | 12–36 | 4 |

Table modified from reference 44

- Life-threatening dermatoses with itching such as bullous pemphigoid may require longer term use of such agents

### Dosage and administration

A dose range of 0.5–1.0 mg/kg/day of prednisone equivalents (Table 11.1) is common for short-term treatment of inflammatory dermatoses.

- Prednisone, methylprednisolone, and prednisolone have minimal mineralocorticoid activity and generally have a sufficiently prolonged action to ensure the sustained effectiveness of a single daily dose

For short-term treatment, some clinicians prefer to taper the dose (for example, every morning take 60mg for 3 days, 40mg for 3 days, 20mg for 3 days) whereas others prefer to direct patients to take continuous dose regimes (e.g. 40 mg every morning for 9 days); there is little objective evidence to substantiate the beneficial aspects of one approach over another.

To minimize hypothalamic–adrenal suppression, for most conditions short-term systemic corticosteroid therapy is best given as a single morning dose. Intramuscular administration of long-acting agents may suppress inflammation better than oral use of shorter acting agents, however these agents are more likely to suppress the hypothalamic–pituitary–adrenal axis. For severe inflammatory conditions, intravenous administration can provide marked, rapid symptom relief.

- Typical adult doses for severe diseases may be the equivalent of 40–100 mg of methylprednisolone every 8 hours
- High-dose intravenous methylprenisolone (20mg/kg/day) for 3 days has been reported to be effective in severe atopic dermatitis unresponsive to standard therapy[45]

### Side-effects

*Short-term administration*

- The majority of patients take these agents for short times without side-effects
- Some of the short-term side-effects include fluid retention, increased hunger, agitation, exacerbation of diabetes or hypertension, weight gain, and psychosis
- Short-term side-effects may be greater in older individuals, and accordingly one should consider decreasing the dose
- Although rare, anaphylactic reactions to systemic corticosteroids have been described in adults and children[46]

*Long-term administration*

- Searching for other systemic agents with anti-inflammatory activity may prove useful
- Side-effects include those mentioned for short-term administration plus hypothalamic–pituitary–adrenal axis suppression, abnormal fat distribution, posterior subcapsular cataracts[47], osteoporosis and numerous other effects

  > Using every other day dosing may decrease the risk of hypothalamic–pituitary–adrenal axis suppression, but posterior subcapsular cataracts and osteoporosis continue to occur[48–50]

- There is little evidence that systemic corticosteroids are harmful in pregnancy

  > Reports exist allegedly linking corticosteroids with stillbirth, spontaneous abortion, low birth weight and cleft palate[51], but solid epidemiologic evidence is lacking

  > There is no adequate evidence substantiating pregnancy risk of topical corticosteroid agents

  > Nevertheless prudence dictates that if effective alternatives exist they should be used

## H₁ antihistamines

$H_1$ antihistamines are probably the most commonly prescribed antipruritic agents. Much of their activity stems from sedation, but some newer agents (e.g. cetirizine and loratidine) may display anti-inflammatory activity that complements their histamine receptor blockade[52]. Side-effect profiles are highly variable.

- Sedative effects are potentiated by benzodiazepines, other neuropsychiatric agents and alcohol
- Anticholinergic side-effects such as xerostomia, urinary retention and impotence are more common with less-specific older agents or with antihistamine-like agents such as amitriptyline and doxepin

- Some patients, particularly children, paradoxically are stimulated by sedating drugs
- Uncommon side-effects include seizures, weight gain, and anaphylaxis

Although not contraindicated, special precautions should be exercised in those operating heavy machinery, or those with sicca syndrome, epilepsy, prostatic hypertrophy, glaucoma and porphyria.

- Caution should be employed in children's dosages[53]
- Although antihistamines may be one of the safest classes of agents to use during pregnancy, whenever possible it is prudent to avoid all agents of marginal efficacy
- Nevertheless, chlorpheniramine, diphenhydramine and hydroxyzine are generally considered safe[54]

### Distinguishing features of antihistamines (see Table 11.2)

- Acrivastine has extremely fast onset and rapidly achieves steady state, but requires frequent dosing[64]
- Fatal cardiac arrhythmias can occur when astemazole and terfenidine interact with macrolide antibiotics including erythromycin and clarithromycin and systemic antifungal agents including fluconazole, itraconazole, and ketoconazole, and these also interact with cisapride and lovostatin[65]
- Of the non-sedating anti-inflammatory agents, loratidine and cetirizine have the fewest known drug interactions[66]
- Cetirizine has specific anti-allergic effects on the leukocytes
- Loratidine and cetirizine, but not astemazole or terfenidine, decrease the itch of non-urticarial conditions[67]
- Cyproheptadine also has anti-serotonergic activity
- Hydroxyzine has mild anxiolytic activity

**Table 11.2** Select H$_1$ antihistaminic agents

| Antihistamine | Adult dose (mg) | Dosing interval (hours) | Histamine blockade | Side-effect profile |
|---|---|---|---|---|
| Acrivastine | 8 | 6–8 | ++ | + |
| Amitriptyline | 10–100 | 24 | ++++ | ++++ |
| Astemazole | 10 | 24 | +++ | + |
| Azatidine | 1-2 | 12 | ++ | ++ |
| Azelastine | 2 | 12 | + | ++ |
| Bromphenirimine | 4 | 8 | ++ | + |
| Cetirizine | 10 | 24 | +++ | + |
| Chlorpheniramine | 4 | 4–6 | ++ | + |
| Clemastine | 1 | 12 | ++ | ++ |
| Cyproheptadine | 4 | 8 | + | + |
| Diphenhydramine | 25–50 | 6–8 | + | +++ |
| Doxepin | 10–100 | 24 | ++++ | ++++ |
| Hydroxyzine | 10–25 | 6–8 | +++ | ++ |
| Loratidine | 10 | 24 | +++ | + |
| Promethazine | 12.5–25 | 6–12 | +++ | +++ |
| Terfenadine | 60 | 12 | ++ | + |

+, minimal; ++++, maximal
Table adapted from references 55–63

- Azelastine is an antihistamine as well as a multifunctional anti-allergy agent capable of inhibiting mast-cell activation and the synthesis and/or release of chemical mediators[68]
- Astemazole and doxepin require the longest time to steady state, but histamine blockade is most prolonged[69]
- Doxepin has the most side-effects of any agent, but is the most potent and has the longest duration; effectiveness has been established in cold urticaria as well[70]
- If sedating antihistamines are used, they are best administered at bedtime

## H$_2$ antihistamines

H$_2$ antihistamines have modest evidence for decreasing itching in select disorders.

- Patients with itching from polycythemia vera may respond to cimetidine (900mg/day)[71]

- Monotherapy with H$_2$ blockers has little efficacy, but cimetidine may increase plasma concentrations of H$_1$ antihistamines[72]
- In urticaria, H$_1$ antihistamines such as chlorpheniramine may be combined with agents such as cimetidine or ranitidine to enhance the therapeutic effect, and H$_2$ agents decrease itching and whealing[73–75]

No published study has compared the addition of H$_2$ agents to the more efficacious newer antihistamines astemazole, cetirizine, and loratidine.

### Herbal remedies

Given the high placebo-response rate, it is likely that most activity in herbal remedies is through the placebo effect.

- Traditional Chinese herbal therapy administered as a daily decoction of a formula containing ten herbs found beneficial in open studies was tested for 2 months in a double-blind placebo-controlled study on adults[76]

> Despite poor palatability, itching and disease severity clearly improved and no side-effects were reported

## Ketotifen

Ketotifen, a mast cell stabilizer, is effective in relieving urticarial wheals and itching and is more effective than clemastine in chronic urticaria[77]. It is also an effective agent in physical urticaria. An additional utility of this agent may be in combination with $H_1$ antihistamines in treatment-resistant disease[78].

- With the exception of neurofibroma-associated pain and itching[79], its activity in non-urticarial conditions has not been well documented

## Lidocaine

Parenteral lidocaine may help the itching of renal disease, and can occasionally be helpful in those undergoing hemodialysis[41,80,81].

## Non-steroid anti-inflammatory drugs (NSAIDS)

NSAIDS inhibit cyclo-oxygenase or lipoxygenase thereby decreasing the formation of prostaglandins and leucotrienes. Although theoretically these agents could ameliorate many inflammatory pruritic conditions and anecdotal case reports suggest efficacy, actual demonstrated efficacy in itching is minor[82,83].

- Aspirin therapy (900 mg/day) failed to reduce itching in 13 patients with chronic, non-urticarial itchy dermatoses[84]; activity may occur through placebo mechanisms
- A controlled study showed that aspirin improves itching in polycythemia rubra vera; this may be related to quantities of prostaglandin E2 and serotonin which are substances produced and released by platelets[85]
- Anecdotal reports have suggested the efficacy of aspirin in other conditions, but one carefully controlled trial failed to demonstrate efficacy

## Cyclosporin

The primary use of cyclosporin is as an immunosuppressive in patients who have received renal, liver and bone marrow allogeneic transplants. Cyclosporin blocks the cell cycle in T-helper cells and inhibits lymphokine production[86,87]. Clinical studies in atopic dermatitis clearly show significant benefit from therapy with decreased itching and disease severity.

- In one study[88] of 10 days' treatment (5 mg/kg/day) of adults with atopic dermatitis, cyclosporin reduced itch intensity, eczema severity, and topical hydrocortisone use
- A second study, also at 5 mg/kg/day, showed that patients experienced improvement in atopic dermatitis involving area, erythema, excoriation, lichenification, itch and requirement for topical corticosteroid
- In another study, after a 6-week treatment period at 5 mg/kg/day, clearance was often attained, but about half of the patients relapsed after 2 weeks, and up to 90% relapsed by week 6 of follow-up

Cyclosporin A is likely to be effective in a broad range of other inflammatory itching diseases ranging from urticaria to lichen planus and psoriasis[89]. This agent can cause significant hypertension, elevated creatinine and blood urea nitrogen, immunosuppression and renal toxicity, and so should be carefully used with appropriate monitoring[90].

## Dapsone

Dapsone, and the related agent, sulfapyridine, is a useful anti-inflammatory agent in dermatitis herpetiformis, urticaria, and other itchy dermatoses[91].

■ The therapeutically innovative physician may attempt to use this agent in inflammatory dermatoses at 50–150 mg per day

■ Side-effect monitoring is indicated because hemolysis with resultant anemia and methemoglobinemia are relatively common; other reported toxicities include bone-marrow damage, peripheral neuropathy, renal damage, cholestasis, and azoospermia

## Thalidomide

This agent has shown great promise in treating itching in renal disease[92], lichen simplex chronicus, prurigo nodularis and primary biliary cirrhosis[93]. Thalidomide is an extreme teratogen and should be used cautiously in women of childbearing age; it can also cause an irreversible peripheral neuropathy and nerve conduction monitoring may be appropriate[94].

## Opiate antagonists

### Naloxone

In spinal-morphine-induced itching, parenteral naloxone (0.2 µg/kg/min) is effective[95]. It may also help in cholestatic itching[96–99].

■ Patients with liver disease may experience an opioid withdrawal reaction on starting the drug

### Nalmefene

Nalmefene, an oral opioid antagonist devoid of agonist activity, helped itching and systemic symptoms in patients with primary biliary cirrhosis, and also helps patients with cholestatic itching[100]. It may well help other patients as well, but only preliminary studies have been performed[101]. Patients with liver disease may experience a severe opioid withdrawal reaction on starting the drug[102].

## Ondansetron

Intravenous administration of the serotonin type 3 receptor antagonist ondansetron induced a marked relief of itching in a small group of itching patients[103].

## Interferon-α

Interferon-α can improve itching in polycythemia vera[104].

■ Patients with refractory itching due to polycythemia vera, were given interferon-α intramuscularly three times a week at a dosage of 3 million units

■ The majority benefited within 2–8 weeks from the start of treatment, but one-third discontinued treatment due to unacceptable side-effects

## Interferon-γ

Daily injection of interferon-γ may also have beneficial effect in severe and treatment refractory atopic dermatitis[105] (see chapter 6: Common dermatitis diseases).

## Intralesional injections

Subcutaneous injection of triamcinolone may be effective in a broad range of locally itchy dermatoses, ranging from anogenital itching to lichen simplex chronicus. The degree to which these agents act locally as compared with systemically is unknown, and long-term use of this modality should be considered the equivalent of systemic administration.

## Physical treatment modalities

### Cool compresses

This is an age old modality that consists of laying wet towels or cloth over a pruritic area. Anecdotal evidence suggests that this is beneficial for short-lived itching.

### Heating techniques

Immersion in hot water may decrease or abolish itching[36,106,107], but may also exacerbate itching[108]. Caution should be exercised, since burning may result.

### Unna boot occlusion

Unna paste boot occlusion can decrease itching and excoriation in select patients with lichen simplex chronicus, neurotic excoriations, and other localized itching[109].

A modification of the original Unna technique, in which medium to potent topical corticosteroid agents are first applied then followed by the paste dressing, may increase compliance.

- This approach works best on the arms and legs, and only should be considered in cooperative patients

### Transcutaneous electronic nerve stimulation (TENS)

- TENS has been reported as beneficial in two elderly patients[110] and one younger atopic patient[111] with severe, chronic itching unresponsive to other treatment
- In a much larger study[112], 41 patients received TENS for 5–30 minutes several times a day for 5–47 days

  63% of the patients benefitted and 20% reported complete relief

  Effects lasted for many hours

  In 15 of the patients who had itching for more than one year, 12 patients were relieved initially, but later only six had a partial relief, and none had the itch resolved – probably due to a strong initial placebo effect

  Only one patient wanted to continue the TENS therapy

TENS effectiveness may be partially the placebo response, which declines with continuing therapy.

### Ultraviolet light

Phototherapy with ultraviolet A light (UVA) and/or ultraviolet B light (UVB) or with psoralen plus ultraviolet A light (PUVA) may help patients with a variety of inflammatory and non-inflammatory dermatoses that are non-responsive to other therapeutic modalities[113–1145].

- Phototherapy primarily has anti-inflammatory effects and these effects are nicely exploited to decrease itching in psoriasis, lichen planus, and other inflammatory dermatoses
- Phototherapy has also been reported to be effective in non-inflammatory skin conditions including the itches of uremia, primary biliary cirrhosis, and other conditions
- PUVA itself may cause itching, but this is relatively minor and uncommon[116]

The mechanism of action of this therapeutic modality is poorly understood.

- UVB decreases the itch response to histamine, but histamine is only secondarily related to itch in the majority of itchy dermatoses[117]
- Cutaneous nerves are ultrastructurally altered by UV, but the significance is unknown[118]

#### Phototherapy applications in itching diseases

- Persistent papular eruption and eosinophilic pustular folliculilitis of acquired immunodeficiency syndrome may respond to UVB[119,120] or PUVA, and is considered quite safe[121]

- PUVA may help patients with aquagenic pruritus, but relapse occurs weeks to months following therapy; maintenance therapy is necessary to maintain remission[122-124]
- Phototherapy is quite effective in atopic dermatitis

  Atopic dermatitis responds best to combined UVA and UVB[125], but some patients respond best to one or the other of these components[126]

  PUVA can also improve disease severity and itching[126]

- Recalcitrant dermatitis herpetiformis may respond to PUVA[128]
- Some patients with chronic hand dermatitis benefit from PUVA[129]
- Hypereosinophilic syndrome may respond to PUVA[130]
- PUVA may induce long-term remission in lichen planus, a notoriously itchy disorder[131]
- Phototherapy with UVA and/or UVB helps pruritus in some patients with primary biliary cirrhosis

  The combination of PUVA with cholestyramine may offer additional benefit[132]

- Phototherapy improves cholestatic pruritus in both adults and children

  Daylight phototherapy treatments may enhance urinary excretion of bile acids[133]

- Mastocytosis, particularly in generalized forms such as telangiectasia macularis eruptiva perstans, may respond to PUVA[134]
- PUVA is particularly helpful with the itch of non-tumor stage mycosis fungoides
- Lichen simplex chronicus and macular amyloidosis[135]

  UVB alone may be helpful in completely macular disease

- Pityriasis rosea

  In one limited study with UVB treatment on one side and sham treatment on the other, UVB decreased disease severity, but the itching and the course of the disease were unchanged[136]

  UVB has systemic effects, thus this trial is not definitive

  Anecdotal experience suggests this modality may be effective in relieving the itching

- Polycythemia vera may respond to PUVA[137]
- The majority of patients with polymorphous light eruption[138] or benign summer light eruption[139] are helped by UVB and PUVA
- PUVA helps select patients with prurigo nodularis[140], and in our center combination UVA and UVB therapy also helps
- Transient and persistent acantholytic dermatosis (Grover's disease) may respond to PUVA[141]
- The efficacy of UVB phototherapy in uremic pruritus has been established in controlled trials[142-146]

  80–90% of those treated respond; remissions may be long-lasting

  UVA is without effect

- PUVA helps induce remission but maintenance therapy is required in chronic urticaria
- UVA or PUVA may help patients with solar urticaria[147]
- PUVA is effective in about one-third of patients with severe symptomatic dermatographism but maintenance therapy is required[148,149]

**Plasma perfusion**

Plasma perfusion through charcoal-coated glass beads was effective in reducing the itching of primary biliary cirrhosis and intractable pruritus; the itch returned to its pre-perfusion intensity by the end of the third week after perfusion[150]. In another study of plasma perfusion through charcoal-coated glass beads, all patients had prompt relief of their pruritus which lasted from one day to 5 months[151].

## Acupuncture

Reports of acupuncture are notoriously unreliable because of the strong placebo effect produced by the effect of needle insertion; nevertheless anecdotal reports suggest efficacy in the itch of chronic pruritus vulvae[152], allergic contact dermatitis[153] and uremic itching[154].

■ Using more rigorous techniques, acupuncture and electro-acupuncture (2 Hz and 80 Hz) were compared with 'placebo acupuncture' (needle insertion at non-traditional acupuncture sites) on experimental itch[155]

   Acupuncture and electro-acupuncture significantly reduced subjective itch intensity when applied intrasegmentally

■ In a pseudo-acupuncture controlled trial of experimental histamine-induced itching, acupuncture decreased itching duration, but did not affect itch onset time or the maximal itch intensity[156]

   Acupuncture also decreased the histamine skin flare

Similar to essentially all other therapeutic modalities, acupuncture may cause itching by allergic contact dermatitis[157].

## Cryotherapy

Anecdotal reports suggest efficacy in prurigo nodularis[158] vulvar lichen sclerosus et atrophicus[159] and chronic pruritus ani[160]. This is an easy, inexpensive, and often effective therapy for prurigo nodularis.

■ In darkly pigmented patients, risks of depigmentation should be considered prior to performing this procedure

## Psychological approaches

Psychotherapy may help in clinical situations in which psychotherapeutic agents are employed, but its use is not limited to these patients[161].

### Atopic dermatitis

■ In the treatment of chronic atopic dermatitis, a randomized controlled trial compared the effectiveness of four group treatments[162]

   At one year follow-up the psychological treatments (autogenic training as a form of relaxation therapy, cognitive–behavioral treatment, or combined approaches) led to significantly larger improvement in skin condition than an intensive dermatological educational program or standard medical care

■ Atopic dermatitis in another study was treated with biofeedback[163]

   Disease severity was helped modestly, and itching severity decreased non-uniformly

Atopic dermatitis may also respond to group psychotherapy[164,165] and to behavioral therapy directed to stopping scratching[166]. Therapeutic success in a large group of children and adults was reported using hypnosis[167].

### Neurotic excoriations

In patients motivated to receive psychologic intervention, modest success can be expected from psychotherapy[168] or behavioral therapy[169]. In some patients, a distinct correlation exists between the outbreak of the disease and the preceding loss of a human relationship, detrimental to self-esteem.

### Chronic urticaria

Relaxation therapy and hypnotherapy are reported as beneficial adjuncts[170].

## Other diseases with reported benefit include:

- Prurigo nodularis[171]
- Guillain-Barre Syndrome[172]
- Hand dermatitis[173]

## Itching and primary psychiatric disease

Itching may be a sign of depression, anxiety, and other disorders which may be helped by psychotherapy and medical approaches[174].

## References

1. Bernhard JD. Pruritus: advances in treatment. *Advan Dermatol* 1991;6:57–71

2. Hägermark Ö, Wahlgren CF. Treatment of itch. *Semin Dermatol* 1995;14:320–5

3. Bromm B, Scharein E, Darsow U, *et al.* Effects of menthol and cold on histamine-induced itch and skin reactions in man. *Neuroscience* 1995;187:157–60

4. Shuttleworth D, Hill S, Marks R, *et al.* Relief of experimentally induced pruritus with a novel eutectic mixture of local anaesthetic agents. *Br J Dermatol* 1988;119:535–40

5. Lever LR, Hill S, Dykes PJ, *et al*, Efficacy of topical dimetindene in experimentally induced pruritus and weal and flare reactions. *Skin Pharmacol* 1991;4:109–12

6. Drake LA, Fallon JD, Sober A. Relief of pruritus in patients with atopic dermatitis after treatment with topical doxepin cream. The Doxepin Study Group. *J Am Acad Dermatol* 1994;31:613–6

7. Bernhardt DT. Topical diphenhydramine toxicity. *Wisconsin Med J* 1991;90:469–71

8. Vidal Pan C, Gonzalez Quintela A, Galdos Anuncibay P, *et al.* Topical promethazine intoxication. *DICP* 1989;23:89

9. Arnold WP, van de Kerkhof PC. Topical capsaicin in pruritic psoriasis. *J Am Acad Dermatol* 1993;29:438–42

10. Ellis CN, Berberian B, Sulica VI, *et al.* A double-blind evaluation of topical capsaicin in pruritic psoriasis. *J Am Acad Dermatol* 1993;29:438–42

11. Green BG, Shaffer GS. The sensory response to capsaicin during repeated topical exposures: differential effects on sensations of itching and pungency. *Pain* 1993;53:323–34

12. Szeimies RM, Stolz W, Wlotzke U, *et al.* Successful treatment of hydroxyethyl starch-induced pruritus with topical capsaicin. *Br J Dermatol* 1994;131:380–2

13. Stoughton RB, Cornell RC. Corticosteroids. In Fitzpatrick TB, Eisen AZ, Wolff K, *et al.* eds. *Dermatology in General Medicine,* 4th ed. New York: McGraw Hill Inc, 1993:2846–50

14. Hägermark Ö, Wahlgren CF. Treatment of itch. *Semin Dermatol* 1995;14:320–5

15. Bodor N. Design of novel soft corticosteroids. In Korting HC, Maibach HI, eds. *Topical Glucocorticoids with Increased Benefit/Risk Ratio. Current Problems Dermatology.* Basel: Karger, 1993;21:11–19

16. Ortonne J-P, Skin atrophogenic potential of methylprednisolone aceponate (MPA). *J Eur Acad Dermatol Venereol* 1994;3(Suppl 1):13–8

17. Zaumseil RP, Kecskes A, Tauber U, *et al.* Methylprednisolone aceponate (MPA) a new therapeutic for eczema: pharmacologic overview. *J Dermatol Treat* 1992;3(Suppl 2):23–31

18. Clement M, Phillips SH, Du Vivier A. Is steroid tachyphylaxis preventable? *Clin Exp Dermatol* 1985;10:22–9

19. Du Vivier A. Tachyphylaxis to topically applied steroids. *Arch Dermatol* 1976;112:1245–8

20. Akers WA. Risks of unoccluded topical steroids in clinical trials. *Arch Dermatol* 1980;116:786–8

21. Lubach D, Bensmann A, Bornemann U. Steroid-induced dermal atrophy. Investigations on discontinuous application. *Dermatologica* 1989;179:67–72

22. Katz VL, Thorp JM Jr, Bowes WA Jr. Severe symmetric intrauterine growth retardation associated with the topical use of triamcinolone. *Am J Obstet Gynecol* 1990;162:396–7

23. Goh CL. Cross-sensitivity to multiple topical corticosteroids. *Contact Dermatitis* 1989;20:65–7

24. Katz HI, Hien NT, Prawer SE *et al.* Superpotent topical steroid treatment of psoriasis vulgaris - clinical efficacy and adrenal function. *J Am Acad Dermatol* 1987;16:804–11

25. Tan CC, Wong KS, Thirumoorthy T, *et al.* A randomized, crossover trial of Sarna and Eurax lotions in the treatment of hemodialysis patients with uraemic pruritus. *J Dermatol Treat* 1990;1:235–8

26. Konstantinov D, Stanoeva L, Yawalkar SJ. Crotamiton cream and lotion in the treatment of infants and young children with scabies. *J Int Med Res* 1979;7:443–8

27. Smith EB, King CA, Baker MD. Crotamiton lotion in pruritus. *Int J Dermatol* 1984;23:684–5

28. Ronayne C, Bray G, Robertson G. The use of aqueous cream to relieve pruritus in patients with liver disease. *Br J Nursing* 1993;2:527–8

29. Lauerma AI, Maibach HI. Topical FK506 – clinical potential or laboratory curiosity. *Dermatology* 1994; 188:173–6

30. Lauerma AI, Maibach HI, Granlund H, *et al.* Inhibition of contact allergic reactions by topical FK506. *Lancet* 1992;340:556

31. Nakagawa H, Etoh T, Ishibashi Y, *et al.* Tacrolimus ointment for atopic dermatitis. *Lancet* 1994;344:883

32. Ruzicka T, Bieber T, Schopf E, *et al.* A short-term trial of tacrolimus ointment for atopic dermatitis. European Tacrolimus Multicenter Atopic Dermatitis Study Group. *N Engl J Med* 1997;337:816–21

33. Haider SA. Treatment of atopic eczema in children: clinical trial of 10% sodium cromoglycate ointment. *Br Med J* 1977;1:1570–2

34. Kimata H, Igarashi M. Topical cromolyn (disodium cromoglycate) solution in the treatment of young children with atopic dermatitis. *Clin Exp Allergy* 1990;20:281–3

35. Fujiwaki T, Furusho K. The effects of rice bran broth bathing in patients with atopic dermatitis. *Acta Paediatrica Jap* 1992;34:505–10

36. Boreham DR, Gasmann HC, Mitchel RE. Water bath hyperthermia is a simple therapy for psoriasis and also stimulates skin tanning in response to sunlight. *Int J Hypertherm* 1995;11:745–54

37. Dannaker CJ, Greenway H. Failure of sodium bicarbonate baths in the treatment of aquagenic pruritus. *J Am Acad Dermatol* 1989;20:1136

38. Meunier L, Levy A, Costes Y, *et al.* Idiopathic aquagenic pruritus treated with the addition of sodium bicarbonate to bath water. *Presse Medicale* 1988;17:962

39. Epstein E, Pinsky JB. A blind study. *Arch Dermatol* 1964;89;548–49

40. Pederson JA, Matter BJ, Czerwinski AW, *et al.* Relief of idiopathic generalized pruritus in dialysis patients

treated with activated oral charcoal. *Ann Int Med* 1980;93:446–8

41. Tan JK, Haberman HF, Coldman AJ. Identifying effective treatments for uremic pruritus. *J Am Acad Dermatol* 1991;25:811–8

42. Stahle M, Hägermark Ö. Effects of topically applied clobetasol-17-propionate on histamine release in human skin. *Acta Derm Venereol* 1984;64:239–42

43. Flower RJ. Background and discovery of lipocortins. *Agent Act* 1986;17:255–62

44. Hardman JC, Gilman AG, Limbird LE. In Goodman, Gilman, eds. *The Pharmacologic Basis of Therapeutics*, 9th edn. New York: McGraw-Hill, 1996:1466–74

45. Galli E, Chini L, Moschese V, *et al.* Methylprednisolone bolus: a novel therapy for severe atopic dermatitis. *Acta Paediatr* 1994;83:315–7

46. Goldstein DA, Zimmerman B, Spielberg SP. Anaphylactic response to hydrocortisone in childhood: a case report. *Ann Allergy* 1985;55:599–600

47. Castrow FF. Atopic cataracts versus steroid cataracts. *J Am Acad Dermatol* 1981;5:64–6

48. MacGregor RR, Sheagren JN, Lipsett MB, *et al.* Alternate day prednisone therapy. Evaluation of delayed hypersensitivity responses, control of disease and steroid side-effects. *New Engl J Med* 1969;280: 1427–31

49. Nugent CA, Ward J, MacDiamid WD, *et al.* Glucocorticoid toxicity: single versus divided daily doses of prednisolone. *J Chron Dis* 1965;18:323–32

50. Reichling GH, Kligman AM. Alternate-day corticosteroid therapy. *Arch Dermatol* 1961;83:980–3

51. Reinisch JM, Simon NG, Karow WG, *et al.* Prenatal exposure to prednisolone in humans and animals retards uterine growth. *Science* 1978;202:436–8

52. Simons FER. New H1-receptor antagonists: clinical pharmacology. *Clin Exp Allergy* 1990;20(Suppl 2):19–24

53. Chan CY, Wallander KA. Diphenhydramine toxicity in three children with varicella-zoster infection. *DICP* 1991;25:130–2

54. Ormerod AD. Urticaria: recognition, causes and treatment. *Drugs* 1994;48:717–30

55. Simmons FE, McMillan JL, Simmons KJ. A double-blind, single dose, crossover comparison of cetirizine, terfenidine, loratidine, astemazole, and chlorpheniramine versus placebo: suppressive effects on histamine-induced wheals and flares during 25 hours

in normal subjects. *J Allergy Clin Immunol* 1990;86: 540–7

56. Rhoades RB, Leifer KN, Cohan R, *et al.* Suppression of histamine-induced pruritus by three antihistaminic drugs. *J Allergy Clin Immunol* 1975;55:180–5

57. Kobza Black A. H$_1$ antagonists in the management of the itch of urticarias. *Skin Pharmacol* 1992;5:21–4

58. Kerdel FA, Soter NA. Antihistamines in dermatology. In Rook AJ, Maibach HI, eds. *Recent Advances in Dermatology,* Vol 6. Edinburgh: Churchill Livingstone, 1983:265–76

59. Kennard CD, Ellis CN. Pharmacologic therapy for urticaria. *J Am Acad Dermatol* 1991;25:176–87

60. Aaronson DW. Comparative efficacy of H1 antihistamines. *Ann Allergy* 1991;67:541–7

61. Monroe EW, Bernstein DI, Fox RW, *et al.* Relative efficacy and safety of loratadine, hydroxyzine, and placebo in chronic idiopathic urticaria. *Arzneimittel-Forschung* 1992;42:1119–21

62. De Vos C. New antihistamines. *Clin Exp Allergy* 1989;19:503–7

63. Krause LB. Shuster S. A comparison of astemizole and chlorpheniramine in dermographic urticaria. *Br J Dermatol* 1985;112:447–53

64. Brogden RN, McTavish D. Acrivastine. A review of its pharmacological properties and therapeutic efficacy in allergic rhinitis, urticaria and related disorders. *Drugs* 1991;41:927–40

65. Katyal VK, Choudhary JD. Occurrence of torsade de pointes with use of astemizole. *Indian Heart J* 1994; 46:181–2

66. Clissold SP, Sorkin EM, Goa KL. Loratadine; a preliminary review of its pharmacodynamic properties and therapeutic efficacy. *Drugs* 1989;37:42–57

67. Langeland T, Fagertun HE, Larsen S. Therapeutic effect of loratadine on pruritus in patients with atopic dermatitis. A multi-crossover-designed study. *Allergy* 1994;49:22–6

68. Grossman J, Halverson PC, Meltzer EO, *et al.* Double-blind assessment of azelastine in the treatment of perennial allergic rhinitis. *Ann Allergy* 1994; 73:141–6

69. Richards DM, Brogden RN, Heel RL. Astemizole; a review of its pharmacodynamic properties and therapeutic efficacy. *Drugs* 1984;28:38–61

70. Neittaanmaki H, Myohanen T, Fraki JE. Comparison of cinnarizine, cyproheptadine, doxepin, and hydroxyzine in treatment of idiopathic cold urticaria: usefulness of doxepin. *J Am Acad Dermatol* 1984;11:483–9

71. Weick JK, Donovan PB, Najean Y, *et al.* The use of cimetidine for the treatment of pruritus in polycythemia vera. *Arch Int Med* 1982;142:241–2

72. Salo OP, Kauppinen K, Mannisto PT. Cimetidine increases the plasma concentration of hydroxyzine. *Acta Derm Venereol* 1986;66:349–50

73. Bleehen SS, Thomas SE, Greaves MW, *et al.* Cimetidine and chlorpheniramine in the treatment of chronic idiopathic urticaria: a multi-centre randomized double-blind study. *Br J Dermatol* 1987; 117:81–8

74. Paul E, Bodeker RH. Treatment of chronic urticaria with terfenadine and ranitidine. A randomized double-blind study in 45 patients. *Eur J Clin Pharmacol* 1986;31:277–80

75. Runge JW, Martinez JC, Caravati EM, *et al.* Histamine antagonists in the treatment of acute allergic reactions. *Ann Emerg Med* 1992;21:237–42

76. Sheehan MP, Rustin MH, Atherton DJ, *et al.* Efficacy of traditional Chinese herbal therapy in adult atopic dermatitis. *Lancet* 1992;340:13–7

77. Kamide R, Niimura M, Ueda H, *et al.* Clinical evaluation of ketotifen for chronic urticaria: multicenter double-blind comparative study with clemastine. *Ann Allergy* 1989;62:322–5

78. Francos GC, Kauh YC, Gittlen SD, *et al.* Elevated plasma histamine in chronic uremia. Effects of ketotifen on pruritus. *Int J Dermatol* 1991;30:884–9

79. Riccardi VM. A controlled multiphase trial of ketotifen to minimize neurofibroma-associated pain and itching. *Arch Dermatol* 1993;129:577–81

80. Joffe P, Andersen LW, Molvig J, *et al.* Intravenous lidocaine in the treatment of pruritus in hemodialysis patients. *Clin Nephrol* 1985;24:214

81. Tapia L, Cheigh JS, David DS, *et al.* Pruritus in dialysis patients treated with parenteral lidocaine. *New Engl J Med* 1977;296:261–2

82. Cronin ME, Wortmann RL. Nonsteroidal antiinflammatory drugs (NSAIDs). Common chemical and clinical characteristics. *Int J Dermatol* 1984;23: 411–3

83. Sowden JM, Berth-Jones J, Ross JS, *et al.* Double-blind, controlled, crossover study of cyclosporin in adults with severe refractory atopic dermatitis. *Lancet* 1991;338:137–40

84. Daly BM, Shuster S. Effect of aspirin on pruritus. *Br Med J Clin Res Ed* 1986;293:907

85. Fjellner B. Hägermark Ö. Pruritus in polycythemia vera: treatment with aspirin and possibility of platelet involvement. *Acta Derm Venereol* 1979;59:505–12

86. Gupta AK, Brown MD, Ellis CN, *et al*. Cyclosporine in dermatology. *J Am Acad Dermatol* 1989;21: 1245–56

87. Kahan BD. Cyclosporine. *New Engl J Med* 1989;321: 1725–38

88. Wahlgren CF, Scheynius A, Hägermark Ö. Antipruritic effect of oral cyclosporin A in atopic dermatitis. *Acta Derm Venereol* 1990;70:323–9

89. Bos JD, Mevinharde MMHM, Van Joost T, *et al*. Use of cyclosporin in psoriasis. *Lancet* 1989;2:1500–2

90. Munro CS, Levell NJ, Shuster S, *et al*. Maintenance treatment with cyclosporin in atopic eczema. *Br J Dermatol* 1994;130:376–80

91. Fry L, Walkden V, Wojnarowska F, *et al*. A comparison of IgA positive and IgA negative dapsone responsive dermatoses. *Br J Dermatol* 1980;102:371–82

92. Silva SR, Viana PC, Lugon NV, *et al*. Thalidomide for the treatment of uremic pruritus: a crossover randomized double-blind trial. *Nephron* 1994;67: 270–3

93. McCormick PA, Scott F, Epstein O, *et al*. Thalidomide as therapy for primary biliary cirrhosis: a double-blind placebo controlled pilot study. *J Hepatol* 1994;21:496–9

94. Aronson IK, Yu R, West DP, *et al*. Thalidomide-induced peripheral neuropathy. *Arch Dermatol* 1984; 120:1466–70

95. Saiah M, Borgeat A, Wilder-Smith OH, *et al*. Epidural-morphine-induced pruritus: propofol versus naloxone. *Anesth Analg* 1994;78:1110–3

96. Bernstein JE, Swift R. Relief of intractable pruritus with naloxone. *Arch Dermatol* 1979;115:1366–7

97. Bergasa NV, Jones EA. The pruritus of cholestasis: potential pathogenic and therapeutic implications of opioids. *Gastroenterology* 1995;108:1582–8

98. Bergasa NV, Talbot TL, Alling DW, *et al*. A controlled trial of naloxone infusions for the pruritus of chronic cholestasis. *Gastroenterology* 1992;102: 544–9

99. Bergasa NV, Alling DW, Talbot TL, *et al*. Effects of naloxone infusions in patients with the pruritus of cholestasis. A double-blind, randomized, controlled trial. *Ann Int Med* 1995;123:161–7

100. Harrison PV. Nalmefene and pruritus. *J Am Acad Dermatol* 1990;23:530

101. Monroe EW. Efficacy and safety of nalmefene in patients with severe pruritis caused by chronic urticaria and atopic dermatitis. *J Am Acad Dermatol* 1989;21: 135–6

102. Bergasa NV, Jones EA. Management of the pruritus of cholestasis: potential role of opiate antagonists. *Am J Gastroenterol* 1991;86:1404–12

103. Schworer H, Ramadori G. Treatment of pruritus: a new indication for serotonin type 3 receptor antagonists. *Clin Investigator* 1993;71:659–62

104. Finelli C, Gugliotta L, Gamberi B, *et al*. Relief of intractable pruritus in polycythemia vera with recombinant interferon alfa. *Am J Hematol* 1993;43:316–8

105. Musial J, Milewski M, Undas A, *et al*. Interferon-gamma in the treatment of atopic dermatitis: influence on t-cell activation. *Allergy* 1995;50:520–3

106. Anonymous. Hot water for itching. *Med Let Drug Ther* 1966;8:50–1

107. Anonymous. Hot water for itching. *Medical Let Drug Ther* 1969;11:60

108. Fruhstorfer H, Hermanns M, Latzke L. The effects of thermal stimulation on clinical and experimental itch. *Pain* 1986;24:259–69

109. Barone CM, Mastropieri CJ, Peebles R, *et al*. Evaluation of the Unna Boot for lower-extremity autograft burn wounds excoriated by pruritus in pediatric patients. *J Burn Care Rehab* 1993;14:348–9

110. Monk BE. Transcutaneous electronic nerve stimulation in the treatment of generalized pruritus. *Clin Exp Dermatol* 1993;18:67–8

111. Bjorna H, Kaada B. Successful treatment of itching and atopic eczema by transcutaneous nerve stimulation. *Acupun Electro-Therap Res* 1987;12:101–12

112. Fjellner B, Hägermark Ö. Transcutaneous nerve stimulation and itching. *Acta Derm Venereol* 1978; 58:131–4

113. Lebwohl M. Phototherapy of pruritus. In *Itch. Mechanisms and Management of Pruritus.* New York: McGraw-Hill, 1994:399–411

114. Monroe EW, Bernstein DI, Fox RW, *et al*. Photochemotherapy. a reappraisal of its use in dermatology. *Drugs* 1989;38:822–37

115. Morison WL. *Phototherapy and Photochemotherapy of Skin Disease,* 2nd edn. New York: Raven Press, 1991

116. Roelandts R, Stevens A. PUVA-induced itching and skin pain. *Photodermatol Photoimmunol Photomed* 1990;7:141–2

117. Fjellner B, Hägermark Ö. Influence of ultraviolet light on itch and flare reactions in human skin induced by histamine and the histamine liberator compound 48/80. *Acta Derm Venereol* 1982;62:137–40

118. Kumakiri M, Hashimoto K, Willis I. Biological changes of human cutaneous nerves caused by ultraviolet radiation: an ultrastructural study. *Br J Dermatol* 1978;99:65–75

119. Pardo RJ, Bogaert MA, Penneys NS, *et al.* UVB phototherapy of the pruritic papular eruption of the acquired immunodeficiency syndrome. *J Am Acad Dermatol* 1992;26:423–8

120. Buchness MR, Lim HW, Hatcher VA, *et al.* Ultraviolet B phototherapy of eosinophilic pustular follicultits in patients with the acquired immunodeficiency syndrome. *N Engl J Med* 1988;318:1183–8

121. Meola T, Soter NA, Ostreicher R, *et al.* The safety of UVB phototherapy in patients with HIV infection. *J Am Acad Dermatol* 1993;29:216–20

122. Menage HDP, Norris PG, Hawk JLM, *et al.* The efficacy of psoralen photochemotherapy in the treatment of aquagenic pruritus. *Br J Dermatol* 1993;129:163–5

123. Smith RA, Ross JS, Staughton RC. Bath PUVA as a treatment for aquagenic pruritus. *Br J Dermatol* 1994;131:584

124. Hautmann G, Teofoli P, Lotti T. Aquagenic pruritus, PUVA and capsaicin treatments. *Br J Dermatol* 1994;131:920–1

125. Midelfart K, Stenvold S, Volden G. Combined UVB and UVA phototherapy of atopic eczema. *Dermatologica* 1985;171:95–8

126. Jekler J, Larko O. UVA solarium versus UVB phototherapy of atopic dermatitis: a paired-comparison study. *Br J Dermatol* 1991;125:569–72

127. Morison WL, Parrish JA, Fitzpatrick TB. Oral psoralen photochemotherapy of atopic eczema. *Br J Dermatol* 1978;98:25–30

128. Kalimo K, Lammintausta K, Viander M, *et al.* PUVA treatment of dermatitis herpetiformis. *Photodermatol Photoimmunol Photomed* 1986;3:54–5

129. LeVine MJ, Parrish JA, Fitzpatrick TB. Oral methoxsalen photochemotherapy (PUVA) of dyshidrotic eczema. *Acta Derm Venereol* 1981;61:570–1

130. Van den Hoogenband HM, van den Berg WHHW, van Diggelen MW. PUVA therapy in the treatment of skin lesions of the hypereosinophilic syndrome. *Arch Dermatol* 1985;121:450

131. Ortonne JP, Thivolet J, Sannwald C. Oral photochemotherapy in the treatment of lichen planus. *Br J Dermatol* 1978;99:77–88

132. Cerio R, Murphy GM, Sladen GE, *et al.* A combination of phototherapy and cholestyramine for the relief of pruritus in primary biliary cirrhosis. *Br J Dermatol* 1987;116:265–7

133. Rosenthal E, Diamond E, Benderly A, *et al.* Cholestatic pruritus: effect of phototherapy on pruritus and excretion of bile acids in urine. *Acta Paediatrica* 1994;83:888–91

134. Fine J. Mastocytosis. *Int J Dermatol* 1980;19:117–23

135. Hudson LD. Macular amyloidosis: treatment with ultraviolet B. *Cutis* 1986;38:61–2

136. Leenutaphong V, Jiamton S. UVB phototherapy for pityriasis rosea: a bilateral comparison study. *J Am Acad Dermatol* 1995;33:996–9

137. Swerlick RA. Photochemotherapy treatment of pruritus associated with polycythemia vera. *J Am Acad Dermatol* 1985;13:675–7

138. Rucker BU. Haberle M. Koch HU, *et al.* Ultraviolet light hardening in polymorphous light eruption – a controlled study comparing different emission spectra. *Photodermatol Photoimmunol Photomed* 1991;8:73–8

139. Leonard F, Morel M, Kalis B, *et al.* Psoralen plus ultraviolet A in the prophylactic treatment of benign summer light eruption. *Photodermatol Photoimmunol Photomed* 1991;8:95–8

140. Vaatainen N, Hannuksela M, Karvonen J. Local photochemotherapy in nodular prurigo. *Acta Derm Venereol* 1979;59:544–7

141. Paul BS, Arndt KA. Response of transient acantholytic dermatosis to photochemotherapy. *Arch Dermatol* 1984;120:121–2

142. Blachley JD, Blankenship DM, Menter A, *et al.* Uremic pruritus: skin divalent ion content and response to ultraviolet phototherapy. *Am J Kidney Dis* 1985;5:237–41

143. Cohen EP, Russell TJ, Garancis JC. Mast cells and calcium in severe uremic itching. *Am J Med Sciences* 1992;303:360–5

144. Gilchrest BA. Ultraviolet phototherapy of uremic pruritus. *Int J Dermatol* 1979;18:741–8

145. Gilchrest BA, Rowe JW, Brown RS, *et al.* Ultraviolet phototherapy of uremic pruritus. Long-term results

and possible mechanism of action. *Ann Int Med* 1979;91:17–21

146. Hindson C, Taylor A, Martin A, *et al.* UVA light for relief of uraemic pruritus. *Lancet* 1981;1:215

147. Bernhard JD, Jaenicke K, Momtaz-TK, *et al.* Ultraviolet A phototherapy in the prophylaxis of solar urticaria. *J Am Acad Dermatol* 1984;10:29–33

148. Johnsson M, Falk ES, Volden G. UVB treatment of factitious urticaria. *Photo-Dermatol* 1987;4:302–4

149. Logan RA, O'Brien TJ, Greaves MW. The effect of psoralen photochemotherapy (PUVA) on symptomatic dermographism. *Clin Exp Dermatol* 1989;14:25–8

150. Lauterburg BH, Pineda AA, Dickson ER, *et al.* Plasmaperfusion for the treatment of intractable pruritus of cholestasis. *Mayo Clin Proc* 1978;53:403–7

151. Lauterburg BH, Taswell HF, Pineda AA, *et al.* Treatment of pruritus of cholestasis by plasma perfusion through USP-charcoal-coated glass beads. *Lancet* 1980;2:53–5

152. Huang WY, Guo ZR, Yu J, *et al.* 56 cases of chronic pruritus vulvae treated with acupuncture. *J Trad Chin Med* 1987;7:1–3

153. Liao SJ. Acupuncture for poison ivy contact dermatitis. A clinical case report. *Acupunct Electro-Therapeut Res* 1988;13:31–9

154. Duo LJ. Electrical needle therapy of uremic pruritus. *Nephron* 1987;47:179–83

155. Lundeberg T, Bondesson L, Thomas M. Effect of acupuncture on experimentally induced itch. *Br J Dermatol* 1987;117:771–7

156. Belgrade MJ, Solomon LM, Lichter EA. Effect of acupuncture on experimentally induced itch. *Acta Derm Venereol* 1984;64:129–33

157. Castelain M, Castelain PY, Ricciardi R. Contact dermatitis to acupuncture needles. *Contact Dermatitis* 1987;16:44

158. Waldinger TP, Wong RC, Taylor WB, *et al.* Cryotherapy improves prurigo nodularis. *Arch Dermatol* 1984;120:1598–600

159. August PJ, Milward TM. Cryosurgery in the treatment of lichen sclerosus et atrophicus of the vulva. *Br J Dermatol* 1980;103:667–70

160. Detrano SJ. Cryotherapy for chronic nonspecific pruritus ani. *J Dermatol Surg Oncol* 1984;10:483–4

161. Koblenzer CS. Psychologic and psychiatric aspects of itching. In *Itch: Mechanisms and Management of Pruritus*. New York: McGraw-Hill, 1994:347–65

162. Ehlers A, Stangier U, Gieler U. Treatment of atopic dermatitis: a comparison of psychological and dermatological approaches to relapse prevention. *J Consult Clin Psychol* 1995;63:624–35

163. Haynes SN, Wilson CC, Jaffe PG, *et al.* Biofeedback treatment of atopic dermatitis: controlled case studies of eight cases. *Biofeedback Self-Regul* 1979;4:195–209

164. Bosse K, Hunecke P. The pruritus of endogenous eczema patients. *Munchener Med Wochenschrift* 1981;123:1013–6

165. Cole WC, Roth HL, Sach LB. Group psychotherapy as an aid in the medical treatment of eczema. *J Am Acad Dermatol* 1988;18:286–91

166. Boddeker KW, Boddeker M. Behavior therapy technics in the treatment of endogenous eczema with special reference to compulsive scratching. *Zeitschrift Psychosomatische Med Psychoanalyse* 1976;22:85–92

167. Stewart AC, Thomas SE. Hypnotherapy as a treatment for atopic dermatitis in adults and children. *Br J Dermatol* 1995;132:778–83

168. Fruensgaard K. Psychotherapeutic strategy and neurotic excoriations. *Int J Dermatol* 1991;30:198–203

169. Welkowitz LA, Held JL, Held AL. Management of neurotic scratching with behavioral therapy. *J Am Acad Dermatol* 1989;21:802–4

171. Valtola J. A psychiatric and psychodynamic investigation of LCO (Prurico Nodularis Hyde) patients. *Acta Derm Venereol* 1991;156:49–52

172. Sampson RN. Hypnotherapy in a case of pruritus and Guillain–Barre syndrome. *Am J Clin Hypnosis* 1990;32:168–73

173. McMenamy CJ, Katz RC, Gipson M. Treatment of hand eczema by EMG biofeedback and relaxation training: a multiple baseline analysis. *J Behav Ther Exp Psychiat* 1988;19:221–227

174. Cotterill JA. Dermatological non-disease: a common and potentially fatal disturbance of cutaneous body image. *Br J Dermatol* 1981;104:611–9

# Appendix: Wake Forest University School of Medicine phototherapy protocols

## Psoralen plus ultraviolet A (PUVA) phototherapy

### Patient instructions

1. All itching patients designated for PUVA will have the basic introduction to phototherapy equipment and safety procedures.
2. Reinforcement of the need for eye protection for all patients and covering of the genital area in males is required.
3. Patients receiving systemic PUVA will be instructed to take the methoxsalen ultra tablets, in the dose prescribed by their physician, one hour prior to the scheduled time of the light treatment.
4. All patients ingesting methoxsalen ultra must wear protective glasses when outside, riding in a car, or next to a window from the time of taking the medication and for the next 18 hours during daylight.
5. Patients are to stand in the center of the light cabinet with arms at rest. A step stool may be used for the patient to stand on when recommended by the physician.
6. A hand-held timer, set by the phototherapy technician, will be given to the patient to have with them during each phototherapy session. The time will correspond with the amount of time calculated for their dose of PUVA that treatment.
7. Instruct patients to come out of the light box when the lights have gone out or within 10 seconds of the alarm of the safety (hand-held) timer. Inform patients that the light box doors are not locked and demonstrate their operation.
8. The current medications will be reviewed by the phototherapist who will ensure that they are contained in the chart. Questions concerning the current medications will be addressed by the attending physician.
9. All patients will be told of the possible complications of PUVA phototherapy, these must specifically include:

    sunburn reaction

    corneal burn if the eyes are unprotected

    photoallergic dermatitis (drug reaction)

    freckling of the skin

    ageing of the skin

    increased risk of skin cancers

11. Patients will be told that additional sunbathing should be avoided the days they receive PUVA. Sunblock (UVA/B) should be used on any sun-exposed areas for the remainder of that day.
12. All patients will be given written information on PUVA phototherapy

### Protocol

1. Obtain signed consent form after patient has been given basic phototherapy education concerning PUVA phototherapy. The patient should be given time for questions.
2. Methoxsalen ultra (8 methoxypsoralen) is to be ingested by the patient at least one

hour prior to UVA therapy. Treatments may be given anytime between 60 and 90 minutes after ingestion.

3. Dosage of the methoxsalen ultra tablets is dependent on the orders of the attending physician and will vary from patient to patient. The standard dosage is 0.4mg/kg.

4. Ask the patient the dose and the time that they ingested their medication.

5. Have the patient undress completely. Male patients should wear an athletic supporter unless otherwise directed or permitted by the attending physician. Patients may apply mineral oil on the plaques prior to the delivery of UV light but this is not mandatory.

6. Eye protection in the form of UV goggles must be worn by all patients when inside the phototherapy unit.

7. Measure the irradiance (mW/cm²) of the UVA light inside the unit. Record this irradiance on the phototherapy record sheet.

8. Determine the initial PUVA dose (J/cm²) according to the patient's skin type as classified by the physician

9. Calculate the time (seconds) to set the UVA light control panel on the light box to deliver the correct dose with the following equation. The initial measurement of the irradiance may be used for subsequent treatments if there has not been any change in the fluorescent lights in the ultraviolet light box.

$$\text{TIME (seconds)} = \frac{\text{DOSE (J/cm}^2)}{\text{IRRADIANCE (mW/cm}^2)}$$

10. The time may also be calculated using the ultraviolet light unit in the following manner: input the DOSE and IRRADIANCE into the computer on the control panel.

11. Set the time on the control panel of the ultraviolet light unit and the hand-held timer to be given to the patient to have inside the unit during a treatment.

12. Verify that the ultraviolet light unit is set on UVA and the time on the control panel and the hand held timer correspond.

13. Turn on the fan and have the patient stand in the center of the ultraviolet light unit with their arms at rest. Double check that they are wearing UV goggles as eye protection.

14. Instruct the patient to come out of the ultraviolet light box when the lights have gone out or within 10 seconds of the hand-held timer alarm. Inform the patient that the light box doors are not locked.

15. Start the treatment.

16. Some patients may receive additional localized ultraviolet light therapy to the legs or trunk as ordered by the physician.

**Subsequent treatments**

17. The frequency of PUVA treatments for the diagnosis of itching is two or three times a week, unless otherwise ordered by a physician. If less than twice a week has been ordered then special instructions as to the advancement of the dose of UVA light must accompany the request.

18. On subsequent visits the patient will be asked about redness and tenderness of the skin during the previous night and this information will be put into the phototherapy record. The patient will also be asked at what time they took the methoxsalen ultra tablets.

**Table 1** PUVA dose increases

| Skin type | Initial UVA dose (J/cm²) | Subsequent treatment UVA increases (J/cm²) |
|-----------|--------------------------|--------------------------------------------|
| I | 1.0 | 0.5 |
| II | 1.0 | 0.5 |
| III | 2.0 | 1.0 |
| IV | 2.0 | 1.0 |
| V | 3.0 | 1.5 |
| VI | 3.0 | 1.5 |

19. If the skin is red the phototherapist will ask that the patient be seen by the attending physician who will make the decision for adjustment in the treatment for that day.

20. Increase the DOSE (J/cm²) of the UVA light by the amount in Table 1 and add it to the previous dose delivered to the patient if the treatment has been within 3 days.

21. Follow steps 6–16 above.

## Combination UVA/UVB protocol for itching

### Background

1. Itching patients designated for UVA/B protocol will have the basic introduction to phototherapy equipment and safety procedures.

2. Reinforcement of the need for eye protection for all patients and covering of the genital area in males is required.

3. Patients are to stand in the center of the light cabinet with arms at rest. A step stool may be used for the patient to stand on when recommended by the physician.

4. A hand-held timer, set by the phototherapy technician, will be given to the patient to have with them during each phototherapy session. The time will correspond with the amount of time calculated for their dose of UVB that treatment. The patient will be told that the first set of lights should go out within 10 seconds of the hand-held timer and the remainder of the treatment will follow.

5. Instruct patients to come out of the light box when the second set of lights have gone out. Inform patients that the light box doors are not locked and demonstrate their operation.

6. The list of current medications should be reviewed by the phototherapist who will ensure that they are contained in the chart. Questions concerning the current medications will be addressed by the attending physician.

7. All patients will be told of the possible complications of phototherapy, these must specifically include:

   sunburn reaction

   corneal burn if the eyes are unprotected

   photoallergic dermatitis (drug reaction)

   freckling of the skin

   ageing of the skin

   increase risk of skin cancers

8. Patients will be told that additional sunbathing should be avoided on the days they receive UVA/B. Sunblock should be used on any sun-exposed areas for the remainder of that day.

9. All patients will be given written information on UVB phototherapy.

### Protocol

1. Obtain signed consent form after patient has been given basic phototherapy education concerning phototherapy. The patient should be given time for questions.

2. Have the patient undress completely. Male patients should wear an athletic supporter unless otherwise directed or permitted by the attending physician. Patients may apply mineral oil on the plaques prior to the delivery of UV light.

3. Eye protection in the form of UV goggles must be worn by all patients when inside the phototherapy unit.

4. Measure the irradiance (mW/cm²) of both the UVA and UVB light inside the unit. Record this irradiance on the phototherapy record sheet.

5. Determine the initial UVB and UVA dose according to the patient's skin type as classified by the physician.

6. Calculate the time (seconds) to set the UVA light control panel on the light box to deliver

**Table 2** UVA/UVB dose increases

| Skin type | Initial UVA dose (J/cm2) | Subsequent treatment UVA increases (J/cm2) | Initial UVB dose (mJ/cm2) | Subsequent treatment UVB Increases (mJ/cm2) |
|---|---|---|---|---|
| I | 3 | 0.5 | 15 | 5 |
| II | 3 | 0.5 | 15 | 5 |
| III | 3 | 0.5 | 15 | 5 |
| IV | 5 | 0.5 | 30 | 5 |
| V | 5 | 0.5 | 30 | 5 |
| VI | 5 | 0.5 | 30 | 5 |

the correct dose with the following equation. The initial measurement of the irradiance may be used for subsequent treatments if there has not been any change in the fluorescent lights in the ultraviolet light box.

$$\text{TIME (seconds)} = \frac{\text{DOSE (J/cm}^2)}{\text{IRRADIANCE (mW/cm}^2)}$$

7. The time may also be calculated using the ultraviolet light unit in the following manner: input the DOSE and IRRADIANCE into the computer on the control panel. This can be done for both UVA and UVB.

8. Set the time on the UVA and UVB control panel of the ultraviolet light unit. The hand-held timer is to be set to the time of the UVB treatment and to be given to the patient to have inside the unit. The patient must be told that the first set of lights will go out within 10 seconds of the alarm on the hand held unit then the remainder of the treatment with the second set of lights will continue.

9. Verify that the ultraviolet light unit is set to deliver both the UVA and UVB light.

10. Turn on the fan and have the patient stand in the center of the ultraviolet light unit with their arms at rest. Double check that they are wearing UV goggles as eye protection.

11. Instruct the patient to come out of the ultraviolet light box when the lights have gone out or within 10 seconds of the hand held timer alarm if the first set of lights do not go out. Inform the patient that the light box doors are not locked.

12. Start the treatment.

**Subsequent treatments**

13. The frequency of UVA/B light treatments for the diagnosis of itching is three to five times a week unless otherwise ordered by a physician. If less than three times a week has been ordered then special instructions as to the advancement of the dose of UVA/B light must accompany the request.

14. On subsequent visits the patient will be asked about skin redness and tenderness the previous night and this information will be put into the phototherapy record.

15. If the skin is red the phototherapist will ask that the patient is seen by the attending physician who will make the decision for adjustment in the UVA/B treatment.

16. Increase the DOSE (mW/cm$^2$) of the UVA/B light by the amount in the table above and add it to the previous dose delivered to the patient if the treatment has been within 3 days.

17. Follow steps 6–12 above.

# Index